THE
PRIMAL CURE

AVOID BEING A SICK STATISTIC

DISCLAIMER: *The Primal Cure* contains plenty of information and suggestions relating to what to eat, when to eat it and how to exercise. This information is not advice, and should not be treated as such. You must not rely on the information in *The Primal Cure* as an alternative to medical advice from an appropriately qualified professional. If you have any questions about any medical matter you should consult your doctor immediately. If you are on any prescribed medicine whatsoever, you should seek advice from your doctor before following any of the information or suggestions in this book. Even if you are not on medication, if any of the information in this book is very different to your current lifestyle, you should sit down and share the information in this book with your doctor and ask them whether they feel it is appropriate for you. The author disclaims liability for any medical or health outcomes that may occur as a result of following the information or suggestions contained in this book.

If you are on medication don't take any of the supplements recommended in this book without consulting your doctor first. If you do take any supplements recommended in this book and suffer any medical condition, or have any signs of diarrhoea, side effects or discomfort, stop immediately and consult your doctor before taking them again. You should never delay seeking medical advice, disregard medical advice, or discontinue medical treatment because of information in the book. It is important to understand that there will be individual variants to arriving at optimal health and you need to uncover the right Primal approach for your own body.

Second Edition: Published November 2018

Book Design: Dan Morris
Cover Design: Theo Johnson

ISBN: 978-1-9999071-3-6

www.bhhpublishing.com
www.primalcure.com

THE GREAT BRITISH HEALTH WARNING

As a nation, we are starving our bodies of good nutrition, and instead poisoning ourselves with mass-produced, artificially-modified, sugar-loaded nonsense. In addition, we are using shampoos, antiperspirants and creams made with substances known to cause harm. Furthermore, we are stressed, don't sleep enough, yet are sedentary.

Our human body was not designed to live like this.
As a result, British adults are now 2.5 stone (nearly 16kgs) heavier than they were just 50 years ago, and it won't be long before 1 in 2 is obese. Alarmingly, half our population at some point in their life will be diagnosed with cancer, and dementia has grown at an epidemic rate to become the biggest killer of women.

How have we ended up here?
Well, much of what we currently believe to be healthy - or at least acceptable - has been shaped by misguided research, corporate greed and outdated governmental advice.

How do we avoid becoming a sick health statistic?
We first accept that we have little evolved since our Primal ancestors and then realign both our diet and lifestyle to the fundamental needs of the human body. Welcome to the Primal Cure.

Steve Bennett, Author

MORE SICK BRITAIN FACTS

Obesity will bankrupt the health service unless Britain gets
serious about tackling the problem
- Simon Stevens, Chief Executive of the NHS

We are the ONLY European country with a declining life expectancy
express.co.uk

Obesity 'to be linked to more female cancers' than smoking
BBC News

The number of people diagnosed with diabetes in the UK has
more than doubled in the last twenty years
diabetes.org.uk

Almost four in five adults in England have a "heart age"
older than their actual age
The Guardian

In the past year, 74% of people have felt so stressed they
have been overwhelmed or unable to cope
mentalhealth.org.uk

A third of elderly patients may be being prescribed unnecessary
medication, putting them at needless risk of side-effects and costing
the NHS millions, a study has shown
telegraph.co.uk

Studies show that up to one in 12 hospital admissions are
medicines-related and two-thirds are preventable
carehomeprofessional.com

Cardiovascular disease kills someone in the UK every 3 minutes
hriuk.org

Neither the message on the cover of this book, nor the Great British Health Warning are designed to cause stress. With a great National Health Service, our chances of living healthily and for a very long time are actually better now than ever before. However, to avoid becoming a sick statistic, it is crucial that you begin to live your life more in line with the needs of the human body. In practice, the more Primal you become, the happier and longer you should live.

All being well, you might even become a centenarian or even a supercentenarian.

Dr Shan Hussain and Dr Dan Maggs

Contents

Acknowledgements 9

How To Use This Book 10

Preface 12

Meet The Author 15

Meet Dr Dan Maggs 16

Meet Dr Shan Hussain 17

Why I Wrote Primal Cure 18

Chapter 1: Life Beyond The Cave 21

Chapter 2: Primal Food Principles 87

Chapter 3: Intermittent Fasting 133

Chapter 4: MOMMS Exercise Principles 157

Chapter 5: Primal Lifestyle 187

Chapter 6: Primal Environment **219**

Chapter 7: Gut Feeling: Taking Care Of Our Microbiome **231**

Chapter 8: Vitamins, Minerals, Herbs, Supplements & Medicine ... **251**

Chapter 9: Food: The Superfoods Through To The Ugly **295**

Chapter 10: Diseases That Plague Britain & How To Avoid Them ... **361**

Chapter 11: The 7-Day Weight Loss Programme **387**

Chapter 12: Primal Living: Conclusion **409**

Primal Scoring System **417**

Primal Cave Card **422**

Index **423**

James Wells' Testimonial **428**

Reader & Journalist Testimonials **430**

ACKNOWLEDGEMENTS

To my personal trainers Sam, Warwick and Ben, for not only getting me in shape, but also for convincing me that age does not put a ceiling on what can be physically achieved. To my entire family, all 27 of you, for always being supportive, especially my wife who has for the past few years had to put up with my obsessive behaviour in researching what is Primal and what is not. To all of the wonderful doctors, authors, nutritionists and medical professionals, for giving up so much of their valuable time. Finally, to my youngest son Louie for being the catalyst, inspiration and on-going motivation to getting the book finished. To Dan for working on the great layout of this book, to Sian for all of her editing skills, to my daughter Jessica for helping me on the index and to Theo for his great work on the cover. Also, a massive thank you to James, the General Manager of Primal Cure and Dr Dan and Dr Shan for all of your hard work in helping me put together this second edition. You are an amazing team and together we WILL make a difference.

To my wonderful grandmother and amazing auntie Avis who both sadly died in their fifties from cancer, you will always be remembered. To my three close friends, who are all undergoing cancer treatment at the time this book goes to print, my thoughts and warmest wishes are with you. I pray that you make a full and speedy recovery. To my incredible dad who earlier this year at the age of 77 was diagnosed with type 2 diabetes, and to my loving mother who is suffering with a neurocognitive disorder, this book is dedicated to you. You may never fully appreciate how your illnesses have driven me spread the word about how to improve the health of our nation and in some small way I hope that you will find some comfort in how it may help others.

To all of the wonderful individuals who have sent letters, emails and provided reviews about Primal Cure and its products. It's your positive success stories that have motivated me to launch this paperback issue, driving down the cover price so that we can wider spread the message. A message that needs to be heard in order to fix our sick nation.

HOW TO USE THIS BOOK

Both to really understand the severity of our sick nation and to also realise that there is an alternative way, please re-read The Great British Warning on page 3 several times. Then, take a photo of it on your mobile and alert as many of your friends and family as you can. My main motivation to writing this book is to help Great Britain once again become healthy, so please feel free to take photos of any page on your mobile and share the information with loved ones. All I would ask you to do in return is also to point them in the direction of **www. primalcure.com**.

The book isn't written with lots of fluffy flowing filler sentences that nicely lead you from one topic to the next, every sentence is designed to deliver a message. I don't make any apologies for this, because if I had written in this style the book would have been a thousand pages long! Plus, to be truthful, I don't possess that type of writing skill.

When a sentence or a paragraph really resonates with you, take a pen, underline it and then re-read it again a few days later. Or take a photo on your smart-phone or tablet so you can easily share it with friends and family.

While reading the whole book is the best way to really understand the Primal way of living and avoid becoming a sick statistic, if at the moment you are a little bit busy, then at the end of each chapter I have also summarised it.

I have also put a lot of effort into the index at the back of the book. The place to start for each heading is the page number in bold. The other numbers are also worth a read too. I don't mention every page the word appears in the book, as for the words 'sugar' and 'cancer' there would be hundreds of references.

We have a great National Health Service and most infectious diseases that once indiscriminately wreaked havoc across our land have pretty much been eradicated in Britain. Yet, we have a declining life expectancy on our small island, due to corporate greed, misinformation and a very unnatural way of living.

About This Edition
The first, hardback edition of this book was designed in full colour to be a coffee table read for the entire family. So why publish this edition?

Recently, in just one week, three close friends of mine were diagnosed with cancer. It made me more determined than ever to spread the word about Primal Cure. Hence, this paperback was conceived. Its lower cover price will help us spread the word more quickly and urgently.

The content is much the same as the first edition, but with an additional chapter called the Primal *7-Day Weight Loss Programme* and an updated section on vitamins and minerals.

PREFACE

"I would rather have questions that can't be answered than answers that can't be questioned."
Richard Feynman

For seventy years now, the answer that cannot be questioned is, "Fats are bad. Carbohydrates are good". Based on this nonsense, dietary guidelines were created by those who knew they had the answer. They didn't need facts - they couldn't have, as they didn't have any. They didn't need to look at the science, they couldn't have, or they would have realised how ridiculous their answer was. They didn't need anything but the pure certainty that they were right. They were going to make us happier, healthier, slimmer. So long as everybody did exactly what they were told.

The food industry and the pharmaceutical industry happily jumped on this bandwagon. The pharmaceutical industry was particularly delighted to see the rates of diabetes go through the roof. 'We have a drug for that' – from which we can make billions. The food industry was delighted to strip out costly fat and replace it with cheap carbohydrates (a fancy word for sugar). 'Fat free yoghurt – hurrah.' It should really be called 'Sugar stuffed yoghurt – designed to give you diabetes.' Well, food must taste of something, and if you take all that fat out, the sugar has to go in.

The public has been meekly accepting of all this utter nonsense. Fat consumption has gone down, carbohydrate consumption has gone up, and guess what? So have the rates of obesity and diabetes; and now the rates of heart disease and cancer are following.

Yes, we have been sold a complete pup. Utter and complete nonsense. However, those who have discovered that this is complete and utter nonsense have been hounded and attacked for daring to challenge the status quo.

You may wonder what corrupt people and interests are behind such prohibitions and behind the witch hunt on honest, open minded and brave people in the medical community as our Dr. Annika Dahlqvist, Prof. Tim Noakes and Dr. Gary Fettke and of course our own present hero who I don't need to mention by name here. What a Kafka world we are living in!

Annika Dahlqvist was almost hounded out of her job in Sweden by the medical authorities for promoting a high fat diet. Professor Tim Noakes, a specialist in nutrition, dared to change his mind about a healthy diet, and began to promote high fat, low carb (HFLC) in South Africa. He has been dragged in front of the medical authority twice. Dr Gary Fettke, an Australian orthopaedic surgeon, advised HFLC to his patients and has been banned from discussing diet with his patients ever again – even if he is proven to be right.

In the UK Dr Aseem Malhotra, a consultant cardiologist and strong supporter of a change in dietary guidelines, unearthed a conspiracy to attack and undermine him – co-ordinated by Public Health England! The very agency whose guidelines have been doing so much harm to the public. Yes, this is a highly contentious arena, and those who dare to stick their head over the parapet need not wait long for the sniper fire.

Into this upward struggling world Steve Bennett has arrived. A bright cookie who has taken the mainstream advice to heart and found that it was doing him no good at all. He has done his own research and realised, as are more and more people, that we have been sold a pup. Steve changed his diet around, he changed his lifestyle around, and he has achieved health and fitness. More than that, he is now bursting to tell the world about how fantastic it all is. He has looked at the lifestyle of our ancestors, how they lived, worked, ate, exercised and recognised that we should do the same. Live the lifestyle that we are designed to live.

I love the enthusiasm, I love the book. There is almost nothing here that I would disagree with – and that is remarkable for me. If you read this book and take on board what is written I can guarantee that you will be healthier and happier – and slimmer and fitter.

Yes, it goes against much of what we are told by 'experts.' So what. My own view, now, is that whatever an 'expert' on nutrition tells you to do - do the opposite. Whatever they say is healthy is in fact unhealthy, and vice-versa. The world of diet and health went mad seventy years ago, this book is a refreshing ray of sanity.

Dr Malcolm Kendrick
Author of *The Great Cholesterol Con* & *Doctoring Data*

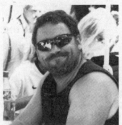 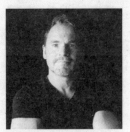

Before Primal   2 Years Living Primally

MEET THE AUTHOR

Steve Bennett is a father of seven children and one of the UK's most prominent business leaders, employing more than 1,000 people around the world. Steve's holding company Bennett Health and Happiness Group works exclusively in areas where they can improve the lives of others. Along with his family, in March 2011 he established the charity The Colourful Life Foundation, which to-date has built schools in countries including India, Tanzania and South Africa.

Steve has spent many years in remote countries and much of the insight in this book has been garnered during his travels. With a keen sense for adventure, Steve and his son-in-law Jake have trekked to the North Pole, and more recently he has walked from the east to the west coast of England with two of his sons Jack and Tom. He has sailed across the Atlantic with six of his family and ran several marathons.

Steve openly admits to spending most of his adult life overweight, but at the age of 50 he decided that enough was enough. This book details the picture as it unfolded for Steve on his journey to restoring his own health and well-being.

Sir Richard Branson

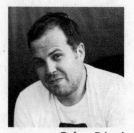 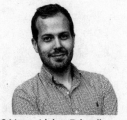

Before Primal   2 Years Living Primally

MEET DR DAN MAGGS

As a General Practitioner (GP), you'd think Dr Dan Maggs would know how to get his weight problems under control. Yet despite several attempts – adhering to a 'balanced diet' as specified in the UK's national dietary guidelines – he found himself clinically obese in his early 30s.

Thankfully, a chance encounter whilst on holiday in 2016 led to him discovering the power of a Primal diet, built around a low carbohydrate intake. In the following six months, he lost an incredible 5 stone (31kg) and rapidly normalised his weight!

Since his remarkable transformation, Dr Dan has developed a love for exercise and well-being and is now in the best shape of his life. Losing so much weight by going against government advice and ignoring mainstream dietary guidelines led him to question much of what he learned during medical training. Quickly, he'd discovered these guidelines aren't based around robust medical evidence at all and that his experiences prove we should be adopting a Primal approach to the way we eat and live.

To avoid weight gain, diabetes, heart disease and other serious illness, Dr Dan is a firm believer in the power of a low carb, organic, Primal diet, enabling us to live longer, healthier, happier lives. As one of our esteemed Primal Doctors and an integral part of the Primal Cure team, he spreads his powerful message both with us and via his own website **www.carbdodging.com**.

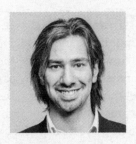

MEET DR SHAN HUSSAIN

Practising as a General Practitioner (GP) for 18 years, Dr Shan Hussain has become a renowned author, health coach, wellness advisor and ambassador to the World Health Innovation Summit.

Dr Shan is founder of The Health Studio, believing in a holistic approach to health, centred around our collective physical, mental and social well-being. As such, he has a special interest in health promotion and disease prevention.

During his career, Dr. Hussain has developed several coaching programmes and mentorship schemes designed to help reverse the symptoms of many stress-related health problems, working with individuals and organisations to help naturally improve health in a sustainable way. His bestselling book, *The Big Prescription*, serves as a guide for readers to learn about evidence-based holistic health practices that create the foundation of his work.

As a firm believer that the top five causes of death in the UK – cancer, heart disease, stroke, lung and liver disease – all have preventable elements to them, he encourages simple lifestyle changes to prevent such illnesses from developing, while also improving levels of health, wellbeing, energy and vitality.

As part of the Primal Cure team, Dr Shan is the perfect fit. Because whilst cure is in our name, prevention is in our nature! See more from Dr Shan at **www.thehealthstudio.net**.

WHY I WROTE PRIMAL CURE

From my late twenties until December 2014, I always carried way too much weight around my midriff, despite the fact that I had strictly adhered to lots of diets and regularly participated in various endurance sports. However, when my wife (after a gap of eight years) announced that she was pregnant with our fifth child, I thought, "Holy crap I am going to be 50 years old with a one-year-old child!" I worried that I wouldn't be able to play sport with my new son or daughter like I have with my other children.

Let me not beat about the bush. The advice I received over the years from doctors and specialists about my excess weight was simply wrong. The low-fat diet I followed on and off led to a life of being constantly overweight. I had ran several full marathons, trekked to the North Pole, sailed across the Atlantic, walked from the east coast to the west coast of the UK, but no matter how much I exercised, I always had a big ugly gut. But I was in many ways lucky – at least it hadn't killed me.

Why call the book *The Primal Cure*? After intensive research and speaking with many experts, I have three core beliefs about how to live a healthy life: we need to eat a diet that is low in carbohydrates and high in quality fats and probiotics (as did Primal man); we should intersperse this food regime with intermittent fasting (as did Primal man); and we should supplement all of this with short sessions of high intensity exercise (you guessed it – as did Primal man). When living Primally, our body can self-heal and numerous aliments and illnesses can be cured.

Is *The Primal Cure* a diet book? That depends on your view of what a diet is. The word 'diet' is derived from the Greek word 'diaita', which means 'way of life', and in this respect *The Primal Cure* is the ultimate diet. But it is definitely not a diet book by the current interpretation of what the word means. As living our daily lives more Primally is enjoyable, it provides a long-term approach to sustainable health.

Does *The Primal Cure* work? Can it make me lose weight forever? Will it reduce my likelihood of dying of disease? The answer is yes, yes, yes. Not just yes to these questions, but to many more as well. However, what this book is not about is what you should do if you are already sick or severely ill, for that we have a wonderful national health service. While cure is in our name, prevention is in our nature.

Enjoy the new 'Primal you' with my guarantee that it works. It might take a little longer for some individuals to start reaping the benefits, but trust me, the benefits will come. Without cutting yourself off from all of your friends and family, it's unlikely that you will be able to follow all of the principles in this book all of the time. Above all I want you to be both happy and healthy, and I also want this-to be a lifestyle change – and for that to happen, you must enjoy it. The more of the philosophies you follow, the healthier you will be, but if after trying some you find that you don't like them, then leave those out.

I have spent 28 years building businesses and charities and have never been afraid to shout out when I see things that I believe are wrong. In-fact I see it as my responsibility; because as Albert Einstein once said "The right to search for the truth implies also a duty; one must not conceal any part of what one has recognized to be true". Our amazing team at Primal Cure, our incredible doctors and I, are all driven by one collective ambition; to reverse Great Britain's decline into ill health, by spreading truth about the food we eat, and the lifestyle choices we make, to every single home in the country.

Are you ready to rock the very foundations of what you believe about food? Are you ready to start providing your body with what Mother Nature created it to devour? Are you ready to reduce, even eliminate the prospect of you contracting many of the diseases we face in Great Britain? Are you ready to stop dieting and learn to eat naturally? Are you ready to prevent yourself from becoming another sick statistic?

Excellent, then let's begin the journey.

01.
Life Beyond
The Cave

This chapter is going to set out the Primal scene. It's part history, part biology and provides background information that will prove useful as you continue throughout the book.

Our environment, our lifestyle and the Great British diet have changed more over the past 100 years than over the past 1 million and there are now more sick Brits than ever. So much for progress!

How would you feel if I told you that most of what we have been conditioned and brought up to believe about food and health is simply wrong? In Chapter 1 we will discuss how these beliefs have formed, but for now feel free to read through the following list full of scepticism and doubt - by the end of this book you will wholly understand the truth about our health, well-being and longevity.

> **"Great is the power of steady misrepresentation." Charles Darwin**

Here are some of the biggest health misconceptions of modern times:

"Don't skip breakfast – it's the most important meal of the day."
Wrong! It's the most dangerous meal of the day and does not set us up properly as we have been taught to believe.

"Our health is predominantly hereditary."
Wrong! It's our diet, our lifestyle and our environment that ultimately shapes our health and longevity.

"We should eat a balanced diet."
Wrong! If you uncover something that's bad for your health you should avoid it. The only place we should occasionally balance is on the bathroom scales!

"Never eat red meat or fat as it causes heart conditions."
Wrong! Organic grass-fed meat is one of the healthiest foods we can consume. In fact, it is what we are designed to eat.

"Never sunbathe as it causes skin cancer."
Yes it can, but there is a far greater chance of developing other internal cancers, osteoporosis or heart conditions by avoiding the sun.

"Eat three meals a day and eat little but often."
Wrong! Eating this way actually triggers disease as our body never goes into repair mode. Intermittent fasting is how we were designed to eat.

"Consume 0% or low-fat everything."
Wrong! We now understand that quality fats are not our enemy. Food labelled as low fat or zero fat are stuffed full of sugars to replace these missing fats, and it's these sugars that are deadly.

"Don't skip meals because your metabolism will slow down."
Wrong! Unless we go a whole four days without food, skipping meals actually speeds up our metabolism.

"Brown bread, brown rice and whole grain cereals are all healthy."
Wrong! They are actually unhealthy foods dressed up in a nutritional outfit. They still turn into poisonous sugar in our body and could eventually cause many to develop type 2 diabetes.

"Educate yourself on what food labels mean."
Wrong! Real food doesn't need a label.

"Prawns, eggs and other food high in cholesterol will raise your cholesterol levels and should be avoided."
Wrong! Just because a certain food type is high in dietary cholesterol has little correlation to what happens when you have consumed it.

"Artificial sweeteners don't make you put on weight."
Wrong! They might not in themselves be very calorific, but they damage our healthy gut bacteria and switch off the satiety hormone, which informs us when we are full.

"Counting calories helps us to lose weight."
Wrong! The body processes calories from carbohydrates, fat and protein differently, therefore using calories as a measure is, in the main, futile. Plus, who wants to spend their entire life doing maths?

"Slogging our hearts out by jogging for endless hours is healthy."
Wrong! It's actually detrimental to our heart and instead we should
learn to exercise in short intervals.

"There is a pill for every ill."
True! But over prescription is responsible for one of the largest
increases in hospitals admission across Great Britain.

This chapter will provide a background to the Primal Cure well-being
principles that I will start to describe in Chapter 2. To truly grasp the
subject of health, we are first going to discuss a little about how our
caveman ancestors survived and thrived, and how we have evolved
since man first set foot on the planet. I will then cover a little biology
to help you develop an understanding of what happens to various food
types when they enter our body. Then we will look at how in a modern
age, with so much research and technology, we are facing a British
health disaster where 2 out of 3 adults are overweight or obese.

How is it that while contagious diseases that caused so much
devastation 100 years ago have been virtually eradicated, we now face
a completely new array of deadly conditions? This book will reveal all.

Major Killers	
100 Years Ago	Today
Pneumonia	Heart Disease
Tuberculosis	Cancer
Diarrhoea	Stroke
Other Killers	
100 Years Ago	Today
Polio	Diabetes
Measles	Alzheimer's
Syphilis	Respiratory Disease
Scarlet Fever	Liver Disease
Typhoid	Influenza
Whooping Cough	Pneumonia

PRIMAL EVOLUTION

To understand the principles of living a Primal lifestyle, we need to first develop a basic understanding of our evolution. Here is a very stripped back timeline of Earth and the progression of our species. Later we will put our flag in the sand and explain at which point our current DNA evolved, which is the same point we should all base our food and lifestyle choices upon.

The Primal Timeline

- Our Earth is 4.5 billion years old
- 3.6 billion years ago, the first microscopic organisms formed
- 230 million years ago, the Herrerasaurus was the first dinosaur to roam our planet.
- 6 million years ago, bipedal apes developed the ability to walk on two legs
- 3 million years ago, some human-like apes began using two legs as their main method of movement
- 2.5 million years ago, humans started to use hand tools, and for many paleoanthropologists and archaeologists this event marks the true beginning of the human race
- 200,000 years ago, Homo Sapiens (Latin for 'wise man') emerged in East Africa
- 100,000 years ago, Homo Sapiens learnt to create fire to heat food
- 70,000 years ago, the cognitive revolution wiped out our Neanderthal cousins and all other human species leaving Homo Sapiens to conquer the world
- 12,000 years ago, the agricultural revolution
- 6,000 years ago, the beginning of agricultural carbohydrates
- 2,500 years ago, the discovery that you could extract and dry the sap of sugar cane
- 300 years ago, sugar still counted for less than 1% of calorie intake
- 75 years ago, the first pesticides were introduced
- 50 years ago, the average adult in Great Britain was 2.5 stone (almost 16 kgs) lighter than today

While the human race can be traced back 2.5 million years ago, for the vast majority of that time we were not at the top of the food chain. For most of our existence, we have been the hunted rather than the hunter. Certainly, for the first 1.5 million years, we lived off foraging, collecting plants, and eating small animals. About the only time we would enjoy feasting on a larger beast would be when an even larger carnivore had moved on from its prey, leaving behind scraps for us humans. While different species of humans have been around for some 2.5 million years ('Lucy' is the skeletal remains of a female of the species Australopithecus afarensis), our ancestral species, Homo Sapiens, only emerged in east Africa around 200,000 years ago.

Around 100,000 years ago, we moved to the top of the food chain when we learnt to create fire and cook our own food. Prior to this, all food that we foraged or killed had to be eaten raw and cold, making much of it hard to digest. When we began to cook, our intestines were able to shrink as we evolved over a period of several tens of thousands of years. 'So what?,' I hear you say. Many experts believe that the shrinking of our intestines, an organ that required a huge amount of energy, provided an extra source of energy that allowed our brains to grow. This led to what Yuval Noah Harari describes in Sapiens as the 'cognitive revolution' that happened around 70,000 years ago.

Both before and after we learnt the ability to heat our food, meat from small animals such as rabbits and wild sheep, bugs, snails and insects were the backbone of our natural diet. But with heat came the ability to eat more fibrous and tough foods.

When meat could not be found or caught, then berries, figs, mushrooms, nuts, roots and leaves were consumed. At this point in our history there were no settlements and human life was nomadic. From season to season our ancestors would travel looking for new sources of food. What they ate in the summer would vary dramatically from what they ate in the cold winters. This brings us nicely to the start of our Primal Cure Principles, in that our early diets were very diverse and provided a wide array of crucial nutrients.

12,000 Years Ago

There were just a few million humans on Earth. That's like the
population of Birmingham spread across the entire planet. With so
much space and freedom, why would any human want to settle down?
When there were plenty of healthy wild animals, nutritious bugs and
organic plants, why would you change anything? But for some reason
they did. As humans migrated from East Africa, they came across
what we know today as Turkey and Iran. They seemed to like it there,
and decided to settle. They started to raise sheep and goats and began
to plant seeds. This was the beginning of the Agricultural Revolution
and the turning point in our evolution. This became our first step
away from eating what we were designed by nature to eat.

6,000 Years Ago

Saw the first development of agricultural carbohydrates. Their arrival
in Southern Europe has been associated with an average decrease
of six inches in height and a shortening of lifespan by 10 years.
The nomadic cultures of America that ate buffalo and the meat-
eating Maasai of Tanzania and Kenya, who all avoided agriculture
carbohydrates, remained tall and lean.

2,500 Years Ago

Humans first discovered that you could extract and dry the sap of
sugar cane. However, until just a little over a century ago, sugar was
still so rare that it was extremely expensive and only affordable by the
rich.

The Speed Of Evolution

As a species we evolve very slowly. Have you ever wondered why it is
that when we get out of the bath our fingers and toes are all wrinkly?
Let me tell you – it's because thousands of years ago we used to catch
fish with our bare hands and feet. Our toes and fingers went wrinkly
so that our feet could grip onto the rocks, and fish did not slip through
our fingers. Do we need to do this today? Of course not! It is, however,
going to take our DNA a very long time to catch up. The principle

of Primal Cure is we have to consume food and undertake a fitness regime in tune with the design of our DNA. It is not about counting calories, or doing what the big food corporations with their misguided and sometimes dishonest research tell us we should do. It's simply doing what nature has designed us to do.

Both our Primal doctors and I believe evolution in the main takes tens of thousands of years, so my starting point for most of my advice is in searching for ancestral precedent. Asking 'how long does it take for us to evolve?', is similar to asking 'how long is a piece of string?' The scientist François Jacob, who won the Nobel Prize in Physiology or Medicine in 1965, said: "Evolution is a tinkerer, not an engineer". So, as evolution is not an exact science, Primal Cure focuses on 'food that is natural to eat'. For that, we should surely look at the period before our ancestors started planting foods and, without question, before we started to genetically mess with them.

Think of evolution in another way. The further we live away from the equator, the paler our skin has become in order to maximise the diminishing amount of sunshine. So, if evolution were a quick process, within a few generations people of African descent would start to develop paler skin. Yet scientists suggest that it can take more than 1000 years to witness even the tiniest degree of change. Still, I would assume that lightening skin tones in order to absorb more sunlight, and therefore create more vitamin D, would not be as big a challenge for evolution as trying to deal with new types of incoming foods!

Today, so many people are on medication mainly because they are consuming foods that the body was not designed to deal with, and evolution hasn't had time to adapt to. An analogy would be that it's like putting the wrong type of fuel in our car and then stuffing it full of additives to try to make it perform!

> **Primal Cure principles are based on the varied diets and lifestyles of the human race, from before the agricultural revolution, which took place 12,000 years ago.**

A New You

Every five or six years, you and I almost become an entirely new person. Our skin is constantly dying and being replaced, in fact our entire outer covering is replaced every single month. Our complete skeleton is regenerated every 10 years or so. Our lungs are replaced every six weeks, our liver in less than six months, and our tongue's 9,000 taste buds are rejuvenated every 10 days. Sadly, the one body part most of us would love to be self-regenerating at high speed – our brain – is, in the main, as old as we are. In fact, most things in our head are permanently ours. The eyes don't replace themselves and once our adult teeth come through, that's our lot. The rest of our body, cell-by-cell, day-by-day, is in a state of continual repair, rebuild or replace... or it should be.

All of this replacing, regenerating and rejuvenating is fuelled by one thing and one thing only: what we consume. Hence the saying, 'we are what we eat'. If we eat junk food, our new body parts will be created by junk and will not be quite as good as the cells they are replacing. That's what causes ageing. Rubbish input equals rubbish output, or 'garbage in, garbage out' (GIGO) as computer scientists say. However, eat the right foods, drink enough water and get the right nutrients, and we are going to make some pretty good body parts and at the same time delay the ageing process.

Dr Shan Hussain

"I believe that you are not only what you eat but also what you absorb and assimilate from your environment."

FAT, PROTEIN & CARBOHYDRATES

Everything that lives – whether it be a vegetable or a human, a dog or a strawberry – is made of the same basic ingredients: fat, carbohydrates (dressed-up sugars) and proteins (amino acids). Fat, carbohydrates and protein are the three macronutrients that, either by themselves or combined, makes up all of the food we eat. The human body needs both fat and protein to survive and flourish but - contrary to popular belief - not a single ounce of carbohydrate is necessary.

Everything we eat - no matter what it looks like, its texture or its taste - is broken down in our gut into one of the three components mentioned above. Later in this book we will learn about micronutrients - which are other foodstuffs such as minerals, phytonutrients, fibre and vitamins - but first we need to get a clear and simple understanding of fat, protein and carbohydrates.

Why do we eat? There are two prime reasons. Firstly, in order to stay alive, from time to time we need to provide fuel to our organs. Secondly, to help repair and replace worn-out parts of our body, we need to consume certain minerals and vitamins. As it turns out, humans need roughly the same balance as all living animals. From koala bears to pigs, from giraffes to lions, from horses to humans, we all have similar needs when it comes to food and nutrition.

Let me start this section on macronutrients with something that came as a shock to me, and something that I still have the hardest time in convincing some of my more stubborn friends. Of the three macronutrients, it's not fat that makes us fat, it is carbohydrates. We could buy the flabbiest cut of meat on sale in our butcher's and serve it with a baked potato, and it would be the potato that makes us fat, not the flabby meat. You see, it's quite simple, our body has no intention of storing fat as fat! Our body has a preference to use fat as fuel.

There are some healthy fats and some deadly fats (especially when it comes to cooking oils), but we will get to these later. We will also learn later that for the body to store fat as fat, it needs the presence of lots of sugar to glue (glycerol) it together, but for now it is important to really understand these two very important and possibly life-changing facts:

1. Eating fat does not make us fat.
2. Carbohydrates and other sugars are the only macronutrients that are easily converted into body fat.

Dr Dan Maggs

"Natural fats are not the enemy. We have demonised and vilified he good guy for more than 50 years, and all the while the sickly sweet kid has been getting away with murder!"

Fat

While proteins and carbohydrates are fairly straightforward to understand, fats are a little more complex. Rather than provide chapter and verse straight away, we will cover just the basics right now and then build up the picture throughout the book.

Let me again state that if we are overweight, fat in food is not our enemy but our friend. Or, more precisely, good fats should become our new best friends. Fats don't make us fat, and never have done. It's carbohydrates and to a far lesser degree protein that causes us to pile on weight, but not fat. I remember how I would always cut the fat off my beef, lamb, chicken and duck in the belief it was the fat that made us fat, when in reality leaving it on meat means we drop it from our waistline.

Quality fats correct our hormones and keep them in balance so that we feel more energetic. Quality fats actually help us burn more energy (not store it) and make us feel fuller so that we stop overeating. And, more importantly, quality fats reduce the likelihood of us falling victim to six out of ten of the most common causes of death in Great Britain!

Sources of good fats include anything rich in Omega 3 such as salmon, flax seeds, nuts, avocado, coconuts, olive and organic butter. Deadly fats to avoid include all trans fats (normally food labels call them 'partially hydrogenated oils') and vegetable oils, which are rarely derived from vegetables.

Protein

This is the basic building block of all life forms. Its name comes from the Greek word 'proteios', meaning 'primary' or 'first'. Protein is the driving force of change within our body. It comes to our aid when we need repairing – it rebuilds many of our organs, body tissue and muscles. It is responsible for growth in the young and is the creator of our hormones.

Protein is made up of amino acids. There are 22 different types of amino acids and they are all created from the elements carbon, hydrogen, nitrogen or sulphur. Our body can actually produce most of the different proteins that it needs, but there are nine that it can't make and these are very important to our health. For this reason they are named the 'essential proteins' and it is imperative that they form part of our diet.

In 2007 the World Health Organisation published a report scoring the quality of proteins from various food sources. As animals contain similar combinations of proteins to humans, it's not surprising that food derived from animals topped the list, with eggs, poultry, meat and fish the clear winners.

Once the body receives amino acids from foods rich in protein or from supplements, using the 22 different incoming varieties it is able to make the more than 50,000 different varieties of protein inside our body (this is known as protein synthesis). Once these new proteins are synthesised they form, among other things, our organs, bones and blood, and replace or repair muscle tissue. They are responsible for the creation of essential hormones such as insulin, melatonin and human growth hormone.

Proteins, along with fibre, make us feel full and therefore less likely to overeat. In Chapter 9 we discuss the healthy foods that should form part of our regular diet, but for now let's state that a good way to take on board protein includes organic meat, organic chicken, organic eggs, oily fish, green vegetables and nuts.

> **PRIMAL HEALTH FACT:**
> **Protein is the building block of all life forms.**

Carbohydrates

Once we start living Primally, our new dietary enemy becomes sugar and processed carbohydrates. Carbohydrates are almost exclusively derived from plants (plus a few dairy products) and are not found in meat, fish or poultry.

Throughout this book you will see carbohydrates written as CARBS. The reason for this is that I want you to see carbohydrates for what they are, with a very apt acronym: 'Carbohydrates Are Really Bad Sugars'. What do I mean by this? Basically, carbohydrates are just sugar in disguise.

Potatoes, pasta, bread and rice all convert to sugar in the body and, to the body, sugar is poison! They might be dressed up in fancy packaging, and often carry labels with misleading health benefits, but we need to realise our body was never designed to consume them.

Whether they are simple or complex, all CARBS are still eventually turned into sugar by our body. The complex ones just take a little longer. Every time we eat any CARBS, complex or not, we are eating sugar. Too much sugar makes us fat, and will eventually lead to a whole host of problems, illnesses and diseases.

THE CARBOCOASTER

With the exception of fibre, all CARBS are converted to sugar, and any excess sugar in the blood is bundled up by insulin and stored as body fat. This can happen so quickly that shortly after a CARB-loaded meal, we feel hungry again. We call this the Carbocoaster.

The Carbocoaster works like this. We eat a sandwich and the body converts the bread to sugar. Our brain summons insulin to quickly grab any excess sugar, which to our body is pure poison, and stores it as fat. Because the bread is now no longer in circulation, we feel hungry again, so consume another. The Carbocoaster effect is enhanced because both the blood sugar levels keep getting topped up and then depleted quickly, and after the initial surge of insulin this too plummets as it finishes hiding the sugar. This rollercoaster only happens with CARBS and other sugars. There is no fatocoaster or proteinocoaster, just the dangerous, highly addictive, adrenalin-rushing, body-crushing, high-speed Carbocoaster. As a nation which is ill, we need to get off this ride as quickly as we can as it is making us hungry, sick and very obese!

Different books, different experts and different doctors tell us how many CARBS we should consume each day if we want to lose weight. Some will say 70g, some 100g and some very specific amounts such as 73g. But the reality is the body doesn't actually need any CARBS at all! Put simply, the fewer CARBS we eat the quicker we lose weight.

When we get down to our ideal weight, if we want a couple of apples or bananas then we can go for it. We won't want bread because once we start living without it, we become as averse to it as we would if we were forced to eat a dead rat! If we start eating too many CARBS in fruits and vegetables and our weight starts to pile back on, we simply just cut them down again. It is that straightforward.

CARBS and other sugars work on the brain the same as cigarettes. We get a craving and we eat a pack of crisps, mints or a doughnut or two.

It satisfies us for a short while, but not for long. Before we know it, we want more. One biscuit becomes two biscuits becomes three biscuits and so on. CARBS are addictive and just like cigarettes they have the power to cause chronic illness and kill us!

TYPES OF CARBS

Let's look at CARBS in a little more detail. Depending on the size of the molecule, they may be known as either simple or complex. As well as breaking down into simple or complex, CARBS are also categorised as refined or unrefined.

Simple CARBS

These are the CARBS with the smallest molecules, so they are quickly absorbed and give a rapid boost in energy, a rapid increase in blood sugar levels and cause a spike in the production of insulin. As they are converted to energy so quickly, if we don't burn off this energy promptly it is quickly stored as fat in our body's favourite fat store. Simple CARBS include virtually all types of sugar. They are also found in natural products such as milk and fruit. But most of all, we are going to find them hidden in all sorts of processed foods, sweets and fizzy drinks.

Complex CARBS

These CARBS are composed of long strings of simple carbohydrates and are therefore bigger. As they are bigger they have to be deconstructed into simple CARBS before they can be absorbed. As a result they provide energy more slowly. Because complex CARBS are digested more slowly, with a slower release of energy, there is more opportunity for our body to use the fuel and they are therefore less likely to be stored as body fat. However, the energy from complex CARBS is still released faster than both protein and fat. Potatoes, peas, whole grain, wheat, rice, pasta and beans are all complex CARBS.

Now before you rush out and eat loads of potatoes, rice, pasta or grains because I have informed you that they are called complex

CARBS, I want you to remember that they still convert to sugar (it just takes a little longer).

Refined CARBS

These are CARBS that have been highly processed in a factory. Any goodness that the CARBS might have been hiding, such as fibre, minerals and vitamins, are normally removed, or at best dramatically reduced, in the refining process. On the packaging of refined CARBS, we will often read that they have vitamins and minerals added, but these are only putting back some of the goodness that resided before being processed.

Unrefined CARBS

As you will have correctly guessed, these are CARBS that have not been processed. As well as vegetables and brown rice, foods labelled as whole grain or multigrain are generally unrefined. Here is the good news: unrefined CARBS from vegetables and fruits (as long as they are organic) come complete with all of the vitamins and minerals that Mother Nature intended for us to consume. That said, if CARBS are over cooked, then their nutritional values start to diminish and in some cases disappear completely.

Complex & Unrefined CARBS

So if someone eats complex CARBS that are unrefined, then surely they won't put on weight – right? It's a nice idea, but unless we are exercising and keeping portion sizes extremely small, then most likely we will. You see, if we consume any more CARBS than we can burn at that time, while the body will store a small amount in the liver and muscles, it will send the rest to our fat stores.

If you are still not convinced that it's CARBS that make us fat with their constant and continual conversion into sugar, and their quick release into the bloodstream causing a spike in insulin, then why s there such a thing called the Glycemic Index? Food labels index all CARBS based on how quickly they perform this task. There is no glycemic index for either protein or fat. Why? Because protein rarely converts into poisonous sugar and fat never does.

GLYCEMIC INDEX

First of all, the name 'glycemic' is derived from the medical term 'glycemia' meaning 'the presence of glucose in the blood'. All CARBS receive a glycemic index (GI) score from 1 to 100. The lower the number the better - or should I say, 'less horrible'. A score of 1 is the lowest and slowest and 100 is the highest and fastest to convert CARBS to glucose (sugar). Therefore, pure sugar obviously scores 100. However, it is not as black and white as the GI score might suggest, as it assumes we are only eating the food being scored in isolation and not combining it with other foods, which when bound together after digested may change the speed of conversion into sugar.

The other limiting factor of GI is that it doesn't look at portion sizes. There are some items with a fairly low GI score, where the portions sizes are by definition big and therefore still not recommended if we are either trying to lose weight or stay healthy. A more reflective index is the glycemic load (GL). While GI is useful to know how quickly glucose will enter the bloodstream, the GL informs us how dangerous that load will be.

The GL index is calculated simply by multiplying the typical grams of carbohydrates in a serving by the GI index for that type of CARB and then dividing it by 100.

Let's look at a few examples. While a watermelon has a high GI of 72 (based on the GI alone we would not touch it with a barge pole), because it has so little carbohydrate in weight per serving, its GL is only 5. Carrots are similar. Their GI is relatively high at 39, but as the CARB density is so low, their GL is only 2.

All brand name data in the following tables was taken from **www.health.harvard.edu** on 12th April 2017.

Food	GI	Serving Size (Gram)	GL Per Serving
Lucozade, original (sparkling glucose drink)	95	250ml	40
Baked potato	85	1 medium (173g)	28
White rice, boiled	64	1 cup (186g)	33
Macaroni and cheese	64	1 serving (166g)	30
Raisins	64	1 small box (43g)	20
Spaghetti, white, boiled 20 mins	42	1 cup (140g)	16
Bagel, white, frozen	72	1 small bagel 70g	25
Rice Krispies	82	1.25 cups (33g)	23
Fanta, orange soft drink	68	250ml	23
Spaghetti, white, boiled, average	46	1 cup (180g)	22
Sweet potato	54	1 cup (133g)	12
Pizza	30	2 slices (260g)	13
Instant oatmeal, average	79	1 serving (250g)	21
Boiled white potato, average	82	150g	21
Coco Pops, average	77	1 serving (30g)	20
Corn Flakes, average	81	1 serving (30g)	20
Dates, dried, average	42	handful (60g)	18
Snickers bar, average	51	60g	18
Sponge cake, plain	46	1 serving (63g)	17
Rice cakes, average	82	1 piece (25g)	17

Food	GI	Serving Size (Gram)	GL Per Serving
Spaghetti, whole-grain, boiled	42	1 cup (180g)	17
Instant mashed potato, average	87	1 serving (150g)	17
Coca Cola, (US formula)	63	250ml	16
Brown rice, steamed	50	1 serving (150g)	16
Sweet corn on the cob	48	1 piece (60g)	14
Oatmeal, average	55	1 serving (250g)	13
Quinoa, cooked	53	1 cup (150g)	13
Cheerios	74	1 cup (30g)	13
Corn tortilla	52	1 serving (50g)	12
Apple juice, unsweetened	41	1 cup (248g)	12
Orange juice, unsweetened	50	1 cup (248g)	14
Potato crisps, average	56	1 bag (40g)	12
Hot chocolate	51	1 cup (28g)	12
White wheat flour bread	75	1 slice	11
Banana, raw, average	52	1 large	14
Bran Flakes	74	3/4 cup (29g)	13
Grapes, black	59	1 serving (120g)	11
Corn chips, plain, salted	42	1 serving (50g)	11
Pita bread, white	68	1 piece (30g)	10
Muesli, average	56	1 serving (30g)	10
Kidney beans, average	34	1 cup (150g)	9
Ice cream, regular, average	62	1 cup (72g)	10

Food	GI	Serving Size (Gram)	GL Per Serving
Graham cracker	74	2 pcs (14g)	8
Microwave popcorn, plain, average	65	1 serving (20g)	7
Chicken nuggets, frozen, reheated	46	4 pieces (100g)	7
Baked beans	40	1 serving (150g)	6
M&Ms, peanut	33	1 handful (30g)	6
Apple, average	38	1 medium size	6
Oranges, raw, average	45	1 medium size	5
Tomato juice, no sugar added	38	1 cup (243g)	3
Milk, full fat, average	31	250ml	4
Milk, skim, average	31	250ml	4
Pear, raw, average	38	120g	4
Watermelon	72	1 serving (120g)	4
Green peas	54	1 cup (80g)	4
Parsnips	52	1 piece (80g)	4
Strawberries	40	1 cup (152g)	4
Grapefruit	25	1/2 slice	3
Chickpeas	10	1 cup (150g)	3
Cashews, salted	22	2 handfuls (50g)	3
Carrots, average	39	1 piece (80g)	2
Beansprouts	25	1 cup (104g)	1
Soy beans, average	15	1 cup (150g)	1
Peanuts	13	2 handfuls (50g)	1

Food	GI	Serving Size (Gram)	GL Per Serving
Broccoli, cabbage, celery, cauliflower, green beans, mushrooms, spinach, almonds, hazelnuts, macadamia, pecan, walnuts, beef, chicken, eggs, fish, lamb, pork, veal, shellfish, lobster, turkey, ham	0	As much as we like	0

HARA HACHI BU

Wait a minute I hear you cry. Don't half of Asia rely on rice for their diet and if it is true that it turns to sugar, then surly they would all be obese. I understand your scepticism. This was the first question I asked when I was told about the evil way of CARBS. But before I tell you about Hara Hachi Bu, bear in mind that in Asia, they tend to be far less sedentary than us Brits, intermittent fasting is also common place and in the main they have far less toxins in their homes than we do in Great Britain. In other words they live far more Primally than we do. But what is Hara Hachi Bu? The Huffington Post summarised it best in a recent article, "The Japanese practice something that makes such sense that I can't believe we don't start teaching this to our kids. It's called "hara hachi bu". It means, eat until you are 80% full. You have probably heard about the Okinawan people and how they often live to 100. They are the longest lived, healthiest people on the planet and they practice hara hachi bu".

The Okinawan people don't eat until they feel full, they eat until they are no longer hungry. Both of these feelings are controlled by hormones, which is the next subject we will take a look at. They also eat a lot more slowly, which also makes them feel like they have consumed more. Eating more slowly has also been attributed to the longer life span of people living in the Mediterranean.

Why do we over eat in Great Britain? Is it simply because we were told by our parents not to leave anything on the plate? Possibly. But more likely it's the supersized portions of sugar loaded takeaways and packaged foods, that have damaged our brains response to a hormone known as leptin.

LEPTIN VS GHRELIN

Armed with a basic understanding of the macronutrients - fat, protein and CARBS - it's time to discuss hormones. First of all, what is a hormone? For now let's think of it in its simplest form: it is a chemical that is released by one part of the body to deliver a memo to a different part. How does the hormone know where to deliver the message? Most biology books suggest that the hormone is like a key and it only opens one lock. In other words, the intended recipient has a shape that only the intended hormone fits into.

If you are guilty of overeating and are overweight or obese, it might not be your fault at all. The guilty party might be a little-known hormone called leptin. After we have eaten a meal, our body is supposed to release this little fella and send him off to our brain to tell us that we're full – to basically tell us to stop eating. Leptin is actually dispatched from our fat stores with a clear message to say we're stuffed, stop sending us more supplies, we're overcrowded.

If something goes wrong with our leptin and it doesn't want to get out of bed and go to work, then we will crave food all day and pile on weight. Not only that, when leptin is having a lie-in, his colleagues in the metabolic department slow down too. It's a double blow for our body. We feel hungry, we consume more food, and our slowed metabolism isn't going to use much of it for fuel.

As Dr Michael VanDerschelden explains in *The Scientific Approach to Intermittent Fasting*, "When we eat a meal under normal conditions, leptin rises, blocks hunger and causes the thyroid to release thyroid hormones to increase metabolism".

When we eat too many CARBS, there is a heightened possibility of developing type 2 diabetes. This is where fat cells can become insulin resistant due to a constant bombardment over a prolonged period of time. Sadly, for those who are overweight or obese, it's the same story with leptin. Over time as you get heavier and heavier, your body cries out for help and dispatches more and more leptin to the brain in an attempt to rein in appetite and stop us from eating. With so much leptin knocking on the door, the brain refuses to listen. It then doesn't realise that it has been fed and thinks it's starving. Not only do you carry on eating, but also the brain warns the thyroid that you are in a period of starvation and tells it to slow down your metabolism. Doubly unhelpful whammy! So now with your slow metabolism, feeling tired and constantly hungry, you sit on the sofa and scoff more foods high in sugar, because they're what's going to make you feel fuller faster. It's a race to the bottom in more ways than one!

If you are overweight, there is every chance that your body has become resistant to leptin. So how do you get the brain to start acknowledging it again? Simply by following four Primal Cure beliefs: eat healthy fats and not CARBS; intermittently fast; get more active; and consume plenty of fibre - as it is known to help repair leptin resistance.

Throughout this book, you are going to discover how vital it is to develop the right type of bacteria in your gut. One way to nurture leptin is to develop colonies of bacteria that support it and remove those that can damage its production. Put another way, some varieties of bacteria can sabotage leptin production, causing us to overeat.

Ghrelin is the opposite of leptin. This hormone is the one that informs us that we are hungry. Ghrelin is essentially our hunger hormone. Before we eat, he runs around screaming to be fed. But after we have eaten, he is sent to the bedroom to wake up leptin and tell him to go to work. What seems to happen when we are overweight is that our ghrelin never goes to sleep. It might slow down the requests for food a little bit while we are eating, but it seems to be ever-present.

Most people go and eat as soon as they hear ghrelin demanding to be fed, but if we can resist its demands, wonderful things start to happen inside our body. First of all, we kick-start our automated repair process, we begin to fight inflammation (which is one of the biggest factors of modern disease) and we stimulate human growth hormones (HGH). What's best is Mr Ghrelin gets a little angry when we don't listen to him, so recruits more and more of his ghrelin family to assist him in trying to get us to eat and the more ghrelin there is in our body the more good it does. Combine this with exercise and we will increase our HGH even more.

As you will read later, there are great gains for most people in skipping breakfast. One of the scientific reasons for this is that there is a lot of ghrelin in our bodies after a good night's sleep and if we can resist its calls for food and exercise in this fasted state, then our health is really going to reap the benefits.

MICROBIOME

For easier comprehension I will keep the explanation brief at this point, but will build on this 'crucial to our health' subject throughout the book.

'Microbiome' is the name given to the collective array of more than 10,000 different species of microscopic living organisms residing in and on our body. Known as microbes, these organisms are too small to see with the naked eye, but rest assured we humans are all home to a colossal quantity of them - in fact, so many of them that they vastly outnumber or own body cells. These microbes include bacteria (good and bad), fungi, protists, archaea, viruses and even microscopic animals.

There is a good reason why I have followed leptin vs ghrelin with a small section on our microbiome. Today, there is much research that suggests it is the type of microbes that are most prevalent in our gut that actually control our feelings of fullness or hunger. In other words, it's not our brain telling us that we are hungry or full, but the colony of microbes that, via our diet, we have allowed to gain a disproportional critical mass.

While there are said to be more than 10,000 different species of microbes in our body, adding up to some 100 trillion in total and meaning that statistically we are 90% microbe and only 10% human – just two groups dominate our guts. I didn't just pluck these numbers out of thin air - there is a fascinating and wonderfully written book by biologist and zoologist Dr Alanna Collen called *10% Human*, which is certainly worth getting hold of. *10% Human* brilliantly details the intertwined lives of microbes and humans and provides an insight into what is happening inside our guts and what a huge contributing factor to body weight and obesity our microbes play.

Let's get back to the two varieties of microbes that play a dominating role in our gut, Firmicutes and Bacteroidetes. These two strands of microbes alone can control whether we stay lean or get fat. When I learnt this, a light bulb went off inside my small brain. I had always wondered why my wife could eat unhealthily for a few days and put on no weight at all, but after just one unhealthy meal I would wake up the next day and scream at my bathroom scales.

First, let's talk about Firmicutes. Even though their name might sound as if they make us firm and cute, they are actually responsible for the total opposite! These bacteria are experts at extracting as much energy (calories) as possible out of the food that we eat. Of course, the more calories that are absorbed, the more weight we will put on. If we can keep our not-so-cute Firmicutes under control, and let our Bacteroidetes flourish, we are less likely to put on weight. Bacteroidetes carry out the opposite task to Firmicutes. After extracting vital nutrients and vitamins from food in our intestines, they let many calories slip through the net and exit the body by catching a ride on the fibre in our poo.

An article in the Huffington Post in December 2014 stated, "Avoid sugars and processed carbs. Firmicutes are so well-suited to grow on sugar that they're known to grow rampantly in factories that process sugar cane into table sugar". There is a lot more to come about our microbiome later on in the book, but for now let's move on.

If you're still not convinced that the difference from being fat or slim could be as simple as taking care of our gut microbiome and ensuring our Bacteroidetes triumph over our Firmicutes, then let me tell you about a recent biological study involving human twins and a group of healthy slim mice. One of the twins had become obese, and scientists injected bacteria from her gut into the gastrointestinal tract of the mice. The other twin had remained svelte and the scientists injected her bacteria into a different group of mice. Guess what happened. Those mice given the bacteria from the obese twin became obese and those that received the bacteria from the slim twin remained lean.

What is this research telling us? If we are overweight or obese, it might not be our fault at all, instead we could have developed a faulty microbiome. It might not have anything to do with a lack of willpower, or genetics, but the fact our bad bacteria are constantly messing with the signals we send to our brain and making us always feel hungry. It's yet another good reason to cut out CARBS and other sugars, and to start eating healthy fibrous foods.

FIBRE

> **PRIMAL HEALTH FACT:**
> It's important to have lots of fibre in our diet as it
> works in partnership with bacteroidetes to literally
> flush our calories down the toilet.

On my last visit to Tanzania, I started to wonder if it was just a lower intake of food that made everyone look so lean and healthy, or whether something else was stopping their obesity rates rising like they are in Great Britain. I asked if anyone had a secret to tell me, but sadly nobody understood that there was any other way to be. When I showed a classroom of children photos of fat British people (just type 'fat British people' into Google and click 'Images' to experience what the kids saw), they burst out laughing and ran around the classroom, sticking their bellies out as far as they could! That night, back in my hotel, I found a report by the National Academy of Sciences of the United States of America titled, 'Impact of diet in shaping gut microbiota revealed by a comparative study in children from Europe and rural Africa'. It began by stating the methodology: "We compared the fecal microbiota of European children (EU) and that of children from a rural African village of Burkina Faso (BF), where the diet, high in fibre content, is similar to that of early human settlements at the time of the birth of agriculture".

The results were staggering, and the whole report is online and worthy of a read. Here is just a small snippet from their conclusion: "Both in the Western world and in developing countries diets rich in fat, protein and sugar, together with reduced intake of unabsorbable fibres, are associated with a rapid increase in the incidence of non-infectious intestinal diseases".

Don't assume this is suggesting that we shouldn't eat fat, protein or sugar, because if it was there would be nothing left to eat. What it is suggesting, is that eating a combination of all three causes problems, especially in the absence of fibre. We will discuss fibre in more detail later.

Dr Shan Hussain

"How important is fibre to our health? According to The American Journal of Clinical Nutrition – consuming 35g of fibre was associated with a lower risk of cardiovascular disease by as much as 54% and death from all causes by 37%."

FROM OUR LIPS TO OUR BOTTOM:
GUT BUSINESS

'A taste on the lips, forever on the hips' goes the saying and, of course, if we are talking about CARBS and other sugars then that is extremely apt. But what we need to develop is a heightened awareness of what happens once food has left our mouth. It's amazing that the vast majority of humans (including me for 48 years) eat stuff every day and only ever think about how it tastes. Most people only ever think about the very first step of the process, because it's the only step that they misguidedly believe they actually experience. The reality of course is very different.

Let's first look at how we digest food. The act of digestion is the breaking down of food by a combination of chemical and physical means. If we can understand the basics, then we will begin to understand how important it is that we eat the right things. When we talk about digestion, it all starts in our nostrils. We rev up our digestive machine the moment we smell the aromas from food. Whether it is sweets, Sunday dinner or a ripe fruit, our mouths begin to produce saliva, our bellies rumble and our intestinal glands set in motion the secretion of various chemicals. Our eyes can also kick-start our digestive system by sending positive messages to the brain.

Then, as we chew our food, our teeth and tongue work in partnership with saliva to break it down for delivery into our body. The mush then travels down from our throat into a 25cm tube called the oesophagus (also called the gastro-intestinal tract or GI tract) and drops into our stomach. It might surprise you that food doesn't just sit still in our stomach, but is churned like a washing machine, with its contents constantly hitting the sidewalls until they break down into much smaller particles. The physical motion is aided by enzymes (molecules that speed up chemical reactions) and acids that are strong enough to dissolve some metals. The length of the stomach spin cycle varies depending on what we have eaten. Simple CARBS virtually pass straight through, but more fibrous foods and meats can take five or six hours before they are ready to leave the stomach on their way to the small intestine.

Our small intestine is a massive 7m (23 feet) in length, and it is way more complex than we might at first imagine. On the inside its surface is not smooth, but looks like a valley full of billions of little cactus plants. These enable the small intestine to create a huge surface area that is bigger than a tennis court! Each square millimetre of our small intestine is filled with 30 or so of these cactus-like structures known as villi. But what purpose does our small intestine fulfil? It breaks down all of the food we eat into the three macronutrients: fat into fatty acids, carbohydrates into sugar and protein into amino acids. The villi then absorb these molecules, placing them into our bloodstream, and dispatch them to the liver to perform a safety check before being passed into the main circulatory system.

If you try to picture the small intestine, you might think that, with its complex cactus-like lining and its job of making all different types of food - from curries to cakes - disappear, it is a pretty smelly and dirty environment. However, at the end of each process, it actually goes through its own cleaning and cleansing routine. The problem is that, if we constantly eat food, it never gets time to finish the job properly. This is one of the many benefits of intermittent fasting – it lets our small intestine finish its cleaning routine properly.

The small intestine passes its goods to the liver for cleansing, however, once it's completed its job, the liver doesn't immediately pass it all into the bloodstream, but actually hangs on to some of the incoming energy molecules and stores them as glycogen. The rest of the molecules finally come to rest in our cells, where the mitochondria (pronounced 'my-toe-con-dria', the powerhouse in each cell) burn them for fuel. Then, like when we burn anything, the process gives off heat, and it is this heat from our cells having their lunch that keeps our body at a regular temperature of 36–37°C.

However, the small intestine has to process fat differently. Fat is insoluble and therefore can't be dispatched into the bloodstream. Instead the small intestine sends fat on a different highway known as the lymphatic system. This works alongside the blood vessels that carry protein (amino acids) and CARBS (sugars). It's like a dual carriageway running alongside the motorways of the body.

Although the two run alongside each another, there is one major difference. While the liver performs a safety check on the sugar and amino acids in our blood before allowing it into the stream, the lymphatic system does not pass its produce through any organ for a safety check. This is one of the reasons why it is important to understand the difference between healthy and unhealthy fats. The fats go straight to the heart to be pumped out into our system. The heart can't perform any detoxification process like the liver does – it can't tell the difference between healthy coconut oil or the deadly highly processed so-called vegetable oils found in packaged food - it just simply injects it into our bloodstream.

Let's recap on the function of the small intestine (also known as the small bowel). It acts like a giant cheese grater and breaks down food into the three main macronutrients and dispatches the energy to fuel our body. Picture it as our internal food processor – it's quick and efficient, and with some types of food gets straight to work after we have eaten. But not everything we consume can be digested by the small intestine, and what it can't cope with is passed into the large intestine.

The large intestine is our well-being centre. Its job is to process all the micronutrients and vitamins that our body requires to operate properly. It is slower and more precise, and sifts through all the leftovers passed on by the small intestine. In terms of length, our large intestine is approximately 1.5 metres long, but it receives its 'large' prefix because of its diameter, which is a gigantic 6–7cm (2.3–2.8in). Yes, we have a pipe inside us that's as long as a pogo stick and as wide as a drainpipe. When we stop and think about how massive these two organs are, our first impression might be to question the reason for their huge size. After all, their role doesn't sound as vital as the lungs that keep us breathing or the heart that pumps blood around our body – both of which are tiny by comparison. But their vast size should act as proof of how vital what we eat is to our overall well-being.

Let's get back to our large intestine's role. Its job is to deal with all of the undigested stuff, and it does this in several ways. Firstly, it tries to reclaim all of the fluids that have been used in the digestive process and put them back into the body. The part of the large intestine responsible for returning water and salts is known as the colon. Another vital role for the large intestine is to process nutrients. It is also home to huge colonies of microbes known as our gut flora, which believe it or not, weighs more than our brain!

Once the entire digestive tract has finished its job, the large intestine signals to the brain that it's home time and together they converse with the final part of the large intestine – the rectum – on the exit strategy for the leftovers, i.e. faeces! The whole procedure of processing food varies in length based on several things including what we have eaten, our age, stress levels and exercise. On average assume it's a 16–24 hour cycle.

In Chapter 7, we will discuss how to maintain a healthy gut in more detail. Hopefully this brief introduction to how we digest food will have highlighted how large a process it is for the body, and later we will discuss how our gut can play a lead role in either the prevention or creation of cancers, Alzheimer's, Parkinson's, inflammation and many more diseases that are epidemic in Great Britain.

METABOLISM

Let's now look at what happens when we eat from a metabolic point of view. Metabolism is a series of chemical reactions that take place inside our body to maintain life. The requirements of life for us humans are things such as reproducing, growing, maintaining a constant body temperature, and so on. All of this can be broken down to the body's ability to utilise four different biomolecules – fats, proteins, carbohydrates and nucleic acids. As we already know, we are designed to eat a certain diet, and the evolution of our species hasn't yet progressed to consume the manufactured and lab created stuff that we all too often put into our body. We were designed to eat free roaming-animals and naturally-growing plants. It's that simple. After all, fresh plants and wild animals were the only food available to our caveman forefathers.

As we eat food, our body digests each meal and breaks it all down to the component parts of these four biomolecules. For example, the smallest component of fat is known as fatty acids, the smallest component of proteins is amino acids (the good stuff that builds muscles), and for carbohydrates they simply become sugar. The fourth is nucleic acids that break down into nucleotides. I won't mention these much in the book, as they are in the main only found in such things as shellfish and offal (organs such as the liver and heart).

The body processes different nutrients in a particular order, based on how easy the task is. Alcohol is absorbed very quickly and around a quarter of what we drink can be transferred into the bloodstream and hit the brain in less than one minute! Next come carbohydrates, which easily break down into sugar, followed by the conversion of protein into amino acids. Fats are left until last, as it is quite a complex task for the body to convert them to fatty acids.

Once the small intestine has finished its work metabolising all of the macronutrients, as mentioned in the previous topic, they follow two different routes. Glucose (the name of sugar when in the bloodstream), amino acids and minerals such as magnesium, calcium and iron, along with soluble vitamins B and C, are transported via the bloodstream to the liver for processing before being dispatched throughout the body. Fatty acids and vitamins A, D, E and K take a different route and enter the lymphatic system where they are passed directly into the blood and sent to cells around the body.

INSULIN

Let's start with a basic understanding of insulin. When glucose
levels are too high - such as what happens after eating sugary foods,
carbohydrates or a huge amount of protein - the pancreas releases
a hormone known as insulin which binds to the liver and muscle
cells, signalling for them to remove glucose (a liquid form of sugar)
from the bloodstream and store it as insoluble glycogen (a solid). The
problem is that, depending on our build, the liver and muscle stores
combined only hold around 300–500g of glycogen, which in terms of
calories is just 1,200 to 2,000, after which all excess glucose becomes
stored as body fat (also known as adipose tissue).

On the other hand, when our blood sugar levels are too low, the
pancreas releases a hormone know as glucagon that breaks down
insoluble glycogen (solid) into soluble glucose (liquid), allowing it to
be released into the bloodstream for use as energy or when it breaks
down glycogen in a muscle that itself needs energy, it uses it as its own
fuel.

Glucagon works in the opposite direction to insulin. The two of them
need to work in partnership to ensure the right amount of glucose is
in the blood.

> ### Energy Sources
> Our body can use three types of fuel. For immediate use, it burns
> glucose. When that's not readily available it calls upon glycogen
> and eventually, when it is out of both glucose and glycogen, it
> consumes fat.
>
> - **Liver** - 100g of glycogen (400 calories)
> - **Muscles** - 300–500g of glycogen (1200 to 2000 calories,
>   enough fuel for an hour or so workout)
> - **Body fat** - 10,000–25,000g of glycogen (40,000 to 100,000
>   calories)

The role insulin performs in the human body is similar to the role of nacre inside an oyster. Pearls are formed in oysters, when a foreign body such as a grain of sand enters the shell and begins to irritate the fleshy little creature inside. In an act of self-defence, the oyster excretes a layer of nacre over the intruder. Trouble is - with its new, shiny, larger coating -this little intruder becomes even more irritating. So the oyster, which obviously isn't overly bright, excretes another layer of nacre over the original layer. This event is repeated over and over again, until eventually the oyster is prised open and a gleaming pearl, often as big as 15mm (0.6in) in diameter, pops out.

The way a pearl is created is very similar to the role of insulin in the body. After we have eaten food with a sugary content, or after the body has converted CARBS into sugar, the body cries out for help in getting rid of the poisonous interloper. Yes, our body sees sugar as a poison. The pancreas steps up and secretes the hormone insulin all over the sugar, in an action not dissimilar to the oyster, secreting nacre over its unwanted intruder. But our body is brighter than the oyster and decides not to leave it in a place where it's going to constantly irritate us, but instructs insulin to march off, carrying excess sugar to our fat stores.

The trouble is, when we keep sending lots and lots of insulin to our fat stores, they get overcrowded and often become what is known as insulin sensitive or insulin resistant. It's a bit like being in a noisy office – we notice the distraction at first, but eventually we just block it out. For those who eat too frequently, and who consume lots of CARBS, the end result might be hyperglycemia (chronically elevated sugar in the blood) or hyperinsulinemia (dangerously high amounts of insulin in the blood).

This is what often causes type 2 diabetes, when overconsumption of CARBS leads to the cells shutting up shop and not letting insulin do its job. Incidentally, type 1 diabetes is much rarer and is a very different condition. For those suffering with type 1, the body isn't able to generate sufficient or any insulin to transport the CARBS and other sugars from the blood and into the body, and therefore most sufferers have to inject themselves with insulin. We won't mention type 1 diabetes again in this book, as sadly it is one of the few things Primal Cure can't help solve.

For those suffering with type 2 diabetes, it is possible for some people to be cured by following the relevant Primal Cure principles. Please be aware that I am not claiming that Primal Cure will reverse everyone's type 2 diabetes, because it will vary from person to person. However, if a sufferer strictly follows a high (quality) fat, medium protein and extremely low CARB eating regime - adhering to the Primal foods that we recommend later - and intermittently fasts (which we also cover later), there is a strong likelihood that Primal Cure can reverse their type 2 diabetes.

Before we start to look down on insulin, we should remember that the hormone is only doing the job nature designed it to do! When we are eating healthily, rather than seeing it as a prison officer escorting a villain to the fat cells, we should view insulin as an usher in a church, accompanying energy to each and every seat. Insulin is one of the most critical hormones in the metabolism of food, and our cells are unable to process glucose without it. As long as we don't consume too many CARBS, just as it has for more than 2 million years, the insulin system functions perfectly. But when we regularly eat a diet too rich in CARBS – a diet that we were not designed to eat, just like a Harley Davidson is not designed to run on diesel – it causes serious damage to our engine. Let's keep it as simple as possible with an equation:

> **CARBS lead to sugar in the blood and the creation of insulin**
> **Too much insulin = insulin resistance**
> **Insulin resistance + overweight = type 2 diabetes**
>
> Looking at the above equation, it's logical to come to the conclusion that type 2 diabetes is in fact the intolerance of too many CARBS!

Let me explain further about hormones. As I mentioned earlier, they are chemicals that send messages from one part of the body to another. The intended recipient of the hormone has what are known as receptors on its surface. Often, the analogy of a key and lock is used to explain their function. The hormone being the key, which floats around the body until it finds a receptor (the lock), which it can open. When cells are constantly offered sugar from the bloodstream, they become insulin resistant. Picture it as the locks freezing up and rejecting the keys. The result is that the sugar can't enter the cell and therefore it stays in the bloodstream. Too much sugar in the bloodstream confuses our immune system - which had worked flawlessly for Homo sapiens in our hunter/gatherer days - so the body instructs the pancreas to keep producing more and more insulin. But that obviously doesn't solve the issue, because once the cells, receptors aren't working, no matter how many keys we throw at the locks, they just won't open and let the glucose in. So now it's a twofold problem. There are now high levels of both glucose and insulin roaming around creating havoc in the bloodstream. For the caveman, at the end of summer stuffing his face full of ripe, sugary apples, this was not an issue. While he would still experience a huge spike in insulin, without refrigerators to keep the fruit fresh, it would all have been consumed over a week or two and then his food would revert back to his normal low carbohydrate staples. But in Great Britain, where we can have whatever food we want 365 days a year, it's not so much a short spike in insulin that causes the problem, but the on-going daily consumption of sugary foods over a prolonged period.

Dr Dan Maggs

"After consuming a meal our blood sugar level will rise and insulin gets to work. While all foods have an effect on insulin, carbs and other sugars cause insulin to work overtime. While insulin is active the last thing our body will want to do is to burn off any energy from our fat stores. Put simply, when sugar is in our bloodstream, no matter how hard we exercise we aren't going to lose weight. Insulin and fat burning work almost exclusively on their own."

CHOLESTEROL

What is cholesterol? Firstly, despite what you have previously believed, cholesterol isn't evil and in fact we can't live without it. Dr Malcolm Kendrick writes in *The Great Cholesterol Con*, "Why do you think that an egg yolk is full of cholesterol? Answer: Because it takes one hell of a lot of cholesterol to build a healthy chicken. It also takes one hell of a lot of cholesterol to build, and maintain, a healthy human being". Although there are many more, let me give just two reasons why we need cholesterol. Later you will read about how vital it is to get out in the sun, as it provides an invaluable source of vitamin D - which among other things helps to prevent certain cancers. The vitamin D delivered by sunshine is actually created (synthesised) by cholesterol. And we would not be here at all without cholesterol, as it is a building block for most sex hormones.

Cholesterol only becomes dangerous, when it builds up inside arteries. More correctly known as Atherosclerosis, this is a disease in which plaque (a combination of cholesterol, calcium and fat) builds up inside our arteries (blood vessels that carry oxygen-rich blood to our heart and other parts of our body). It starts off with a gunk-like substance that can eventually calcify, making the arteries stiff and narrow. Nobody knows how long this takes, but it is believed to be a couple of decades. However, the most dangerous period seems to be before the arteries calcify. This intermediate stage is known as unstable plaque. These plaques don't just build-up in arteries leading to the heart (the coronary arteries), but in many other areas of the body too. When plaques build up in the carotid arteries in the neck they often break off into chunks and are carried in the arteries towards the brain. As they get into the smaller arteries they get stuck, and the result is often a stroke.

If we simplify it a little, it appears there is good cholesterol and bad cholesterol. In fact, there are four main measurements we might get from our doctor:

- The good cholesterol (HDL – high-density lipoproteins)
- The bad cholesterol (LDL – low-density lipoproteins)
- The ratio between our good and bad cholesterol
- Total cholesterol

> **Technical Stuff**
>
> Sterols are a group of molecules with a specific shape and structure. In plants they are called 'phytosterols' and in animals 'zoosterols', of which the most well-known is cholesterol.
>
> Lipoproteins are made of fat (aka lipo) and proteins. Our body produces three main types of lipoproteins: Very low-density lipoproteins (VLDL), low-density (LDL) and high-density (HDL). The amount of lipid (fat) in a lipoprotein is what affects its density. Fat is less dense and lighter in weight than protein and as a result LDLs contain more lipid relative to protein. Fundamentally, LDLs carry cholesterol into blood vessels, while HDLs transport them out of the body.

Let's use an analogy to explain this a little better. Imagine cholesterol as a life raft travelling through our body. On it are our fats and proteins. The fats are big and take up a lot of room and as the life raft continues its journey they get knocked overboard. The extra space is taken up with heavier, denser proteins and eventually it becomes so full, so highly dense (HDL), that it sinks and falls out of our bottom. In reality there is only one type of cholesterol, it just depends what has jumped on or off the raft that determines what state it's currently in. Effectively, once a cholesterol becomes too dense, it is unable to pass through arteries and blood vessel walls and exit the body.

So the burning question is not what causes cholesterol per se, but what causes the bad guys - VLDs and LDLs. It appears that it's not by avoiding certain foods that are themselves high in cholesterol. It turns out that the biggest preventative measures we can take are to lose weight, exercise and avoid excessive levels of stress. I confess that when I was diagnosed with high levels of LDL cholesterol, I was the heaviest I had ever been and after launching a new company just several months before my medical examination, I was so stressed out, and working such long hours that I had no time to exercise. From personal experience I fully agree with the current thinking on the causes of elevated LDL cholesterol.

Throughout this book we repeatedly learn that CARBS pile on the weight, and constantly scoffing rather than giving our body a break from eating prevents the body from going into self-repair mode - so, indirectly, LDL is fuelled by CARBS and by not fasting. All that said, it appears obsessing about cholesterol levels, whether it be total cholesterol or bad LDL, might actually be barking up the wrong tree. A tree that is making the pharmaceutical industry super rich. Statin business is big business. It's now a £23 billion industry, with more than 40 million people around the world currently being prescribed the drug.

An interview with cholesterol expert Barry Groves PhD, which can be found online, indicates that there is more evidence to support that an overall low cholesterol level is actually more harmful than overall high cholesterol. He cites recent research, which suggests that a low cholesterol increases the risk of numerous other diseases and, overall, leads to an earlier death. He explains that we are more likely to get infectious diseases, cancer or Alzheimer's if our cholesterol is too low. And in the same vein Dr Malcolm Kendrick finishes his book, *The Great Cholesterol Con*, by suggesting that avoiding heart disease is actually far more about managing stress levels than it is about obsessing about cholesterol levels.

So now you know some of the basics about cholesterol, you can almost understand why virtually the entire medical professional arrived at the same hypothesis about how to avoid it. The hypothesis went something like this: "When we consume too much food containing cholesterol, the cholesterol levels in our blood will rise too. This then gets deposited in our artery walls, causing them to gradually narrow and thicken. Over time this will stop blood getting to our heart, and can cause a stroke or a heart attack."

But the hypothesis is wrong. It is now believed that, just like eating fat does not make us fat, reducing our intake of cholesterol does not lower blood cholesterol. So avoiding eggs, prawns and meat, all of which are high in cholesterol, isn't necessary even if you have an issue with cholesterol. As Dr Malcolm Kendrick writes in *The Great Cholesterol Con*, "And boy, is the cholesterol hypothesis wrong. To adapt a quote from Blackadder, 'it is wronger than a very wrong thing'. Yet it has mesmerised scientists, doctors and the general public for years".

If you are already on statins for high cholesterol, one of the best things you could ever do for your health is to quickly go out and buy *The Great Cholesterol Con*, and form your own opinion whether the £23 billion statin industry may have led you up the wrong path. If you are not on statins, then following the Primal Cure principles and getting your weight down, intermittently fasting and trying to live as stress free as possible, should suffice.

Let's close this section on cholesterol with some words of wisdom from Dr Aseem Malhotra, interventional cardiology specialist at the Croydon University Hospital in London, who wrote, "Scientists universally accept that trans fats – found in many fast foods, bakery products and margarines – increase the risk of cardiovascular disease through inflammatory processes. But 'saturated fat' is another story.

The mantra that saturated fat must be removed to reduce the risk of cardiovascular disease has dominated dietary advice and guidelines for almost four decades. Yet scientific evidence shows that this advice has, paradoxically, increased our cardiovascular risks. Furthermore, the government's obsession with levels of total cholesterol, which has led to the overmedication of millions of people with statins, has diverted our attention from the more egregious risk factors".

If you want to reduce your bad cholesterol (LDL), then, before making a lifelong commitment to funding the pharmaceutical companies, why not first try a Primal Cure? Here are 10 foods known to reduce cholesterol:

- Oily fish
- Broccoli
- Spinach
- Nuts (especially walnuts and almonds)
- Avocado
- Coconut and coconut oil
- Olives and olive oil
- Tea
- Garlic
- Dark chocolate

Dr Dan Maggs

"Cholesterol is an area in which it is very easy to get confused. What is cholesterol? What is LDL? If cholesterol is something you are concerned about, then a great place to start would be to watch the Primal Cure interview with Dr Malcolm Kendrick on YouTube, or to purchase his book."

CARDIOVASCULAR

Ask anybody in the gym flogging their guts out on a running machine why they are doing it, and most will respond that it is to improve their cardiovascular system. In Chapter 4, I will explain why, according to research, endless hours on the treadmill are just not necessary. But first, let's start with a basic understanding of what cardio or cardiovascular really is.

Our cardiovascular system refers to the way our heart and blood vessels transport approximately five litres (eight pints) of blood around our body - all day, every day. Cardiovascular originates from Greek 'kardia', meaning heart, and 'vasculum' from Latin for 'small vessel', which relates to the blood vessels. Driven by the heart (which is not much bigger than our fist), blood is used as a vehicle to transport nutrients, oxygen and hormones to every part of the body. Our arteries carry blood away from the heart and our veins bring it back. The heart has a left side (left ventricle) and a right side (right ventricle). The left ventricle pumps blood out of the heart. People that are sedentary tend to have a smaller left ventricle than those who exercise. Put simply, those who exercise regularly can turn their low-powered engine from a Mini into a Ferrari. Obviously, the more powerful the engine, the better it deals with stress, such as going up inclines.

Let's assume we are now training regularly, and our heart has increased in size and power, the next thing we want is our transport system, (aka our arteries), to enlarge, so that pressure doesn't build up. If we can become less stressed, and therefore more relaxed, then our arteries won't be uptight and our blood pressure will therefore drop. Both sprinting and weightlifting are what we call interval training, which helps the heart to grow strong and arteries to become more elastic. In contrast, we now understand that - despite what was originally believed - the endurance sports we were encouraged to do, such as running (the very activity that was first called aerobic), do not help strengthen the heart after all and instead completely stress out our hormones and immune system. Sorry joggers, but it's true. There is a lot more to come on the dangers of endurance sports later.

CELL POWERHOUSE

Each cell in our body is made up of trillions of atoms. In each cell there are various tiny cellular structures that perform specific tasks and functions. These groups are known as organelles. Their name explains what they do very well – what organelles perform inside the cell is similar to the role organs perform in our body. One of the most important organelles within each cell is the mitochondria, which are found in all cells with the exception of red blood cells. Their job is to create life and to provide energy to the rest of the cell. If each body cell were a city, mitochondria would be the energy plant or electricity board. If a cell were a toy, the mitochondria would be the battery that brings it to life. Alongside the nucleus (another vital organelles that holds our DNA), maintaining healthy mitochondria is vital to our health and wellbeing.

While mitochondria organelles can use glucose as an energy source, they actually prefer to use fat. Although it might sound a little far-fetched, as long as we take it at a gentle pace, most of us could walk from Land's End to John o' Groats without taking in any food at all. As long as we drank plenty of water and stayed hydrated, our fat stores, which typically hold around 40,000 to 100,000 calories, could provide sufficient energy for us to fuel our muscles for the duration.

It is now believed that looking after these key components to each cell and feeding them what they like to eat – healthy fats – is of paramount importance to a healthy body. By example let's consider multiple sclerosis (MS), which is thought to be an autoimmune disease where the body's immune system breaks down and starts attacking the central nervous system. When Dr Terry Wahls became wheelchair-bound, she decided to take matters into her own hands and began researching the effects of nutrition. In her brilliantly insightful book, Minding My Mitochondria, while introducing her readers to what they do she says, "If those little maintenance workers don't have all the proper nutrients, like amino acids, then they can't build according to the DNA blueprints". In other words, the mitochondria, the powerhouse of each cell, must receive the right nutrients.

Some cells have just a handful of internal mitochondria, while others like those in our brains can have hundreds. In fact, it is estimated that 10% of our entire body weight can be attributed to mitochondria. One of their most vital tasks is their role in informing the rest of the cell when it is time to die. If cells don't die at the appropriate time, and instead continue growing, they can become a cancerous tumour.

IT'S IN THE GENES - OR IS IT?

If our parents suffered from a heart condition, Alzheimer's or cancer, does that mean that our fate is sealed? Is it just destiny that we will fall victim to the same bad luck? In this topic I want to demonstrate that, through the choices we make and the actions we take, it is us who are in control of our destiny - and not our genes. Let's start with a little caution, and then move on. There is an elevated risk that we might be more susceptible to the same conditions as our parents and grandparents. In Patrick Holford's brilliant *Optimum Nutrition Made Easy*, he says, "In studies tracking the health of 44,000 sets of twins, 27% of the risk was due to inherent factors. That means that in 73%, the risk is due to external factors such as diet and lifestyle. Alzheimer's is another good example. Only one in 100 cases of this debilitating disease is caused by genes".

What Holford is trying to tell us is that, while our genes might be predisposed to a certain condition, it means we need to follow a healthier lifestyle to balance our odds. By eating well, fasting intermittently and exercising, any rogue genes we might have inherited should stay dormant for our entire life. Our genes don't dictate our future, but instead increase our *susceptibility* to various diseases. If I tell you that sugar can cause cancer, it might be the case for some and not for others. It also doesn't mean that sugar is the only cause of cancer. What it does mean is that consuming sugar, just like smoking cigarettes, increases our chances of getting cancer – just as it does with most of the other almost exclusively Westernised diseases we will discuss later. If cancer, Alzheimer's, gout, diabetes, thyroid problems or heart disease runs in your family, then it's your susceptibility that rises. If we have a heightened susceptibility to a modern disease, then living Primally, reducing our intake of CARBS and other sugars, and intermittently fasting and exercising are actions we should take to mitigate our susceptibility.

We discussed earlier in the chapter that it takes thousands and thousands of years for evolution to take effect and hence the need for us to eat the food that our Primal ancestors used to eat. Anything else is most likely to cause an imbalance and lead to ill -health or disease. Anyone who has accidentally put diesel in a petrol car (or vice versa) will know what happens. As soon as the wrong fuel is sucked into the engine, it splurts, struggles and eventually stops. Yes, genes play a background role, but what's leading the rapid growth in modern diseases are the actions and choices we humans are making. If it was all the fault of our genes, then common sense says cancer rates could not have exploded in the UK, from one in 20 people a century ago, to one in two people now contracting the disease during their lifetime.

Dr Mark Hyman provides a great analogy in the foreword of *Hashimoto's Protocol* by Dr Izabella Wentz: "Genes are not your destiny is something I truly believe in. I tell my patients that genetics load the gun, but environment pulls the trigger. The way you eat, how much you exercise, how you manage stress and your exposure to environmental toxins all contribute to the formation and progression of chronic diseases".

> **PRIMAL CURE POKER ANALOGY:**
> **Our genes deal us our hand, but it's how we play**
> **our cards that defines our outcome.**

If ill-health runs in your family, and you are of the mindset that it is futile looking after yourself because you're doomed anyway, then check out the website epigenetics.com. The word 'epi' is Greek for 'over' or 'on top' and genetics of course relates to that which we inherit, something transmitted from one generation to another. Those who study epigenetics are trying to discover how much of who we are is actually inherited or induced. After spending a lot of time researching epigenetics for myself, I believe we have far more control over our outcome than we realise. It is worth remembering that, many of the diseases we fear – Alzheimer's, heart disease, diabetes etc – are all fairly modern illnesses. Just a century ago they virtually didn't exist. Three of my four grandparents, plus my wonderful auntie

Avis, all died from cancer. But several decades ago, when they passed away, they weren't fully aware of what caused the diseases. On paper it might look like the dreaded cancer is a very probable outcome for my family, but I believe that it isn't. I believe that genes have very little influence over modern diseases. Sure, they govern the colour of our eyes, hair and how tall we become, but are they really that responsible for passing on diseases that have come about because we have changed our lifestyle so much from that which nature designed for us? If we subscribe to Dr Hyman's analogy that, 'genetics load the gun, but environment pulls the trigger', that still leaves us in full control. Or as I teach my children, 'If it's to be, it's up to me'.

What about being overweight, surely that is in the genes? Apparently not. We can understand why people believe this, as we will often see entire families being overweight or obese. However, in 2010 it was proven that our genes do not predetermine our weight. In that year, in order to try to discover what genes were associated with being overweight, more than a quarter of a million people had their DNA analysed. Of the 21,000 genes in our body, only 32 appeared to play any role in weight gain. Such a small number led scientists to suggest that the difference in weight between those with the very lowest genetic likelihood and those with the absolute highest likelihood was just 7.7kg (17lbs). That means, even if we are extremely unlucky and the permutation of our genes is the very worst possible outcome, then at most we can only blame our parents for a little more than one stone of our weight. The realistic chances of all of our DNA lining up in this combination is lower than winning the jackpot on the National Lottery!

As Dr Jeffrey S. Bland writes in *The Disease Delusion*, "We are not hardwired to come down with the diseases that undermined the later years of our parents or grandparents". His outstanding book also states, "The bottom line is that genetic inheritance is not fate. Your lifetime health was not predetermined at your conception. On the contrary: You have the opportunity – and the power – to shape your own pattern of health and longevity".

> **STEVE'S THOUGHT:**
> When I was born in 1966, only 1.5% of Brits were obese, yet less than two generations later 28% of the population are obese. Therefore obesity is invented and not inherited.

THE VICIOUS OBESITY CYCLE

The obesity equation is not as simple as many would have us believe, and it is not as I read the other day where it was described as, 'Greediness + Laziness = Fatness'. Of course, we have to take some responsibility for occasionally overindulging, and sitting on the sofa watching TV when we could be outside walking in the park, but this is only part of the story. There is a lot more to the obesity epidemic than meets the eye. If it were as simple as cutting back on our food and moving a little more, then I am confident that we wouldn't be in our current predicament, where two out of three British adults are overweight!

Later I will discuss the secret to why, in my opinion, governments are not really motivated to help us eat food that will allow us to live longer, and how easily research can be manipulated to say almost anything the researchers want it to. I firmly believe that most people who are overweight or obese have just become trapped in what I call the vicious obesity circle.

It revolves like this: big food corporations, just like the cigarette companies, fill their produce with ingredients that are addictive. We see the misleading adverts, showing beautifully fit and healthy people consuming these goods, and go out and purchase them. The more we buy, the more the supermarkets feature them in what they call 'end caps' and at the checkout, which further leads to more purchases. We then consume all these unhealthy products and get fatter, but as we are still exposed to the adverts of slim models pretending to eat them, we assume it can't be their produce that is making us fat... so we carry on buying. The government at this point are earning loads of tax from the sales and therefore either turn a blind eye, or even worse sometimes endorse the wrong stuff!

How do we bring a halt to the vicious obesity circle? We need to get a better understanding of what makes us healthy and what does not, and then tell the big corporates where to stick their evil produce. We need to kick their CARBS and sugary produce into touch. Together we need to stop buying their hugely profitable packaged foods stuffed full of dangerous oils and infused with chemicals. Breaking the vicious obesity circle will mean that I won't get to write another book, but it will mean our kids will all live longer, happier and healthier lives.

Under the topic of insulin, we have already mentioned the work of Jen Whitington, the author of the brilliant book *Fixing Dad*, in which she writes, "So do we still believe that the responsibility for this disease [type 2 diabetes] lies with the individual sufferers or do we share Professor McGregor's opinion that it lies as much if not more with the food industry? Or is it that the government has seriously let us down? After all, how many people knew that government nutritional guidelines had, for years, been funded by industry and had nothing to do with World Health Organisation [WHO] recommendations?"

When I was born in 1966, only 11% of the British public were overweight and only 1.5% were obese. Today those numbers have risen to 64% being overweight and 28% obese. The average weight of an adult in the UK is approximately 2.5 stone heavier than it was 50 years ago. If we keep expanding our waistline at this rate, a few generations from now everyone in Britain will weigh more than 30 stone!

Now here is an interesting point. With more than half of the British population being overweight, should we not recalibrate the scales and change what constitutes as overweight? Currently, if more than 25% of our body mass is fat (a Body Mass Index – BMI – of 25) we are described as overweight, and if it is more than 30% we are obese. Some people are suggesting that now is the time to change the qualifying criteria, but I believe we shouldn't! Make no bones about it: being overweight shortens lives. Being overweight can cause diabetes, cancer and much more. We must not just accept this epidemic. We must not simply accept the unacceptable.

> **PRIMAL THOUGHT:**
> If our Primal ancestors had put on weight at the same rate as we have over the last two generations, each human would weigh more than the planet itself! Of course that's nonsense, but it demonstrates that something has gone very wrong in recent decades and something must be done about it.

SHOULD WE MEASURE WEIGHT, BMI, OR BODY FAT %?

This is a really good question and the answer will be different for different people. Personally, I feel the best measure is our percentage of body fat, but let's go through the four main measurements that people use to determine if they are a healthy weight.

Weight

In isolation, this is a pretty useless measurement. If you are six foot tall and weigh the same as your mate who is four foot eight, then the likelihood is one of you is not a healthy weight for your height.

Body Mass Index (BMI)

Devised in the 1830s by Belgian mathematician, statistician and sociologist Lambert Quetelet, the Body Mass Index is just one measurement that can provide a rough indication of how healthy we are. However, it only considers our height compared to our weight, and therefore it might incorrectly tell us that we are overweight, when we have a big frame or lots of muscle mass. It is important to remember that muscle weighs more than fat. Actually, that's not strictly true as a ton of feathers weighs the same as a tonne of lead. But what is true is that three extra stones of fat will undoubtedly make us look fat, but if they were three stones of muscle, we would look lean and ripped!

Let's use me as an example. I am 1.73m (5 foot 8) tall (or short depending on your view) and I currently weigh 81.3kg (12 stone 8lbs). To calculate BMI we divide our weight by our height squared.

$$BMI = 81.3 / (1.73 \times 1.73)\ 2.99 = 27.19$$

The BMI Index is as follows:

<18.5 - **Underweight**
18.5 to 24.9 - Normal
25 to 29.9 - Overweight (fat)
30 to 34.9 - Moderately obese
35 to 39.9 - Severely obese
40 plus - Morbidly obese

Based on BMI only I am overweight and halfway to becoming obese! In addition, BMI does not differentiate between males and females, which is a little strange as women tend to carry less muscle than men and have more slender frames. Therefore, overall it is likely to underestimate females and overestimate males.

Waistline

Call it what you like: 'beer belly', 'spare tyre', 'jelly-belly', 'muffin top' or 'love handles', they are all nicknames for **visceral fat**. Measuring visceral fat via our waistline might be more beneficial than it first appears. While it is only one measurement, it's by far the most important. Without doubt, the fat we carry around our waist is considered to be the most dangerous of all. While we might be desperate to reduce our bingo wings, oversized buttocks or large hips for appearance reasons, it's the size of our belly, regardless of our height, that is an important indicator of our overall health.

The size of our waist reflects the amount of fat deposited around our heart, kidney, liver, digestive organs and pancreas. Fat around these vital organs can lead to a wide range of illnesses including heart diseases, type 2 diabetes, cancer and strokes. It is said that a waistline of more than 37 inches (94cm) for men, and 31.5 inches (80cm) for women, indicates that there is too much fat surrounding organs, and the NHS website would describe you as 'at risk'.

The same website states you are at very high risk and you should contact your GP if your waist is:

- 102cm (40ins) or more for men
- 88cm (34ins) or more for women

To better understand the correlation between our waistline and health, over a period of nine years researchers across the Mayo Clinics in America studied more than 600,000 patients between the age of 20 and 83 years. Their findings suggested that the risk of mortality increased by 7% in men and 9% in women for every 5cm (2in) in waist circumference!

What's more startling is that men who had a waist of more than 109cm (43in) had a 50% increase of mortality compared to those with a waist of 89cm (35in) or lower. Even worse is that women with a waist of more than 94cm (37in) had an 80% increase in mortality than those with a waist of less than 68cm (27in).

Just as BMI is inaccurate as it doesn't take into account muscle mass or frame, the problem with just looking at waistline is it doesn't look at any other factor. While it's an accurate indicative measure for those of a fairly normal height, it might not be terribly precise for those that are very short or very tall.

> ▶ **Technical Stuff**
> The waist measurement is taken just above the belly button
> and is often referred to as an anthropometric measurement.
> Anthropometry is derived from Greek 'anthropos' for 'human'
> and 'metron' meaning 'measure', suggesting that just this one
> measurement provides an overview of an individual's health.

Measuring Body Fat Percentage

One of the most useful indicative measurements of a healthy body is
to find out what our percentage of fat is, compared to our total body
mass. There are several ways to measure this. First, there are lots of
websites where we can enter multiple body facts and stats, and they
will perform a calculation for us. We could invest in a pair of digital
scales that send a pulse through our body and estimate the amount
of fat we have. Alternatively, we could go to our doctor and have
them analyse our fat for us. Then there are a whole range of callipers
and various other devices we can purchase that we place on various
parts of the body, and they provide a measure of the body fat in that
particular region.

The calculation is very simple. For example, if you weigh 81kg
(180lbs) and have 8kg (18lbs) of fat, then your body fat percentage
is 10%. However, getting an accurate measurement is surprisingly
challenging. Obviously, if we put on more weight our percentage goes
up, and if we lose fat our percentage goes down. But also, increasing
or decreasing muscle or retaining or losing water content can
dramatically alter the measurements. For example, if I measure my
body fat as soon as I get out of bed I get a reading of around 16%, but
this can drop dramatically to 13% just two hours later if I have been to
the gym or played tennis.

The key thing if you are going to measure your percentage of body fat
is to do it at exactly the same time each day. My recommendation is
to get out of bed, go to the toilet and then take your measurement. On
mornings when we get out of bed much earlier than normal or have a

long lie-in, then we shouldn't weigh ourselves that day as the body fat percentage reading will be misleading.

> **GREAT BRITISH HEALTH WARNING:**
> **For every two extra inches on our waistline, we increase**
> **our chances of dying prematurely by 7–9%.**

NATURE DIDN'T DESIGN US TO BE FAT

Other than animals that are raised and nurtured to feed us humans, when was the last time you saw any overweight or obese animal in the wild? In their natural habitat, it's a case of catching food or being caught as another creature's meal. To prove this point, I took my family to South Africa where we stayed at Ulusaba, in the Kruger National Park. During our adventure, we saw lots of lions, elephants, leopards, hyenas, wild dogs, zebras, giraffes and much more - none of which were overweight or obese. Now, before you start to question me by saying what about whales and buffalo, let me counter that with a question – do you ever see skinny whales? The answer is no! The point is these species were designed by nature to carry excess fat to fight the cold when they migrate. Bears in the Arctic Circle are designed to store a huge amount of fat so they can draw on it during hibernation. As us humans don't hibernate, we were not designed to carry the fat so many carry today.

Why Calories In/Calories Out Isn't The Answer

'Move more, eat less'. 'Just ensure that the calories going in are less than we burn, and then we will lose weight'. You must have heard this before, and it's an over-generalisation that's very misleading. Firstly, the body utilises the calories it receives from CARBS, fat and protein in different ways. While it is true that, in a test tube known as a calorimeter, we can burn different types of food and measure the amount of heat they give off (remember that calories are measurements of heat/energy), it's only loosely relevant to how the body utilises food calories.

By the gram, it's true that CARBS have fewer calories than fat. Per gram CARBS contain four calories, protein sits in the middle at five and the previously vilified enemy, fat, possess a much larger nine calories per gram. Looking at the maths you can see how so many people have reached the wrong conclusion for so long, blaming fat for making us fat, and not CARBS. But the human body does different things with all three macronutrients. For example, it pretty much uses protein to grow our hair and replace blood, skin and nails, so these calories aren't exactly going to make us fat. Likewise, it uses fat not just as energy, but to create vital hormones and acids that we need to survive. But with CARBS, unless we are burning more than we consume each day, the body just doesn't use them for anything other than storing energy, i.e. they make us fat. If we're not planning on getting marooned on a desert island, or going into hibernation for six months, we don't actually need to consume a single CARB to survive.

Most importantly, as you are going to read repeatedly through this book, insulin plays a vital role in our health, or lack thereof. What really makes us put on weight is insulin and Primal Cure is going to show you how to be the master of it. What we should be focusing our attention on is whether the body is more likely to store the calories that we consume or burn them. This primarily comes down to two things – what we eat and, almost as importantly, when we eat it. Any conversation regarding 'eat less – move more' is futile without an understanding of both the role insulin plays in the body and the bacteria in our gut.

What does the gut have to do with it? A lot! You see, calories are only relevant if we absorb them. If I told you a secret that, by balancing the bacteria in our gut, we were able to let a lot of our unwanted calories pass straight through our body and out in our faeces, you might think it was a load of rubbish. But as you will read later, it's not just possible to reduce calorie absorption, it's also fairly straightforward too. Let me labour this point for a moment because it's very important if we are looking to lose weight. As certain species of bacteria strip more energy from food than others, if we allow them to dominate the space in our gut, then losing weight becomes extremely difficult. It is for this reason that subscribing to the basic law of thermodynamics – energy in = energy out – is just plain wrong!

Medical research now suggests that by getting a better balance of microbes in our stomach, even consuming the same amount of energy, we can absorb 50 calories less each day. Over three years that equates to a stone in weight and over 10 years to more than three stone. That's enough to turn someone who's obese into a streamlined specimen!

One calorie = the amount of heat it takes to raise the temperature of one gram of water by one degree Celsius.

Don't Count Calories

It's not just calories in/calories out that's a waste of time. Counting calories consumed in isolation is pretty meaningless too. Let me tell you a short story. A few years back I was skiing with my uncle Dave. A really nice guy, but ridiculously accident-prone. His house once burnt down and when, a week later, he went back to evaluate the damage, in the process he disturbed a wasp nest and got multiple stings!
On the mountain we rounded a corner on the slope and 100m below us was a class of small children enjoying a skiing lesson. I turned to Dave and as we descended I kept repeating, "don't-hit-the-kids-don't-hit-the-kids-don't-hit-the-kids-don't-hit…" and you can guess what he did – he took out every single one of them. By the time he came to a stop there was not a single child left standing. After a number of apologies and 15 minutes helping them put their skis back on, luckily without injury, they were on their merry way.

Later that night I tossed and turned in bed wondering why Dave had ploughed into them and then it struck me. It is like what happens when we get told not to think of a pink elephant. I kept yelling "don't hit the kids!" and all Dave could focus on was the kids. If I had said "ski left, keep left," then he most likely would have done it and avoided them all together.

So here lies the problem with most diets: they focus on food, food, food. In reality, when we count calories we're thinking more and more about food. What Primal Cure is about is stopping us from overthinking about what we eat. When we fast we are not thinking about it. When we are eating natural food, we're not thinking about having to read food labels, we just enjoy our meals. It's easy once we get into Primal Cure – we don't have to read heaps of diet and fitness magazines every month, we don't need to go to slimming clubs and instead of reading labels we just avoid them!

Plus, as we discussed in the previous topic, there is a gross misunderstanding with those who count calories in that no two calories are the same. On paper, the same number of calories from bread or meat should provide the same amount of fuel for the body. Wrong! Wrong for so many reasons. For example, protein is thermogenic, which means it produces heat as we digest it. When our body creates heat, we burn more calories. Therefore, for this reason alone (and there are many more) it is incorrect to assume that calories are an accurate measurement at all.

By the way, if you are counting calories are you calculating kilocalories (kcals) or the international standard for energy kilojoules (kJ)? While kilojoules are more accurate, most people and food labels in the UK count kilocalories, which are the equivalent of 4.18 kilojoules. Confusing hey?

Okay, there is one other calorie number that we might want to take note of and that's 2,000 calories. That is the approximate number of calories from CARBS and several other food types that our body can store in the liver and muscles in the form of glycogen. Any further intake of calories that aren't immediately used to fuel activity just increases the waistline, love handles and several other fat stores.

My advice to Religious Calorie Counters: If you insist on counting calories, then you should take a helicopter view. One pound of body fat is 3,500 calories. Therefore if we want to lose a pound of body fat, we must burn 3,500 more calories than the combination of what our human body and the trillions of micro-organisms in our gut extract from what we consume.

When we start evaluating the nutritional value of food that we eat, we want as high a percentage as possible to be in the form of vitamins, minerals and phytonutrients (much more on these later), as well as plenty of fibre and oils such as Omega 3.

FOOD LABELS

Cigarettes kill us, it even says it clearly on the packets. CARBS and other sugars kill us too, but as of yet the warnings are not that explicit on food labels. Cancer, Alzheimer's, gout, tooth decay, heart attacks, obesity and many more nasties can be attributed to the wrong diet.

When we struggle to pronounce all those added chemicals on food labels then we can, with a fair degree of certainty, assume that our body will be just as confused by the ingredients once we have consumed them. Long shelf-life packaged foods are often so full of complex preservatives and chemicals that they could survive a nuclear war.

We won't find a label on organic steak or celery. If we want to get our health on track, we should keep our food choices simple and avoid as much labelled food as possible. This includes sauces, ready meals, tinned beans and almost anything with a label. On the occasion when we feel the need to buy something to complete a meal and it has a label on it, or if it contains long words that we don't understand, we can bet our bottom dollar that it's not going to be good for our health. And, of course, here we are talking about what goes on the label. What's often just as frightening is the information they leave off.

PRIMAL CURE LABEL PRINCIPLE:
If food has a label it has most likely been engineered for addiction and manufactured for overeating.

DISEASES VS. SELF-INFLICTED HARM

I remember once, when working with the Colourful Life Foundation in a tiny village outside of Moshi in Tanzania, we visited a young man named Eric in his tiny mud-built home. Eric had been receiving nutritional flour from our foundation after he was diagnosed with AIDS. As we talked, he explained that he also had tuberculosis, and the previous week had contracted malaria. That evening I was having dinner with Jo Waddington, whose magnificent charity Ace Africa we partner with for projects in Tanzania, and we started discussing how terrible a hand Eric had been dealt. Jo was born in England but has now been in Africa for more than 15 years, and she started to explain her view on diseases. Jo explained that in Africa, almost without exception, every person her charity was treating had caught his or her illness. Most of the conditions they suffered from were virtually cured in the modern world through vaccinations or avoided through education. But while people suffering from syphilis, meningitis, malaria, tuberculosis and AIDS were seen on a regular basis, they virtually never came across a patient with high blood pressure, Alzheimer's, cancer or diabetes.

As different as the way of life is from rural villages in Africa to that in a British city, so are the illnesses people suffer. Together, Jo and I arrived at the conclusion that virtually all of the diseases in the modernised world must come down to a combination of lifestyle, pollution and diet. Since that dinner, having researched health extensively and since beginning the Primal Cure movement, I have found many experts also believe that the food we consume in Great Britain is the catalyst for virtually all diseases in this country.

The medical fraternity have done a brilliant job of virtually wiping out cholera, dysentery, smallpox, diphtheria, whooping cough, polio, meningitis and many more deadly infections that we might have caught in the past. But they have simply been replaced with new diseases such as cancer, Alzheimer's, heart disease, obesity, diabetes, ADHD, multiple sclerosis, Parkinson's and a host of other illnesses.

As I have been extremely privileged to spend time in so many different countries, both wealthy and those that sadly even today experience extreme poverty, I tell you the following with absolute certainty. Not from research, not from science, not from statistics, but just from witnessing it with my own eyes – the cause of death in Great Britain is completely different to that of the developing world. It's not marginal, there are no fuzzy lines, and it is as clear as night and day. In the developing world people prematurely die from transmittable infections and diseases. In Great Britain, we die in the main from a combination of what we eat and the lifestyle choices we make. Understanding this differentiation is so fundamental to our health - and the health of our loved ones - that I am going to ask Dr Shan to repeat it one more time.

Dr Shan Hussein

"In the developing world, people die prematurely from contagious infections and diseases. In Great Britain we die prematurely mainly because of our food and lifestyle choices. The top five causes of death, namely cancer, heart disease, stroke, lung and liver disease, all have preventable elements to them."

Don't forget that, 100 years ago, the killers in Great Britain were more similar to those in the developing world, but through advancements in science we have eradicated most of them. But eight of the top ten causes of death in our country today were virtually unheard of a century ago! Therefore, without question, modern illnesses have to be connected to the food we eat, our lifestyle choices and the environment in which we are living.

CAN GOVERNMENTS BE THAT WRONG?

Sure they can, they even have a track record of it! Back in 1998, Labour's Gordon Brown was so convinced that diesel cars caused less pollution that he gave the people of the UK a lovely tax break for buying one. They made the fuel more affordable than petrol, and did everything they could to move us all away from dirty petrol to their lovely clean diesel! Less than 10 years later, they told us that they got it completely wrong and it is in fact diesel that is the devil in disguise, and were going to emulate the Dutch and French and offer us incentives to scrap our diesel cars! The government screwed up on one source of energy and they are, in my opinion, still screwing up on another – food. Or is it that they don't want us living beyond an age where we are a financial contributor to the wealth of the nation and therefore continue to recommend food that silently reduces the life expectancy of its citizens?

For many years, and against mounting evidence, the governments still did not take a stance against cigarettes. Even today, with full knowledge of the fact that one in two smokers die of a smoking-related illness, they still allow them to be sold. Why? It is a well-known fact that governments, make heaps of revenue by putting hefty taxes on cigarettes. But I believe there is an even bigger reason. Take the Russians. When I was there in 2016, it seemed that everyone smoked. I did some research and the life expectancy of the average Russian male is only 64. Contrast that to Canada where very few smoke and men live on average to the age of 81. If that 17-year difference was the reality in the UK, it would cost the government hundreds of thousands of pounds per person in pensions. Now you could argue this idea is nonsense. Surely if someone suffers from cancer then the hospitals bills will be huge? But they are still very small compared to supporting someone for another 17 years with a pension.

In 2015 pensions cost the taxman £74 billion in the UK and the number is set to grow rapidly over the next 30 years. In 2015 the NHS cost a little more than £100 billion to run, but when we consider that expense covers people of all ages, we realise that extending our lifespan might not be in the government's best interest. Maybe they are better off putting us up in hospital for a short period and demonstrating lots of care and compassion, while prescribing lots of tablets that often do more harm than good (plus the government gets considerable tax from the pharmaceutical companies) and then freeing up the hospital bed for the next unfortunate.

Put simply, in my opinion, governments that pay out pensions have little motivation to help us live beyond retirement age. Once we turn from an asset into a governmental liability – in other words from a taxpayer into a drain on resources – they secretly would prefer for us to no longer be around. Even if in the short-term we become a burden on the healthcare system, it's more economical than us living for two or possibly three more decades. The same goes for food. If governments know CARBS and sugar cause obesity, cancer, Alzheimer's and many more life-shortening diseases, we can understand why they are not entirely motivated to let everyone know about it. Plus, just consider how huge the packaged food industry is and all that lovely tax it gives to the government.

Imagine what would happen if the government forced manufacturers to put health warnings on all food containing sugars and dangerous chemically-enhanced oils. It would result in a huge drop in sales and lead to the closure of so many 'get fat quick' factories that the government would lose huge amounts of tax revenue. We can understand from their perspective why it's best to remain in denial and just keep quiet.

MISREPRESENTATION AND RESEARCH

In 2012, Derren Brown flipped 10 coins in a row and all were heads – everyone thought it was pure magic. However, it took thousands of coins to be flipped and nine hours for it to happen. On TV we saw only the final minute of Derren Brown's attempt and not the previous nine hours of failure. Why is this relevant? Simply because much of today's governmental advice is based on research funded by the food industry. And as we can see, if you take snippets of information in isolation, you can manipulate research to show only the results you want to show. If you want 10 heads in a row, then just isolate and measure the last 10 flips to prove your case. If you produce cereals and want to demonise fat and praise sugar, you can always twist research to support your case. If you can't, then keep on doing more and more research until a small selection can be isolated to back up your claim.

Still don't believe me? In the 1940s, cigarette manufacturers were still using research papers proving that smoking had health benefits! One advert even claimed 'More doctors smoke Camels than any other cigarette', while another stated its product was 'for your throat's sake'. And in 1949, if you really wanted to be healthy and at the top of your game then you simply needed to 'smoke a Lucky to feel your level best'. Even though by this time there was evidence that smoking was harmful, they were backed up by the type of statistics Mark Twain warned us about and the coin flicking techniques of Derren Brown.

In 2016, news broke that, 50 years previously, the sugar industry funded Harvard University scientists to conduct research that downplayed sugar's role in heart disease and to instead put the spotlight on dietary fat. Globally, the food industry spends millions of pounds on so-called nutritional research. One recent report in America suggested that as much as 90% of the studies that food giants fund, result in outcomes that favour the sponsor's interests. Lobbyists, in-house laboratories and misguided research is both big business and it is rife. I'm not normally a sceptical person, but when it comes to any nutritional or biological research, if it is in any way funded by someone with vested interests, I just don't believe it's of any substance. There is a great book by our good friend Dr Malcolm Kendrick called *Doctoring Data*, it's a fascinating insight into how we - the general public of Great Britain - have been misled and misguided over recent decades. One of the things that Malcolm tries to stress is how so many pieces of research come to the wrong conclusion by linking correlation with causation. Maybe you read a newspaper headline that says something like "Eating Red Meat Causes Heart Disease", yet what the article doesn't state that is that it reduces the chances of other diseases. Or another headline "Wine Increases Cancer Rates By 12%", yet what it doesn't tell you that moderate consumption decreases the chances of heart disease and that in hotspots in the world where there are more centenarians than normal, red wine consumption is partly credited with their longevity! Plus, these studies are nearly always anecdotal and based on surveys and questionnaires, not controlled trials. For example there was once a survey that said, "Eating Bacon

Kills". What a load of rubbish. These type of negative headlines are just to sell newspapers and the research is often supplied by someone who is trying to sell the opposite of bacon, i.e. the cereal companies. One of two things might have occurred in this research: firstly, the correlation might be that people who eat bacon might be most likely to never fast, or might always have it with bread, or use it as a hangover cure, or are eating breakfast when others are exercising, are you with me on this? Secondly, it might be just fake news!

The only research you should ever listen to, is when thousands of very similar people are recruited for a trial, are then split into two random groups and the only thing that changes and I mean the only variable, is the thing you are testing. Then, the trial must last many years and the rate of illness or death between the two groups measured. Do you really think, anyone will ever fund that type of research to see if bacon is unhealthy? Of course not. These types of properly researched studies are known as controlled, randomised and interventional, and they are very rarely behind any breaking news article. Please promise me one thing, if you ever read a newspaper headline again, ask yourself 5 questions.

1. Were thousands of similar people involved?
2. Was the study over many years?
3. Was the study group properly controlled?
4. Was it randomized? (This means that there are at least 2 different groups in the trial and the people taking part are put into one or other group at random.)
5. Was it truly interventional?

If you feel even just one of these five didn't happen, just take no notice of the article at all. It's just large corporates trying to manipulate your future spending habits using a Derren Brown type technique or newspaper companies using negative stories (sadly bad news still sells more papers than positive) to sell more newspapers. Oh and one more thing. The Internet. Sadly, when one of these crazy stories break, it spreads like wildfire on the internet. Within days you do a search to see if there is any substance behind the headline and you get back thousands of results saying the same thing. So much so, you believe it must be right. The reality it's just that one bit of (probably fake) research that everyone is regurgitating and claiming as their own!

SEVEN ROOT CAUSES OF BRITAIN'S DECLINE INTO ILLNESSES

I believe the root cause of nearly all illnesses in our modern society, including diabetes, rheumatoid arthritis, Alzheimer's, Parkinson's, multiple sclerosis (MS), depression, asthma, obesity, heart disease, cancer, bipolar disorder, gout, high blood pressure, migraines, ADHD and many more can be traced back to:

1. Imbalance of macronutrients (fat, CARBS, protein)
2. The poor state of our gut's microbiome
3. Toxins (not just eaten but absorbed through the skin or inhaled)
4. Lack of fasting
5. Lack of certain vitamins and minerals
6. Sedentary or incorrect exercise
7. Stress and lack of sleep

All seven of these are because we no longer live our lives in the way us Homo Sapiens have been programmed. We are no longer staying true to our Primal design.

PRIMAL STEVE:

Don't submit to illness: Some say that most of the modern diseases that finish us off are because we are simply living longer. Others say 'we have to die of something' and while, of course, they are right, I don't buy the fact that cancer, Alzheimer's, heart disease, diabetes and others are simply a result of longer lifespans, as centennials in places such as Ikaria and Okinawa rarely die from these conditions.

Chapter 1 Highlights

- We must live the life we were designed for.
- Primal Cure principles are based on the varied diets and lifestyle of the human race, from before the agricultural revolution, which took place 12,000 years ago.
- By eating a diet based on CARBS, sugar and packaged foods, deficient in essential nutrients, many people trigger their own chronic degenerative diseases.
- CARBS and other sugars are the only macronutrient (rarely protein and certainly not fat) that is easily converted into body fat.
- Deadly fats to avoid include all trans fats and vegetable oils, which are rarely derived from vegetables.
- Our hormones leptin and ghrelin control our satiety and hunger signals from the gut to the brain. To help them work properly, we should avoid CARBS and other sugars, exercise and take care of our microbiome.
- We must get the gut working on our behalf rather than against us. We do this by consuming more fibre and, of course, reducing CARBS and other sugars.
- Insulin's role is to escort excess sugar out of the bloodstream and store it as body fat.
- Feeding the body with junk food high in CARBS, which leads to subsequent undernourishment due to a lack of minerals and vitamins, is causing a profound effect on our mitochondria, resulting in an epidemic of modern, Westernised diseases.
- Focus your mind and efforts only on the things you can change - and don't fear your genes.
- Measuring the calorific value of CARBS, protein and fat, is like saying 100 American dollars, 100 British pounds and 100 Euros are all the same amount of currency. While they are identical mathematically, their actual realisable values are all totally different.

02.
Primal Food Principles

In this chapter we dive into more detail about which foods we are designed to eat, and which ones are responsible for Great Britain's sick statistics.

OVERVIEW

The DNA in our cells is principally still hard-wired to process the diet of our Primal ancestors. They are still programmed to digest and derive benefit from a similar diet to that of our hunter-gatherer forefathers, and not the manufactured foods that we consume today. Since the agricultural revolution around 10,000 BC, our food has steadily become less and less rich in nutrients, vitamins and minerals, and progressively manufactured with more and more starches, unhealthy sugars, hydrogenated oils and fake food ingredients that we are simply not designed to consume.

If you are heavily overweight or obese, then there is no doubt about it – getting your weight under control is the most important step you can take to a healthier, longer and more enjoyable life. So let's get to one of the most important principles of Primal Cure.

Today, more people are going to gyms, jogging and cycling than at any point in the history of mankind, yet as a nation we are the fattest we have ever been. The same goes for most of Europe and America – in fact the whole modern world! Look at the statistics. In the UK, more than 9 million people are now paying for gym membership, and as a result there are now more than 6,500 gyms. Yet, even with our new gym obsession, according to the NHS, "Obesity levels in the UK have more than trebled in the last 30 years".

Let's get this straight. More people are going to the gym and yet we are getting fatter and fatter. Before you jump to the wrong conclusion, it is not the gym that is necessarily making us fatter, it's that more people are believing that getting fit is the best way to lose weight, when in reality we must first tackle what type of fuel we are putting in our tank.

Dr Shan Hussain

"You can't out exercise a poor diet."

Avoiding CARBS

We don't need to write too much about it in this chapter, because hopefully by now you realise that excess CARBS (other than fibre) are just terrible for our health. Just as we realised decades back that there was an undeniable link between smoking and cancer, in the same magnitude we are now aware that there is a direct link between CARBS and obesity. And, just as I sent this edition of this book to print, the BBC ran an article on its website on the 24th of September 2018 titled, "Obesity 'to be linked to more female cancers' than smoking", and states, "Obesity is set to overtake smoking as the biggest preventable cause of cancer in UK women by 2043". It doesn't matter which CARBS we are talking about, they all get entirely broken down into sugar in the body and too much sugar causes a spike in insulin - and the health effects are devastating.

> **PRIMAL STEVE:**
> **The case against carbs and other sugars should be made
> as strongly as the case against cigarettes.**

Eat Plenty Of Protein – But Not To Excess

Remember it's protein that creates life. It is protein that repairs the body. After a big session in the gym, if we don't consume sufficient protein (amino acids), then our muscles won't repair themselves and they won't complete their anabolic duties. Plus, as we get older our ability to process proteins declines – meaning that we need to consume more to achieve the same results.

But it's important that we don't go all-out on protein consumption. While CARBS are quickly turned into sugar, excess protein can also be converted too. Therefore, if we overdose on protein there is a chance we might put on weight. Plus, a by-product of protein is nitrogen. When we consume too much protein, the nitrogen can cause problems for our liver and kidneys. However, when we get the balance right this nitrogen just passes through our system and exits in urine.

CONSUME PLENTY OF GOOD FATS, BUT AVOID THE UGLY ONES

We have already discussed that it is not the consumption of fat that makes us fat, but CARBS and other sugars. However, while some fats are healthy for us, others are outright dangerous. At first the subject of fats can be overwhelming and appear difficult to comprehend, so I have decided to simplify the matter by breaking it down into a few subheadings and to only focus on the information that makes the biggest difference.

No wonder the subject of fats is so bewildering. For the past 50 years or so the government, backed by inaccurate research, has informed us that saturated fats are bad for us and we should eat polyunsaturated fats instead. That meant meat got a bad rap, as about half the fat found in cattle, sheep and pigs is saturated. The demonisation of saturated fats led to the decline of many breeds of British cattle such as the Hereford and Shorthorns and the import of leaner breads of cattle from the continent. And the poor pigs, which to keep them warm in the winter are very fat indeed, have had their natural diet dramatically modified so that they, the modern pigs, are much leaner. If we look at photos of pigs from 50 years ago to those reared today, we will notice they are far skinnier in comparison. We have basically changed our breeds and reared them differently because we once thought saturated animal fats caused diseases. Today, we know that as long as the meat is organic, consuming their fat is actually healthy.

How did the government get it so wrong? When the deadly trans fats started to appear en masse, some misguided and ill-informed individuals lumped all fats under the same heading, and deemed them all unhealthy. Yet, natural animal fats vs factory-created, chemically enhanced fats is like comparing chalk and cheese.

In the incredibly insightful book *Smart Fats*, written by Dr Steven Masley and Jonny Bowden PhD, CNS, they write, "We've been so concerned with 'saturated fats vs. unsaturated' and 'animal vs.

vegetable', that we've lost sight of a far more important distinction: toxic vs. non-toxic fat – or, as we call it, dumb fat vs. smart fat".

For more info, go to the PrimalCure.com website or visit our channel on YouTube to watch our interview with Dr Malcolm Kendrick, author of _The Great Cholesterol Con_.

Not only are most fats healthy for us, they are so much better at making us feel full. Unlike deadly CARBS, which spike our glucose and insulin levels, and then bring them crashing down shortly afterwards making us crave even more food, fat leaves us feeling full for longer – much longer. In fact, it is exclusively fat that has zero effect on our blood sugar levels; remember, even our beloved protein can spike both blood glucose and insulin if over-consumed.

One of the reasons fat makes us feel fuller for longer is that it isn't processed in the stomach, but instead has to wait until it reaches the intestines. Fat, just like a balloon, floats on water. The enzymes that break down fat are lipases. Lipases struggle to get at the fat in the stomach while it's floating on top of the watery mush being tumbled in our internal washing machine, and patiently wait for it to drop into the intestines. While the body is busy processing carbohydrates and protein, the sidelined fats make us feel fuller for longer.

Oils & Fats Are The Same Thing

While I mentioned earlier that trying to understand fats can be a little bit daunting, there are two fat facts that once known help put the rest of the more complicated stuff into perspective.

1. The only difference between oils and fats is that oils are liquid at room temperature.
2. All fats and oils fall into one of two categories – they are either saturated, or unsaturated.

The following chart shows the main groups of fats and oils and how they relate to one another. It's important to understand that many foods that we eat contain more than one type of these fats.

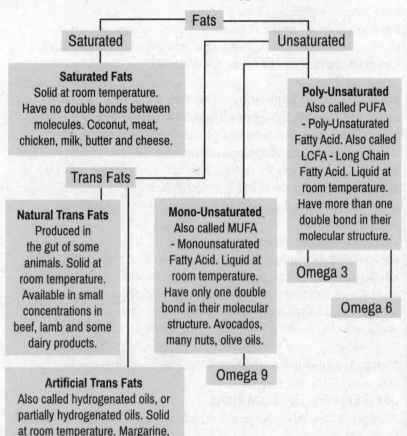

Fats

Saturated

Unsaturated

Saturated Fats
Solid at room temperature. Have no double bonds between molecules. Coconut, meat, chicken, milk, butter and cheese.

Poly-Unsaturated
Also called PUFA - Poly-Unsaturated Fatty Acid. Also called LCFA - Long Chain Fatty Acid. Liquid at room temperature. Have more than one double bond in their molecular structure.

Trans Fats

Natural Trans Fats
Produced in the gut of some animals. Solid at room temperature. Available in small concentrations in beef, lamb and some dairy products.

Mono-Unsaturated
Also called MUFA - Monounsaturated Fatty Acid. Liquid at room temperature. Have only one double bond in their molecular structure. Avocados, many nuts, olive oils.

Omega 3

Omega 6

Omega 9

Artificial Trans Fats
Also called hydrogenated oils, or partially hydrogenated oils. Solid at room temperature. Margarine, packaged foods, pizza, donuts etc.

Omega 3
You need to fall in love with this fat, as it is the answer to so many prayers. It is the solution to so many problems and carries the key to health, happiness and longevity. We will discuss the merits later, but for now start eating plenty of nuts (especially macadamia nuts), organic oily fish, olives, dark chocolate, avocados or go out and source a quality Omega 3 supplement.

Why is Omega 3 so beneficial? For a start, it makes platelets, which are microscopic particles in our blood, less sticky. As a result, it reduces the likelihood of blood clots, which among other side effects lead to heart attacks.

Omega 3 also reduces the risks of cancer, arthritis and makes our brains brighter too. And that's just for starters! If you're of my generation, your mother might have given you cod liver tablets as a child. Although they didn't have a nice taste, even 40 years ago our mums knew more about health than most do today. I personally recommend Omega 3 supplements to almost everyone I meet.

Omega 3 vs Omega 6

Nature designed us to consume Omega 3 and Omega 6 in roughly the same quantities. Our body ideally needs this 1:1 balance for us to function properly. However today, it is estimated that those who consume a lot of fats via fast foods, packaged foods and vegetable oils actually consume a ratio closer to 1:20. That means the balance is out by a massive 2000%. Is this a worry? You bet! Omega 6 causes inflammation and inflammation is the root cause to many deadly diseases.

It's not that Omega 6 is a bad fat, it's just that it behaves like a reckless child in the absence of its sensible sibling Omega 3. On a diet primarily based on CARBS the balance can be as far out as 25:1. That spells danger. If you love your meat but always buy your beef from corn-fed, hormone- and antibiotic-enabled cows, then you are probably at about 7:1, rather than 1:1 from organic grass-fed cows. For better looking ratios of Omega 3 to Omega 6, look no further than some of the items in the Top 20 Superfoods on page 297.

Why all the talk about Omega 3 and 6 – aren't there more? Yes there are. They have some pretty special siblings that are quite advantageous for more niche health benefits, but as our body can create them naturally they are not essential in our diet. Omega 3, 5 and 6 are all poly-unsaturated fats, while Omega 7 and 9 are mono-unsaturated.

> ### ▶ Technical Stuff
> How did the word 'Omega' and a bunch of numbers come about? Omega is the last letter in the Greek alphabet. The various numbers associated with them refer to how far from the end of the molecule chain the first double bond occurs. For example, in Omega 6, the double bond occurs on the sixth carbon atom from the end (the Omega).

Saturated Fats

Firstly, not all saturated fats are exclusively from animals. Coconut oils are saturated too. While there is no need to take any precautions with the holy coconut, saturated animal fat is slightly different. With saturated animal fat, most beliefs have shifted from them being the cause of cardiovascular diseases to somewhere between healthy to neutral fats. However, this is only the case if the meat, dairy and poultry is from an organic source. If we are talking about meat from a cow forced to eat corn and pumped full of drugs, then the resulting fat is very bad indeed.

What Oils To Keep In Our Primal Pantry

Let's look in detail at some of the oils we will find on supermarket shelves, from the great through to the deadliest.

Coconut & Medium-Chain Triglycerides (MCTs)

MCTs, also known as medium-chain fatty acids (MCFAs) are the really good fat guys, and the King of the MCT jungle is the coconut. MCTs are the fats that just keep on giving! When consumed they turn almost immediately into fuel, help the body convert body fat into energy and help suppress hunger. Because they have a shorter chain length, they travel rapidly from the digestive tract to the liver, where they can be quickly converted to energy or morphed into ketones.

When we live Primally, MCTs help increase our energy levels and, while I don't subscribe to endurance sport as part of a healthy lifestyle, on the odd occasion when playing a long game of tennis or if I do get roped into going for a run, I will consume a few serving spoons of coconut oil as my fuel. It provides energy just as fast as CARBS and other sugars, but without any of the negatives.

Although we don't count calories when living Primally, it's interesting to know that MCTs have a lower caloric content than other fats. Not only are they low in calories and provide almost instant energy, they actually help the body burn its own fat stores in a process called thermogenesis. In the absence of sugar, MCTs encourage our body to create ketones (much more on ketones coming up).

Other than coconut oil, smaller concentrations of MCTs can also be found in other saturated fats including organic butter, palm oil and full-fat yogurt. However, around 98% of all other fats, whether they are derived from animals or plants, are long chain fatty acids (LCFA). MCTs are so good for our body that they are starting to be used in the treatment of cancer, obesity, Alzheimer's, Parkinson's and many other diseases.

> ### Technical Stuff
> MCTs are a saturated fat. Let me explain something about their complicated name. Triglycerides are a type of fat (lipid) found in our blood and in certain foods. MCTs are beneficial triglycerides that have a reduced chain length, meaning that they are more able to quickly enter through the membrane of our mitochondria. This rapid absorption by our cells means they almost immediately become fuel for our brains, organs and muscles.

Coconuts

Grant Petersen in his book *Eat Bacon, Don't Jog* preaches, "Olive Oil is Good but not God: God is a coconut!" The mighty coconut is my favourite flexible friend in the kitchen. I use it as an oil, as milk to thicken curries, as a flour, as flakes in a salad... in fact I use it in every way I possibly can. I add it to smoothies and I put it in my morning coffee, I use it as a moisturiser, sunscreen and even as a mouthwash.

Understanding The Types Of Coconut Oils

Sadly, unlike the labelling of olive oils, which are heavily regulated by the IOC (International Olive Council), there isn't currently a body that regulates the naming of coconut oils. For example, there is no official difference between extra virgin coconut oil and virgin coconut oil. It appears the 'extra' is just an invention of the marketing departments.

Virgin coconut oil, sometimes labelled as 'pure', means that the raw flesh (known as copra) of the coconut has been naturally dried and then cold pressed, maintaining the maximum amount of nutrients and beneficial oils. Virgin coconut oil should not be refined, and should be processed without heat and exposure to sunlight. Regular coconut oil may have been dried artificially, boiled, bleached, deodorised or otherwise chemically treated.

Even though the labelling of coconut oil isn't strictly regulated, as long as you select a brand that you trust, don't let the lack of regulation put you off consuming it. Not only is it great to cook with, it is also fuel for the brain and medicine for the body. Here are just some of the benefits associated with coconut oil:

- Helps to prevent Alzheimer's
- An instant source of energy that won't get stored as fat
- In the winter it helps to stop us feeling cold by boosting circulation
- Helps improve the quality of sleep
- Great as a mouthwash and whitens teeth
- Increases the absorption of magnesium and calcium
- Accelerates weight loss
- Boosts hormone production

Algae (Aka Algal) Oil

A friend recently asked me about algae oil. My immediate reaction was that, although it would be great if we could buy it in a bottle, I hadn't yet seen it on a supermarket shelf or in a health store. So I did some research and lo and behold, we can now get algae oil in a bottle – and a glass bottle to boot! Double goodness! You will discover later why I love glass bottles, or more importantly why I loathe and discourage the use of plastic in their manufacture.

Why is this so exciting? Have you ever stopped to think why fish are such a rich source of Omega 3? The reason is they eat algae, or if they don't eat algae, they eat other fish that eat algae. Or if they don't eat other fish that eat algae they… well, you get my point. Even when we eat fish towards the top of the food chain, such as tuna, we still get the benefit of some Omega 3. Now algae oil is derived directly from algae, which is predominantly made up of the Omega 3 – docosahexaenoic acid (DHA). DHA is said to make up almost all of the Omega 3 in our brains. Put simply, consuming algae oil (or the smaller fish in our oceans that eat algae) is going to give us a higher dosage of the fats that fuel our brain.

Butter & Ghee

Here is another u-turn, in fact I should say a full 180 degrees about-turn. For the last few decades, margarine has been masquerading as a healthy alternative to saturated butter. We now know that it is full of deadly hydrogenated fats. It might spread nicely on our toast (not that you will eat much toast after turning Primal), but it is just not good for our health. Its smoothness might not put holes in our bread, but will put holes in the lining of our gut.

Butter, which has been demonised over recent decades, is in fact super-healthy as long as it originates from organic grass-fed cows. Yes, the fat is saturated, but we now know that saturated fat is no longer the enemy.

But even better than butter is ghee. Until recently, I never entertained having ghee in my Primal pantry and assumed it was just for cooking Indian dishes. But then, while researching how to get my fitness back on track, I read an article singing the praises of its miraculous health benefits. To make ghee, water is evaporated (clarified) out of butter, leaving behind a higher concentration of fat and making it more suitable for cooking at higher temperature. As a by-product of the simmering process, the ghee often becomes more aromatic and can sometimes develop a pleasant light nutty flavour. Many remote cultures around the planet use ghee as a natural medicine and some even make it from human breast milk.

Olive Oil

We all know that olive oil is good for us, and is said to make all those Mediterranean people healthy, but when you're standing in a supermarket aisle looking at a plethora of olive oil nomenclature on labels, no doubt you're wondering, 'which ones do those Mediterranean people actually consume'? To answer this, I studied the International Olive Council's (IOC) website and, whilst there was some confusion, I got some help from a lovely lady in their office. To class as a virgin olive oil, the IOC insist that, "virgin olive oils are the oils obtained from the fruit of the olive tree solely by mechanical or other physical means under conditions, particularly thermal conditions, that do not lead to alterations in the oil, and which have not undergone any treatment other than washing, decantation, centrifugation and filtration". The following is to clarify the choices:

- **Extra virgin olive oil** – this is the Rolls-Royce of olive oils, as it is the richest in antioxidants and polyphenols. To achieve its 'extra' status, it has to have an oleic acid level of not more than 0.8g per 100g, and this provides it with a better taste and maximises its health benefits.
- **Virgin olive oil** – to achieve its 'virgin' status, it must have an oleic acid level of not more than 2g per 100g.
- **Ordinary virgin olive oil** – to have an 'ordinary virgin' status, it must have an oleic acid level of not more than 3.3g per 100g.
- **Refined olive oil** – this is obtained from virgin olive oils by refining methods that must not alter the initial glyceridic structure. It must have an oleic acid level of not more than 0.3g

per 100g. It's important to note that refined oils often lack the antioxidants and anti-inflammatories that are found in virgin olive oil.

- **Olive oil** – a blend of refined olive oil and virgin olive that must have an oleic acid level of not more than 3.3g per 100g.

In addition to the above, you might come across olive pomace oil. These are second-class oils that can be produced with the use of solvents and can be blended with all sorts of other oils. With such stringent IOC governance over what constitutes the different grades, it's about finding a brand of oil that tantalises your taste buds and still fits your budget.

What about first cold press? Why is this not listed above? Simply put, it is not an IOC nomenclature. Many years ago, when they used mats to press olives, there was such a thing as first press and second press, but this is no longer the case these days. Today, it's just pure marketing hype. Speaking of marketing, don't be fooled by those who label their oils as 'light'. It's not an approved IOC description, and has nothing to do with calories. If anything, they tend to be lighter in flavour only. Another useful thing to understand is that olive oil, unlike red wine, does not get better with age. Therefore, look at the labels and try to find those with the most recent harvesting dates. They should also be stored in cool, dark places - so even in the UK, during the summer, we might want to store it in the fridge. Once you have opened the bottle, really use it generously and try to consume it within a month or two. Regardless of the bottle's expiry date, regardless of how nice its aroma remains, the longer it's open and the more it's exposed to warm air and sunlight, the fewer health benefits we will receive from it. And, as always, go for a glass bottle so that it doesn't leech nasty chemicals into what should remain a bottle bustling full of pure healthfulness.

Peanut Oil & Almond Oil

While nuts themselves are a Primal Superfood, when their oils are extracted without all of the other nutrients and fibres, they become exposed to air and sadly oxidise – and oxidised oils are detrimental to our health. Plus, just like seed oils, the process used to extract nut oils is often extremely un-Primal. Nut fans should look for cold-pressed and unroasted.

Seed Oils: Sunflower, Safflower, Sesame, Cotton & Rapeseed Oils

They sound healthy, don't they? Sadly, they're often not. Their Omega 3 to Omega 6 ratios can be out-of-kilter by as much as 1000:1. But an even larger danger lies in how the oils are extracted. The method is often less about nature and nurture, and more about science, technology and highly toxic processes. While our body thrives on olive oil, coconut oil, and fats from meats, seed oils are often chemically extracted, bleached and deodorised in a way that just isn't fit for human consumption.

Soybean & Corn Oils

I am pretty sure you have already guessed that oils from soybeans and corn are not good for our health. Not only are they extracted from genetically modified crops, but they are extremely high in Omega 6. When we heat these oils, they become easily damaged, and as a result can clog up our arteries.

Peanut Oil & Almond Oil

While nuts themselves are a Primal Superfood, when their oils are extracted without all of the other nutrients and fibres, they become exposed to air and sadly oxidise – and oxidised oils are detrimental to our health. Plus, just like seed oils, the process used to extract nut oils is often extremely un-Primal. Nut fans should look for cold-pressed and unroasted.

Trans Fats (AKA Hydrogenated Oils): Toxic, Ugly And Deadly

In the early 1900s, German chemist Wilhelm Normann discovered that you could add hydrogen to some cheap fats and make them even cheaper. Plus, when added to almost any packaged food, this deadly chemical cocktail massively extended the product's shelf life.

In *Smart Fats*, Dr Steven Masley and Jonny Bowden PhD, CNS, write, "Artery-clogging trans fat, which we have likened to embalming fluid that turns our tissues to plastic, is a killer, pure and simple… great for shelf life, but not for your life". Why are they so unhealthy? Because, by raising the level of the bad type of cholesterol LDL (low-density lipoprotein), while diminishing our good guys HDL (high-density lipoprotein), they start to block our arteries. Before being hydrogenated or partially hydrogenated to solidify these nasty oils, they are often infused with chemicals. These cause havoc with our immune system, raise insulin levels and are most likely responsible for many types of cancer.

Where are these life-shortening oils used? Breads, cakes, junk food/fast food/fried food, biscuits, crackers, microwave meals, soups, donuts, microwave popcorn, margarine, coffee creamers, crisps and virtually every type of packaged or processed food we can buy in a supermarket. Hopefully, by the time you finish reading this book you will be put off purchasing packaged food and fast food for life. However, if occasionally you wander from the Primal path, please read the labels carefully and make sure you avoid these poisonous oils at all times.

Vegetable Oil

Remember the guessing game we played as kids, where we had 20 questions to guess what someone was thinking of? Remember how the first question was always 'animal, vegetable or mineral'? As it turns out, vegetable oils don't actually come from vegetables, but to differentiate them from fats derived from animals (and of course they are not minerals), they became known as vegetable oils. But be sure about one thing, they neither contain or are derived from vegetables! Even worse they are created from corn and soybeans, two ingredients that are in no way Primally acceptable. The oil industry has misled us into believing that vegetable oil is made of vegetables and therefore must be healthy. Wrong! As in, really wrong!

Ever since the birth of the low-fat diet – a diet I sadly followed for more than two decades, the diet that kept me overweight and gave me a foggy brain – vegetable fats have been praised for being unsaturated, and therefore good for the heart. This is simply incorrect. It is just as wide of the mark as when the government told us to purchase diesel cars, as they were supposedly better for the environment.

Vegetable oils are rich in Omega 6 which, on its own without the balance of Omega 3, causes inflammation. And, as you will discover later, inflammation is the catalyst to nearly all Western diseases. In his book *Toxic Oil* (which on the cover states, 'Why vegetable oil will kill you & how to save yourself'), David Gillespie writes, "Vegetable oil makes you exceedingly vulnerable to cancer. Every mouthful of vegetable oil you consume takes you one step closer to a deadly (and irreversible) outcome. Every mouthful of vegetable oil you feed to your children is doing the same to them".

Maybe think about it like this. Around 100 years ago vegetable oils did not exist and cancer was very rare. Today one in two people living in Britain will develop cancer and it's almost impossible to avoid vegetable oils in packaged foods. If all this talk on fats was a little too much, then here is quick guide. Be sure to only consume the good fats listed below.

The Good & The Ugly	
The Good	The Ugly & Deadly
Avocado	Trans fats
Coconut	Hydrogenated oils
Coconut oil	Partially hydrogenated oils
Dark chocolate	Vegetable oils
Fatty fish	Oils from soybeans
Meat (only organic)	Oils from corn
Olives and olive oil	Hidden fat in packaged food
Organic butter	Hidden fat in fast food
Organic ghee	Fats from force-fed cows

The Smoking Point Of Fats

If we overheat certain fats and oils then, not only can we kill off their goodness, we turn them toxic. As a general rule of thumb, we don't want to make our fats and oils smoke. Therefore, depending on what we are cooking, we are going to need a few different healthy oils in our cupboard or fridge. And as oils are sensitive to light, make sure you keep them in the dark.

Fat/Oil	Smoke Point °C	Smoke Point °F	Good For
avocado oil	271°C	570°F	Use for frying, searing and roasting or as a tasty salad dressing. 70% mono-unsaturated fat
ghee (clarified butter)	252°C	485°F	62% saturated fat, has a distinctive flavour, excellent for frying, especially Asian dishes
olive oil (extra light)	242°C	468°F	Use for frying, searing and roasting or as a tasty salad dressing
coconut oil (re-fined)	232°C	450°F	Great for everything! 86% healthy saturated fat, and a powerful antioxidant. Contains 66% MCTs
macada-mia oil	210°C	450°F	Can be expensive, but a great all-rounder for both cooking and applying to the skin
olive oil (virgin)	199°C	391°F	Use for frying over medium-high heat or as a salad dressing. Rich in vitamin E and antioxidants

Fat/Oil	Smoke Point °C	Smoke Point °F	Good For
olive oil (extra virgin)	191°C	375°F	Use for frying over medium heat. Or as a salad dressing. Rich in vitamin E and antioxidants
lard	188°C	370°F	Made from the fat surrounding a pigs stomach, lard is most definitely a Primal fat. Makes the best fried chicken
coconut oil (extra virgin)	177°C	350°F	86% saturated fat, a superfood, use for everything except for frying
butter	120-150°C	250-200°F	Use to add flavour in low temperature cooking
flax seed oil	107°C	225°F	With its low smoking point, not to be used for cooking. An excellent source of Omega 3 (4:1 Omega 3 to Omega 6 ratio) and tastes great over salads or add to a smoothie

MEAT

Let's start by reaffirming that Primal Cure is not a diet - we're simply going to commit to eating as close to what Primal man ate, and eat what our body has evolved to thrive on.

When it comes to animal produce, it is critically important to buy as natural as we can possibly afford. I am sure you have heard the saying 'we are what we eat' but, when it comes to animal produce, the saying should be extended to 'we are what our food eats'.

Free-range eggs, free-range chicken and grass-fed cows all provide us with heaps of benefits. They are rich in vital vitamins, and have a really healthy Omega 3 to Omega 6 balance. Cows, pigs, chickens and lambs that are allowed to live naturally, in their natural habitat, feeding on their native Primal diet, are really good for our health. But those that are forced to eat corn and grains, foodstuffs that we now understand turns to sugar in the gut, are nowhere near as healthy for us to consume. Remember, one of the core principles of Primal Cure is that we should only eat what we are designed to eat. It's exactly the same for cattle. They were designed to eat grass, not mass-produced cheap corn full of Omega 6. The food is so unsuited to them that their stomachs bloat like a hot air balloon, and often the factory farmer has to stuff their feed full of antibiotics.

The antibiotics are not just used so that the cattle can digest food that they weren't designed to eat, but also to supersize them. The antibiotics kill off all of the bacteria that inform the cow that they are full, so it keeps on eating and becomes obese. As we are what we eat, there is a lot of research to suggest that if we eat meat or poultry that has been enhanced with antibiotics, a certain amount of it makes its way onto our dinner plate. So if we are constantly eating meat produced in factories and not fields, we will undoubtedly damage the helpful bacteria in our gut and our hormones too.

We are not just talking the odd cow that is being stuffed full of drugs. In the USA, more than 75% of all antibiotics sold are consumed not by humans, but by factory-grown animals that make their way into the American diet. It's not just antibiotics, some cows are on hormones and steroids too! Add all of this to the immorally cramped conditions of the factories they live in, and we start to realise that factory meat has virtually nothing in common to the meat our Primal ancestors once hunted.

In the excellent book written by Dr Mark Hyman, *Eat Fat Get Thin*, he informs us, "The ratio of Omega 6 to Omega 3 fats in grass-fed beef is about 1.5 to 1. In grain-fed beef it is about 7.5 to 1". Dr Hyman then further promotes the virtues of organic grass-fed meat, saying, "It also has two or three times as much conjugated linoleic acid (CLA) as grain-fed beef, a potent antioxidant that is protective against heart disease, diabetes and cancer and even helps with weight loss metabolism". So, next time we read a newspaper article saying meat is not good for us, it probably either stems from misinterpreted research or the article is just referring to chemically injected, industrialised factory-produced meat!

If you are still not convinced that we should go organic for everything we consume, then get hold of a copy of *Eat Your Heart Out* by Felicity Lawrence. The book's subtitle is, 'Why the food business is bad for the planet and your health'. Felicity goes behind the scenes of milk production, cattle and pig farming, and much more. When I read the book, it concerned me so much about the produce we were consuming as a family that I told my wife, under no circumstances, was she ever to buy non-organic food again. It's a brilliantly insightful book, however the thing that took me most by surprise was SalmoFan. Felicity reveals, "I have personally never felt the same about farmed fish since discovering the SalmoFan – a little fan of colour charts that look for all the world like a sheaf of Dulux paint charts. The SalmoFan specify how much food dye a salmon farmer should administer with his feed depending on how strong a pink colour he wants his end product to be".

> **Visit PrimalCure.com for lots of healthy Primal recipes.**

AVOID GRAINS

If it was a bit of a challenge to get you to realise that potatoes, pasta and bread make us fat and shorten our life, surely grains with all of their fibre can't be bad for us? Sadly, yes they are. Just like CARBS, grains get easily converted into sugar in our digestive tract. But aren't they full of healthy fibre? Yes they are, however, just like the strawberries in strawberry ice cream might be good for us, there are other ways of getting our strawberries without eating bucket-loads of sugary ice cream. We should get our fibre from nutritionally rich sources such as nuts, seeds and greens, but not from grains. Grains, just like CARBS, spike our insulin levels and turn to fat on our waistline faster than you could possibly imagine.

Hang on a minute, what about whole grain and brown rice – aren't these proven to be good for us? Sorry, no. They might be marginally less bad for us than their heavily processed brothers, but they still aren't Primal and therefore our body is not designed to eat them. At the end of the day, while they might have a little more nutritional value, it's still just mutton dressing up as lamb.

One more thing. I hate to be the bearer of bad news, but corn isn't a vegetable – it's another form of grain. While corn on the cob might not be as unhealthy, as most of it normally passes straight through the body - popping perfect little yellow cubes out in our poo - just like other grains and CARBS, those pieces that do become digested are converted into poisonous sugar. In fact, stop and think about this for a moment. Since the mid 1960s, scientists in America have been able to genetically modify corn so much, that it is now used across the globe as a sugar (high-fructose corn syrup) in packaged foods. Corn syrup will most likely one day in the future be regarded as an even bigger killer than cigarettes.

THE COLOUR OF OUR FOOD

In the main, edible white stuff is not healthy. Bread, rice and wheat not only turn into sugar in the body, but also have most of their beneficial nutrients sucked out of them during their manufacturing process. So, with a broad-brush approach, if we avoid the white stuff then we are on our way to a healthy life. The only whites we want to consume come in the form of vegetables, such as onions, garlic and cauliflower.

Colourful Cure

When you read through the list of Primal foods in Chapter 9, you will notice the appearance of some phytochemicals such as lutein, carotenoids and curcumin. A phytochemical (from the Greek word 'phyto' for 'plant') is a chemical compound normally produced by plants to help protect them. Several of these phytochemicals are associated with a colour, and when consumed in food they will provide similar benefits to our health. All fruit and vegetables contain phytochemicals (which I tend to refer to as phytonutrients as it sounds nicer), and they are so beneficial to our well-being that many of them can now be bought as a supplement.

Orange & Yellow Fruit & Vegetables

Tend to contain carotenoids (I will let you figure out where this phytonutrient gets its name), which are known to slow down the ageing process and reduce the risk of various cancers. Foods such as carrots, apricots and bananas all get their colour from carotenoids. Yellow spices such as turmeric and mustard don't get their colour from carotenoids but from curcumin, which also has many health benefits, such as being a natural painkiller and a potent antioxidant.

Green Fruit & Vegetables

Normally contain the phytochemical chlorophyll, which is known to protect against cancer and to help heal wounds. Most dark green vegetables and seaweed contain high doses of chlorophyll.

Blue & Red Fruit & Vegetables

Such as blueberries, strawberries, cranberries and red onions contain quercetin. This gets to work in the body fighting off inflammation, and battling with free radicals (more on these bad boys later). As inflammation is the root cause of many diseases (some experts believe it is the root cause of all diseases), then consuming plenty or red and blue fruit and vegetables could be the most important colours to include in our daily diet.

Purple Fruit & Vegetables

Contain an antioxidant called anthocyanin. Blueberries are rich in anthocyanin, which has been linked to the prevention of neurological diseases such as Alzheimer's and Parkinson's. Other healthy purple foods include blackberries, plums and radishes.

AVOID DEADLY SUGAR

It is thought that Primal man developed a bit of a sweet tooth by occasionally finding fruit, and in some regions, honey. When he did, he gorged on them. Remember, he didn't have a way of refrigerating food, so he just sat there and scoffed down as much as he could. It is therefore our early ancestors fault, if you like, that we are programmed through our DNA to enjoy gorging on sweet things. But before you start thinking that it is therefore Primal to eat loads and loads of sugar, remember that for our ancestral caveman, the fruit would only be available once a year!

When we eat sugar, we are not consuming anything helpful. Sugar does not possess any of the vitamins or minerals our body requires. Zero! Although we don't count calories when living Primally, I shall use them here to highlight a point. Let's say we have on average six cups of coffee a day, with two spoons of sugar in each. Chances are each spoon has 30 calories heaped upon it. So that's 60 calories per cup, multiplied by our six coffees a day and all of a sudden, we are consuming 360 empty calories a day. Now, even the largest person who will ever read this book will have a limit to the amount of calories they can consume in a day, but to keep it simple, let's assume we consume above average and that we are currently ingesting around 2880 calories a day. That means that one eighth of our intake is from empty calories. That means that one eighth of our intake, even if it wasn't doing us any harm (while of course by now we know it's wreaking havoc inside our body) isn't providing us with any of the vital stuff we need.

Now let's add on the cakes, biscuits and fizzy drinks and before we know it, more than half of what we are eating and drinking is having zero positive effect. Plus, if you like the idea of intermittent fasting to lose weight (which we will discuss the merits of later), on the days where you are eating, you are going to need to bank some vital vitamins and good nutrients. We simply can't fast if on the days we eat normally we are eating empty calories. Lastly, if we do eat a diet high in sugar, we'll find fasting miserable as we will be craving food.

Just like cigarettes and booze, sugar is addictive. Just like cigarette manufacturers stuff their cancer-causing products full of addictive nasties, food manufacturers put sugar into almost everything these days. From baked beans to canned meats, from sauces to even bottles of supposedly healthy water. Make no bones about it - food manufacturers attempt to get us addicted to their products by adding sugars.

While these food manufacturers are really clever and have all sorts of marketing spins, with a little knowledge we can spot the deadly white stuff even if it has been well hidden. On food packages, pretty much every word that ends in '-ose' is a sugar. Maybe it's a subliminal acronym for something like 'other sugar exposed', or buyer beware – 'obesity sugar exists'.

Dextrose, fructose, galactose, glucose, lactose, maltose and sucrose are all simply different types of sugar. As well as watching out for the deadly '-ose', treat all syrups with the same contempt. They are all high in sugar, with heaps of calories that offer minimal nutritional value.

PRIMAL ANALOGY:

It is said that if a frog is put into a jar of boiling water, it will jump out immediately, but if the frog is put into cold water which is then brought to a boil slowly, it will not perceive any danger and will be cooked to death. It's the same with sugar. It doesn't kill you immediately, but both poisons and ages you, just a little bit every time you eat it.

THE FIZZY EQUATION

On 17th March 2016, the BBC reported that in the UK alone, we got through 14.8 billion litres last year of fizzy drinks, or 233 litres per person. To keep it simple, if we assume the average fizzy drink contains 10g per 100ml of sugar and therefore 100g per litre; that means the average person in the UK received 23,290g of sugar just from fizzy drinks. Grams are hard to visualise, so let's keep it simple. Most dieticians agree that there are 4g of sugar in an average teaspoon, so in the UK the average person is consuming 5,822 teaspoons full of sugar each year, just from fizzy drinks.

According to Coke's own website, they sell more than 1.9 billion drinks per day and, according to coca-cola.co.uk on the 18th February 2017, in a regular 330ml can of Coke Classic there are seven teaspoons (35g) of sugar. They also state, "Our original and iconic cola is still our top-seller. However, 43% of the cola we now sell is made up of Coca-Cola Zero Sugar, Diet Coke or Coca-Cola Life, which have less or no sugar". (Please note that more recently Coca-Cola Life has been removed from sale in the UK.) Interesting isn't it that they want to let us know that a lot of people are moving to the no- or low-sugar options? So, let's assume the UK is similar to the rest of the world and that all countries are consuming 57% Coke Classic. How much sugar is that? It works out as 1,080,000,000 drinks per day, which is approximately 37,800,000,000g of sugar. If you're struggling to visualise this number, here is a comparison: the amount of sugar consumed in Coke Classic around the world each day weighs far more than the weight of 1000 London double-decker buses.

To keep it simple, I have created the chart on the next page. It shows how many sugar cubes (or teaspoons as they are approximately the same weight) of sugar we consume in each standard-sized 330ml can. Admittedly some of the brands don't actually do a standard can, but I felt it the fairest comparison.

Drink	330ml Grams - Cubes
Mountain Dew	46g - 12
Cherry Coke	40g - 10
Pepsi Cola	39g - 10
Red Bull	39g - 10
Monster Energy Drink	39g - 10
7up	39g - 10
Coca-Cola	35g - 9
Vimto Regular	32g - 8
Lucozade Energy Original	31g - 8
Dr Pepper	26g - 6
Fanta	24g - 6
Sprite	23g - 6
Schweppes Tonic Water	18g - 5
Lilt	16g - 4
Tango Orange	15g - 4

Dr Dan Maggs

"If you take just one thing away from this book, it would be don't drink sugary drinks!"

BREAKFAST, THE BRITISH CEREAL KILLER

For more than 25 years I got annoyed with myself if on a hectic day, with a busy schedule, I skipped breakfast. After all, we have been taught that breakfast is the most important meal of the day. We were taught that it sets us up properly for the day ahead; others told us that we can't function without a good breakfast; while marketers of cereals told us that it kicks starts our metabolism. And then there is the old saying 'breakfast like a king, lunch like a prince and dine like a pauper'. So, on days when I just couldn't fit in time for breakfast, I got angry with myself. Now, however, I have learnt that those days of skipping breakfast weren't doing me any harm - they were making me healthier. No longer are the low-fat yoghurts, cereals and large glass of orange juice the healthy breakfast option. They are in fact a recipe for disaster.

Now there are several reasons why breakfast is dangerous. I am only going to touch lightly on the subject, but for a detailed explanation I highly recommend reading Terence Kealey's book, *Breakfast is a Dangerous Meal*.

First, it's important to say that I don't recommend that you stop eating breakfast until you have broken free from eating CARBS and other sugars. Don't start this Primal Cure principle until you have turned yourself into a fat-burning machine. You see the problem is this: when our body is used to eating lots of CARBS, after sleeping for seven to eight hours there is very little sugar left in our bloodstream (as it has all been sent to reside in our waistline and other fat stores) and we will wake up feeling hungry. Just like the smoker needs their next nicotine rush, the sugar eater desires their insulin spike.

What's more, as Terence Kealey demonstrates in his book, any sugar consumed within the first couple of hours of waking cause the body to create an even bigger insulin spike than normal, which of course is highly dangerous, especially for type 2 diabetes sufferers. Breakfast really is a cereal killer.

So, let's assume you have taken to the Primal Cure movement. Your body will become used to burning its own excess body fat as energy (see ketosis - page 146), and therefore when you wake up you don't need to fill your face with stuff that quickly turns into sugar. Remember from Chapter 1 that the body treats sugar (or glucose as it is called once it is in the bloodstream) as a poison. It doesn't matter if it's sugar in our tea, fructose in our orange juice, a donut or a bagel, a cereal or literally anything made of wheat or grain – it's all going to be turned into sugar before we reach our school or place of work.

But once you begin living Primally, you rarely feel hungry in the morning and therefore simply don't need to eat. For me, since I started to eat this way I seldom have breakfast. I don't even miss it! Occasionally, when I want to get my children to try out something new (they actually like being my guinea pigs so please don't complain to the authorities), I might eat with them, but the rest of the time I just love a simple coffee. Pretty much the only other occasion I have anything else at this time of day is when I'm on holiday with my family, and I will join in with their ritual of blending fermented yogurt with lots of different berries. It's a brilliant way to get the healthy gut bacteria back on track, and the berries come loaded with amazing micronutrients.

You have already read in Chapter 1 how corporations mislead us. If you want to learn more about how they screw up your breakfast, then read Felicity Lawrence's insightful book *Eat Your Heart Out*, which carries the subtitle on the cover, "Why the food business is bad for the planet and your health". In this book she reveals how Kellogg's went against government suggestions on labelling and instead pioneered a revolution with other food manufacturers, particularly those who formed part of the Association of Cereal Food Manufacturers (ACFM), to create labels that have mislead us for decades.

> ▶ **BREAKFAST IS NOT PRIMAL:**
> Have you ever stopped and thought about where breakfast gets its name? It is named after its function – it breaks the fast.

FIBRE

So if we are going to skip breakfast and cereals, are we not missing out on a source of fibre? Yes we are. But fear not, we can get plenty of fibre from shirataki, nuts, seeds, vegetables, fibre supplements and certain fruits.

For those who juice, stop right now! Juicing is one of the most ridiculous trends of the last 50 years. When we extract juice from our fruits and vegetables, we lose all of their great fibres, miss out on most of their nutrients (healthy nutrients are normally bound to the fibre) and often end up with a glass full of fructose (sugar). Orange juice is possibly the worst of them all. If you don't like fruit the way nature designed them, don't juice the goodness out of them, but instead retain all the benefits by liquefying or blending them. We need to throw the entire fruit into the blender, or we are missing out on the best bits. Sure, we will want to peel the skins off our oranges and bananas, but then it's essential to throw the whole fruit in our high-powered blending machine.

Take apples. Eating apples reduce our chances of type 2 diabetes, but drinking just the pure sugary juice, the type that is transparent, increases our chance of diabetes.

What is fibre? It's the rough guys who hang around with macronutrients. They can either be absorbed in water (soluble) or not (insoluble). Fibre is great at making us feel full without taking on lots of calories. In fact, insoluble fibre tends to pass through the system without leaving any calories behind, and even soluble fibre is extremely light in calories. For example, there are pastas, spaghetti and noodles that have been consumed in Japan for thousands of years that have zero calories and zero CARBS! How is that possible? Known as shirataki (meaning 'white waterfall') and made from glucomannan which is found in the root of the konjac plant, these transparent insoluble fibre noodles are edible, but not digestible. They absorb water so well that, while what is eaten might look identical to normal wheat noodles, they are actually made of 95% water temporarily suspended in fibre. The great news is they are now starting to become available in UK supermarkets.

Why tell you about glucomannan? Because it's a great example of what fibre does. It can fill up our stomach, and at the same time be used as a vehicle to transport micronutrients around our body. There are numerous health benefits for making sure we eat plenty of fibre in our diet, and I felt it right and proper to feature at least one quote from our amazing National Heath Service in this book. The NHS website states, "Fibre is an important part of a healthy balanced diet. It can help prevent heart disease, diabetes, weight gain and some cancers, and can also improve digestive health". Glucomannan is also the only ingredient recognized by the European Food Standards Agency (EFSA) to aid weight loss. Recently there have been several slimming products to hit the market based glucomannan, including our very own Primal SlimShotz.

WATER: THE MIRACLE CURE

Different experts and different medical professionals all seem to have different perspectives on how much water we should drink, and even on what constitutes water! Some suggest we get enough of it in our sodas, coffee and tea to live a healthy life. But Dr Fereydoon Batmanghelidj's book, *Your Body's Many Cries for Water*, which has sold more than 1 million copies, suggests something very different: "Caffeine is a natural diuretic, forcing more water out of the body than is contained in the caffeinated beverage".

As someone who historically has been rubbish at drinking plain water, I have read many books and white papers on the subject and have come to the conclusion that we need between 1.5 to 2.5 litres of water a day. If you are petite and don't exercise much then 1.5 litres might be fine, but if you are well-built or exercise a lot you might need closer to 2.5 litres. Bear in mind that we shouldn't count water in coffee or alcohol towards our daily intake, as both actually dehydrate rather than hydrate. If you find water 'boring' try adding a slice of lemon, lime or ginger to improve the taste. Also, if you regularly have more than half a dozen cups of coffee or tea each day, you might find that it is the warm water that you are drawn to, rather than the coffee or tea itself. Try a glass of warm water with nothing added, then try it with blackberries, blueberries, strawberries, or lime to see if you prefer it.

I remember a good friend of mine called Edward, who was previously in the Royal Air Force, but who's career after leaving the military was that of a wine expert. He is someone that you wouldn't naturally expect to believe in the virtues of water, but he always preached the following message to his colleagues. If your urine is clear then it is a healthy sign that you are well hydrated. If it is a pale yellow then you are reasonably hydrated, but if the colour is dark yellow to orange then you are seriously dehydrated. I remember him telling me that the brain is made up of 85% water and that it was important to keep it topped up, and to flush it regularly. Since then, I have read many books that say good hydration can help prevent Alzheimer's disease, and possibly even reduce its symptoms post-diagnosis.

I remember once, near Wamba in central Kenya where we were building a library in a remote village, we came across two Maasai tribesmen many miles from the nearest settlement. We pulled our Jeep over and offered them a ride. It turns out they were walking more than 80km (50 miles) to take part in a spiritual ceremony. One was carrying a really old and dirty plastic 1-litre Coke bottle, and I asked him where they refilled it en route. He explained that they didn't, there was plenty for them to share on their 20-hour walk! It was a baking hot day and these tribesmen were not drinking at all! They went on to say that they didn't actually drink it much as it made them sweat, and they only used the water to stop their lips from drying out.

My observation is that skipping water occasionally like these Maasai doesn't necessarily mean a lack of performance immediately, but there is growing evidence that water might cure far more conditions than many doctors and medical advisors realise. If the Maasai can go a day without water, it means that the body is not very good at notifying us when we are dehydrated, and therefore we must not wait until we are thirsty before sipping water. I bet you're similar to me in that there are days when you get into the late afternoon and realise you haven't had a glass of water all day. Try to do everything you can to make consuming sufficient water part of your Primal routine.

On the cover of Dr Batmanghelidj's book, *Your Body's Many Cries for Water*, there is the subtitle: "You're Not Sick; You're Thirsty, Don't Treat Thirst with Medication". He goes on to say, "The simple truth is that dehydration can cause disease". In this brilliant book, full of insightful information about how the human body uses water, he explains how dehydration can be a cause of rheumatoid arthritis, lower back pain, neck pain, migraines, hypertension, Alzheimer's and much more, all backed by lots of scientific research. In fact, talking of Alzheimer's, Dr Batmanghelidj goes on to state: "The primary cause of Alzheimer's disease is chronic dehydration of the body"; later in the book he says, "people with Alzheimer's disease and children with learning disabilities should not drink anything but water. Definitely no caffeine-containing beverages should be consumed". He delivers the message with great clarity and some great analogies: "In prolonged dehydration, brain cells begin to shrink. Imagine a plum gradually turning into a prune. Unfortunately, in a dehydrated state, many functions of the brain cells begin to get lost". If you read his book, I guarantee you will increase your daily intake of water.

When it comes to exercise, keeping hydrated is really important as dehydrated muscles are weak muscles. During a one-hour workout we can easily lose a litre of water by sweating, and when it's hot it's possible to lose as much as three litres in just a single hour. Ever wondered why, if you jump on a pair of scales after a workout or a game of tennis, you are lighter than you expected to be? There is an old saying that goes, 'A pint's a pound the whole world round'. In a litre there is close to two pints, therefore in a normal one-hour workout we are going to temporarily lose around 0.9kg (2lbs) in weight - and if it's midsummer we could drop close to 2.7kg (6lbs) in water. By the way, if we lose around 2–3kg of water after an exercise session and don't promptly replace the fluids, then it's extremely dangerous!

Exercising isn't the only time we will need to increase our intake of water. By the time you finish reading this book I am sure you will be consuming a lot more fibre with your meals. While fibre is hugely beneficial to our health, it acts like a sponge and absorbs lots of water. Therefore as we increase our fibre intake, we must ensure to take on board more water.

Finally, I didn't know where to mention cellulite. I don't want to put it under diseases as it is not really a disease, so I thought I would put it under water, as keeping our skin hydrated helps to repair cellulite. There are two other major factors in having healthy skin, and keeping the body's inbuilt 'cellulite criminal' at bay – they are getting our weight under control and exercising. When we are overweight, we have to distort our skin to cover the enlarged surface area. Sadly, yo-yo diets can leave us with excess amounts of skin. Interval training, both sprinting and weightlifting, produces hormones that enhance the levels of both collagen and elastin within the skin.

> **The weight of the human body is approximately 20% fat (well, it should be), 20% a combination of predominantly protein, minerals, carbohydrates and vitamins, and a massive 60% water. This just shows how vital it is to keep ourselves properly topped up.**

Is All Water Equal?
Sadly not. The best water is natural mineral water supplied in glass bottles, or filtered tap water. What is least healthy is bottled plastic water and unfiltered tap water. Let me explain why.

Tap Water
Don't get me wrong, in the UK tap water is extremely good for us, but it should be filtered to reduce the level of chlorine. While chlorine

acts as a highly efficient disinfectant - killing off harmful bacteria that grows throughout the entire water supply system, from the reservoirs to the pipe network - it can also kill off healthy bacteria in our guts. Chlorine is a necessary evil in the supply of water to our homes, as without it water could carry deadly diseases and harmful bacteria. Of course, all governments will tell us that chlorine in water is so low in concentration that it is totally harmless. However, as you will read throughout this book, it's critical that we look after the healthy gut bacteria in our microbiome and it's therefore just common sense that, no matter how low the concentration, we should do everything possible to filter out harmful chemicals.

If you want to know how harmful chlorine is, spill some bleach on your jeans (most household bleach is normally made of chlorine) and watch the colour disappear, quickly turning white and eventually burning holes in the material. Our delicate gut lining is only one cell thick, and therefore you can easily imagine what damage even a tiny amount of chlorine could potentially do to it. Don't fall for the 'concentration smokescreen' – poison is poison, regardless of its concentration.

> **PRIMAL CURE TAP WATER TIP:**
> Be sure to fit a water filter at home, or alternatively purchase a water filter jug. If you find yourself in a hotel room, and aren't sure if the water is filtered, be sure to boil it before you drink it.

Glass Bottled Water

A few years back, I was sitting in a hotel room in the Maldives, enjoying the glorious views of the turquoise Indian Ocean as I talked to my children about how fortunate we were to be enjoying our holiday. I explained that, due to global warming, sea levels are predicted to keep rising and that, sadly, 50 years from now these beautiful islands are predicted to be lost forever. I picked up a lovely shaped glass bottle and begin to sip the cool water. It tasted great. On it there was a label that read, "Four Seasons Resorts Maldives support sustainability. This water has undergone a unique seven-stage purification process. The bottle is re-usable, saving the resort from disposing around 140,000 plastic bottles every year".

A few years prior to this, my family and I had sailed across the Atlantic in a small boat and were distraught at the amount of plastic debris we witnessed floating on the surface of the water. A few months after arriving home, my brother and I discussed the state of the oceans and how some companies such as the Four Seasons were doing their bit to help the planet, but wondered what else could be done. So we funded the wildlife and environmental charity Earthwatch to conduct a study to discover the effect humans were having on our oceans. The findings were shocking. There is so much plastic floating around, that if you gathered it all together, turned it into dust and covered the entire land mass of our planet – including the two currently frozen Poles – the dust would almost be up to our knees! That's more than 300 billion pounds in weight. Across all of the oceans there is an average of 46,000 pieces of man-made plastics per square mile, and it will take between 500 to 1000 years for each piece to degrade. The effect of all of this is that we are unnecessarily killing millions and millions of fish and birds each month!

In the UK, it is estimated that every day we use more than 35 million plastic bottles, and more than half don't get recycled. That means they either end up in landfill sites - where it takes the Earth up to 1,000 years to decompose - or, even worse, in our oceans. That's right, what we drink in minutes, only use once and then throw away, required millions of barrels of oil to produce and takes up to 1,000 years to then get rid of! And the situation is getting worse. On 2nd October 2017 the Guardian's website revealed, "Coca-Cola increased its production of plastic bottles by a billion last year, says Greenpeace".

Plastic bottles are not just harmful as waste, as the cost to the environment of their creation and transportation is equally as damaging. All in all, water in one-time use plastic bottles is just damn stupid. But this book is not primarily about saving the environment – it's about saving you! So let me stop my rant about plastic and its effect on our planet, and tell you why drinking water out of plastic bottles is bad for our health.

Drinking from one-time use plastic bottles is not as healthy as you might think. Some of the toxins from the plastic can leech into the water and potentially harm our body. The main culprit is a compound called BPA (bisphenol A), which the European Food Standards Agency (EFSA) have already banned from being used in polycarbonate infant feeding bottles, but as yet neither the UK's Food Standards Agency nor the EFSA have banned it from being used in other products. Why not? I am sure you can guess by now. Could it be that preventing the death of babies before they can become tax payers is bad news, but slowly and silently poisoning the rest of us, so that the effect is not felt until after we retire, is commercially and financially very efficient? If I am going a bit far with this let me apologise, but could BPA really be the industry's secret acronym for 'Bottles to Poison Adults'?!

I am sure in the coming years the government will have no choice but to ban the use of BPAs, which I am convinced leech poison into the water and cause damage to our gut's friendly bacteria. Studies have also shown that BPAs can mimic the hormone oestrogen, which is used in the female body to develop breasts, regulate periods and maintain pregnancies. Researcher Dr Jianying Hu of Peking University in Beijing says, "In recent years, BPA was shown to have [oestrogenic] activity, linking BPA to endocrine diseases and to an increased incidence of endocrine-related cancers".

Some plastic bottles are now being produced that are free of BPAs, but often these contain other chemicals such as fluorene-9-bisphenol (BHPF). It now appears that these can mess up oestrogen in a different way to BPAs, and in tests carried out on mice they caused them to have smaller wombs and smaller babies. Of course none of this should shock us, because plastic bottles only came into mass production during the 1960s and, as we have already learnt, most things that have been invented for our consumption during the past few centuries are almost guaranteed to be something that we were never designed to consume.

Stop for a moment and think about how much of a nonsense this is! Something that is dressed up as a health product, often costing more than petrol, is anything but healthy due to it leeching BPA. Costing up to 10,000 times more than tap water, some of the biggest brands actually contain very much that – glorified tap water! In fact in 2004 the BBC revealed, "Soft drink giant Coca-Cola has admitted it is selling purified tap water in a bottle. It says the source for its new Dasani bottled water is the mains supply at its factory in Kent". Branded bottled water is one of the cleverest marketing campaigns ever invented and one of the most successful bluffs ever!

One last thought. To prove that British tap water tastes s good as branded water, we conducted a blind water taste test with the teams in our TV studios, warehouse and call centre – not once but twice. The first time we took five leading branded bottled waters and chilled them to the same temperature as the filtered tap water in our office. We served them in the same glasses as the tap water, and simply asked our team members to say which one they preferred. We added the results and were completely blown away by the findings. The tap water came out joint first, scoring as much as 11 times more preferences as one of the brands. The next week we repeated the experiment, but without telling the participants we served the tap water at slightly lower temperature than the bottled water. This time the tap water triumphed massively – 77% of all participants preferred the filtered tap water over five of the top water brands on sale in the UK.

The conclusion? Filtered tap water is not only 10,000 times cheaper than leading brands of bottled water, and it not only helps protect the environment for our children's children, but it tastes better too! Don't fall victim to bottled water advertising, further lining the pockets of corporations whose motives are driven by shareholder value and not our health.

> **PRIMAL THOUGHT:**
> **According to a report by the Ellen MacArthur Foundation, by 2050 there will be more plastic in our oceans than fish!**

THE PROS AND CONS OF BEING A VEGETARIAN

Through my involvement in the jewellery industry, I have spent many years travelling back and forwards to visit our factories in India and have many wonderful colleagues who, due to their faith, are strict vegetarians. I also have other friends who are vegetarians for what they believe are ethical, moral, environmental and/or health reasons. While Primal Cure principles suggest that meat and poultry should be consumed as part of a healthy lifestyle, I have no intention of trying to convert any vegetarian into becoming a meat eater. While I do have many overweight and obese vegetarian friends, I also have several that are extremely fit. So, if you are vegetarian the two pieces of advice I would give are to try to pay even stricter adherence to all other Primal Cure principles, (as for sure you are certainly missing out on some good healthy proteins, fats and micronutrients) and to take appropriate supplements.

If you are avoiding eating quality organic meat and animal produce for health reasons, then you have simply been mislead. We are designed to eat meat. It has numerous health benefits and has been the staple diet of humankind since day one.

If you are avoiding eating meat on ethical or moral grounds, then I admire your restraint and motives, but before committing yourself to a life of abstaining, I would recommend you read a book by Lierre Keith called *The Vegetarian Myth*, where she explains why being vegetarian may not be as kind to animals and our planet as you might think. After spending 20 years as a vegan, she explains how she concluded that cultivating land is the biggest and worst effect man has made to the planet, and how the ploughing of fields destroys complete ecosystems, dislodging and killing many kinds of animals and birds.

Planting vegetables and other items of the vegetarians' conscientious menu are mass killers in their own right.

However, if you are a vegetarian because you realise that there is not enough land on our planet for the growing population to all be meat-eaters, then I thank you from the bottom of my heart for your sacrifice. To deal with the challenge of feeding our overcrowded planet, I see there are but two options: one would in fact be to encourage more people to turn vegetarian, but that would not be fair to their health. The second would be to limit our meat consumption with intermittent periods of fasting. Lots more on this coming up later.

> **PRIMAL THOUGHT:**
> **If you are avoiding eating quality organic meat and animal produce on health reasons, then you have simply been misled. We are designed to eat meat.**

THE FEEDING CONUNDRUM

There are already some researchers predicting that the planet will run out of space to feed everyone when the global population hits 10 billion, and that's probably a lot closer than we realise. The problems of our planet are growing, and growing very quickly indeed. Around 2000 years ago the population of our planet was just 200 million, and by the time Henry VII took to the throne in 1485, the population had grown to around 500 million.

When I was born in the sixties, the world population was still only 3 billion. Yet today there are 7 billion of us, and by the end of this century there is every chance it could be 15 billion. We already use most of the arable land on our planet to produce food, yet we still have 2 billion people who are starving and 1 billion who have to search for drinking water on a daily basis. So we already don't seem to have enough to go round, and if we do, we certainly don't distribute it fairly!

A growing population will probably mean on-going urbanisation and deforestation. I was recently in the forests of Oregon, USA, with a great forager called Derek. He explained how researchers have found that, within the next 60 years, we will have made more than a third of the species on our planet extinct. That's one of the biggest mass extinctions our small globe has ever seen, and this time it's man-made. I was in Kenya last year, and Professor Nick Oguge of the University of Nairobi explained to me how global warming is the driving force behind the fact our weather patterns are changing. In the past, they could have counted on the rainy season being much longer, and the rain falling at a fairly constant level at a particular time of year. Today, however, today the rain is anything but predictable. The precipitation in inches is still the same, but now it comes in flash floods, making it far more difficult to capture.

When we see three young children digging a dried-out riverbed searching for water when they should be at school, we realise the world is really unfair. We caused their heartache in the Westernised world. The more we have, the less they have. Every time we drink from that plastic bottle of water, there is a huge negative impact somewhere else in the world – usually in a region that really doesn't need any more devastation.

Of course, as we continue to deforest areas, we are wiping out the very thing that eats up all of those nasty gases that we in the modern world produce on a daily basis. I truly believe we are in a lot of trouble, and we cannot hope that the politicians will sort it all out for us, because they won't. They are too busy trying to get re-elected to take a long-term view on anything. Whether or not you believe it is their responsibility to rebalance the world's distribution of wealth and food, or whether you feel they should sort out issues of starvation and AIDS, they simply are not going to do it.

By the time they do wake up and really try to make a difference, it is going to be too late. When it comes to food, here is the challenge: The likes of you and I have got to figure it out.

It takes 10 times more space to create the same amount of food energy from meat, eggs and milk than it does from CARBS. So if we had a population of just 1 billion, then you would probably have the governments of the world give each and every person a copy of this book!

Is it really that much of a problem? Does producing meat really occupy that much more land? Here is what Felicity Lawrence has to say in her book *Eat Your Heart Out*, "Farm an acre of decent land and you can produce only 20lbs of beef protein from it, but give the same acre over to producing wheat, and you'll get 138lbs of protein".

Now don't get me wrong, wheat is undeniably bad for us, however if you are worried about feeding the world and growing enough protein to go round, I am afraid we shouldn't be eating meat daily either. Even though our Primal ancestors might have done so, we just simply no longer have the capacity. Other than the immense health benefits, this is another reason why I heavily promote intermittent fasting.

DAIRY PRODUCE

Part of the secret to avoiding many diseases lies in the maintenance of our healthy gut bacteria. Some 2,500 years ago Hippocrates, the father of modern medicine, taught, 'All diseases begin in the gut'. Okay, so that part of the secret is already in the public domain, but here is the bit – my hypothesis – to health, happiness and longevity that I believe governments know, but are keeping a lid on. Yes all three – health, happiness and longevity – can be unlocked by understanding one secret!

I believe Hippocrates was in fact way ahead of his time, and that many diseases really do begin in the gut. There is something in our modern society that is causing mass murder of certain bacteria in our stomach. As you will discover later, our gut is one huge ecosystem. Our bodies contain more than 10,000 different species of microorganisms and together they and us exist in harmony. The fact is that we need them more than they need us. For every one human cell, there are nine non-human creatures living on or in our body! We are therefore only 10% human, as already noted! This isn't a new phenomenon, it has been that way ever since we descended from apes. More accurately, the harmony and balance has been mutually beneficial for more than 2.5 million years, but over the past 50 I believe it has started to fall apart. Just like the destruction of a glorious rainforest can happen when just one or two species become extinct, or a coral reef can become completely barren after a short period when sea temperatures rise too quickly, something is destroying the microbiomes of those of us living Great Britain.

Whether it is diet, pollution, pesticides, starch, microwaves, fast food, fizzy drinks, ready meals, overly prescribed medicines, hydrogenated oils, incessant snacking, sugar or any one of the multitudes of modern world problems, something is upsetting the balance of our ecosystem at an alarming rate.

It might just be that nearly every disease and disorder we face in modern civilisation can be tracked back to the reduction or total elimination of just one or two varieties of necessary bacteria in our guts. Remember back in science lessons at school where we learnt Newton's third law (for every action there is an equal and opposite reaction)? I believe that while the action might be too many CARBS, or toxins entering our body from a plastic water bottle, it is actually the gut's *reaction* to these events that is causing us harm. While to live healthily and happily the key lies in preventing the negative actions in the first place, meaning that purely focusing on the gut is not necessary, the issue lies in the fact that we probably have already accidentally wiped out some species in our ecosystem. What's more, because of the environment we live in we will continue to do so.

This is where dairy enters the scene and where Primal living takes a divergence from those following a strict Paleo diet. In order to defend and indeed rebuild the body's ecosystem – the microbiome – it's beneficial to eat a diet rich in fibre and fermented foods. While fibre is taken care of with choices such as nuts, seeds and lots of leafy greens, in the modern diet fermented foods are generally absent without leave! In Chapter 9 we will detail which fermented foods will help rebuild our gut's microbiome, but let's briefly just mention that three of the top five are derived from dairy – probiotic live yoghurts, fermented milk known as kefir and certain cheeses.

While yoghurts and cheeses start out as milk, milk itself is not necessarily as healthy as we were brought up to believe. The sugar it contains is known as lactose and it is estimated that, once we pass infancy, more than two-thirds of the world's population become lactose intolerant. What does this mean? It means that for two out of every three people it is not beneficial to drink milk. When we think about it logically, nature designed milk to help newborns grow rapidly. Whether it be human, cow, goat or dog, nature didn't intend us to rely on milk as we matured.

According to the US National Library of Medicine, "Lactose intolerance in adulthood is most prevalent in people of East Asian descent, affecting more than 90 percent of adults in some of these communities. The prevalence of lactose intolerance is lowest in populations with a long history of dependence on unfermented milk products as an important food source. For example, only about 5 percent of people of European descent are lactose intolerant".

Lactose (a sugar) is normally broken down by cells found in the lining of the small intestine with the assistance of an enzyme called lactase. However, once past infancy there is normally a reduction of lactase in the gut and if the reduction is severe, the result is that we become lactose intolerant. If shortly after drinking milk you experience abdominal pain, flatulence, bloating, nausea or diarrhoea, then you are likely to be lactose intolerant.

Is drinking milk Primal? Not really. Research suggests that civilisations only started drinking animal milk around 8000 BC. For the following millennia, consumption appears to have been sporadic and non-commercial. Then in the 1800s the calcium and phosphorus in milk became heavily promoted as good for our bones. As a result a whole industry emerged and as demand grew, cattle started to get shoehorned into smaller and smaller milking sheds.

As overcrowding escalated these sheds became dirty and before long milk production became very unhygienic. In an attempt to make milk safer, dairy farmers responded by sterilising bottles and having doctors test cattle for disease. This did little to solve the problem and eventually lead to the heating of milk to 62°F (145°F) for around half an hour, killing off any viruses and bacteria in a process that became known as the pasteurisation of milk.

▶ Understanding The Milk Label

HTST – created in the 1930s, High Temperature Short Time (HTST) pasteurisation is where milk is heated to 71°C (161°F) for 15 seconds, which provides a shelf life of several weeks. The process is often marketed as pasteurised.

UHT – first used in the 1970s, Ultra High Temperature (UHT) pasteurisation is where milk is heated to 138°C (280°F) for just two seconds. This provides an extended shelf life of approximately nine months, and is often marketed as ultra-pasteurised.

Homogenisation – after pasteurisation, some milk goes through a separate process called homogenisation. This process breaks the molecules down into tiny pieces and prevents a layer of cream from forming on the top of the milk.

Semi-skimmed and skimmed milk – when milk is skimmed it means that the level of fat has been reduced through filtering. In the UK skimmed milk has around just 0.1% fat and semi-skimmed milk is typically around 2.5%.

When you consider whole milk is around just 4% fat and especially when we start to understand that natural fat has never been the real enemy, why would anybody use skimmed milk? Plus when we remove the fat, we dramatically reduce the fat-soluble vitamins A, D, E and K. This has a double negative effect, because one of the health benefits of milk is its concentration of calcium, yet to truly absorb calcium you need vitamin D. In other words, if we skim the fat off milk, we remove most of the health benefits of drinking it in the first place.

As we can get all the beneficial vitamins and minerals that milk possesses through other means that are more in line with what we are designed to eat and drink, I personally avoid the white stuff. However, if you enjoy the odd glass of milk (and assuming you aren't lactose intolerant), let me offer a little advice. As with all meats and dairy product, going organic is crucial. Think about this for a moment – in America the number of dairy cows halved between 1960 and 2005, yet the total output grew by nearly 50%. How did they achieve this? Mainly via injecting cows with antibiotics, force feeding them grains and several other unnatural additives, all of which makes the end product very cheap to create yet unhealthy for human consumption. The safest milk to drink is whole organic pasteurised milk. There is an argument that suggests raw milk is more beneficial than pasteurised, but of course being raw it carries a slightly higher risk of carrying infection.

To conclude this chapter, let's get back to how I started this section on dairy by discussing our gut. While I am not a big fan of milk, I feel there are huge advantages in consuming yogurt and certain cheeses. While they both originate from dairy, these two products are super healthy. Yogurt achieves its creamy thickness as bacteria convert the lactose (sugar) to lactic acid. Cheese making follows a similar process, where the end result can be a product with various varieties of bacteria that are wildly beneficial for our guts. So much so, that by consuming just a small portion on a regular basis we might assemble a little army of helpful bacteria that help us lose weight! More to follow.

Chapter 2 Highlights

- Fats are either healthy, neutral or killers! Our longevity depends on us understanding the difference between the good and the ugly and following the right path.
- As our body can't produce Omega 3, it's crucial that we get plenty from our diet.
- The balance between Omega 3 and Omega 6 plays a crucial role in our health and longevity.
- Organic grass-fed meat and dairy fats, plus coconut fats, are not demons and devils, but delightfully delicious and good for our health.
- Caveman ate organically and so should we. We were not designed to consume meat, poultry or dairy produce full of antibiotics and other dangerous toxins. The food in our fridge must be organic or outlawed!
- Despite what we previously believed about grains, they should be avoided like the plague. We must get our fibre elsewhere.
- Avoid most white foods and instead cook colourfully.
- Fibre is only found in plants. We don't acquire any dietary fibre from meat, poultry, fish, eggs, milk or cheese. That's why it's essential to add shirataki, nuts, seeds, vegetables, fibre supplements and certain fruits to our daily menu.
- According to The American Journal of Clinical Nutrition, a daily consumption of 35g of fibre is associated with a lower risk of cardiovascular disease by as much as 54% and death from all causes by 37%.
- For the sake of both your health and the planet, don't drink water from one-use plastic bottles. Instead, filter your water at home, put it in a glass or stainless steel container and take it with you wherever you go.
- Avoid crap food and live healthier for longer.

03.
Intermittent Fasting

In this chapter we discover how having periods without food is something that the human body has developed to both endure and appreciate. And how, if we are to reverse Britain's decline into ill health, intermittent fasting is something that most people should partake in.

INTERMITTENT FASTING

During the Second World War, when food was rationed, a common saying gained traction: 'eat little but often'. It might have been born out of necessity, but you still occasionally hear people saying it today. Sadly, from a medical perspective, it now appears to be very bad advice indeed. If you subscribe to our views on evolution – that we must both eat what we were designed to eat and eat to a frequency we have evolved to digest – then ask yourself whether caveman ate little but often! Of course not. He was constantly going from feast to famine. As it turns out our body is not designed to eat little but often.

I first got into intermittent fasting when a good friend of mine, Nick Davies, gave me a book called *The 5:2 Diet Book*, subtitled: 'Feast for 5 Days a Week and Fast for 2 to Lose Weight, Boost Your Brain and Transform Your Health' by Kate Harrison. Both Nick and his wife had been on it for a while, and both had dropped a lot of weight and looked fantastic.

When we fast, we are changing our food source from incoming sustenance to consuming our own body fat. It's a myth that we lose muscle doing this. The only time the body would consume our muscle is when there's too little fat left to use.

Balance Feeding With Fasting

If you want to lose weight quickly – and there is very little else in life that feels so rewarding than rapid weight loss, especially if you are seriously overweight – then you would be best to not just cut out CARBS, but start cutting out entire meals too. If you work in business then I am sure you have heard about the 80/20 rule, an idea coined by Italian economist Vilfredo Pareto, whereby 80% of your profits are generated by just 20% of your top customers. When it comes to our health, preventing diseases and finding cures, 80% of it comes down to food and 20% from environment and lifestyle choices. Of that 80% we believe it's a fairly even split between what we eat and when and how we eat it.

Eating Regularly Is Not Normal

We aren't designed to eat regularly. Caveman and the hunter-gatherer didn't have fridges or freezers. They couldn't store an apple for a year like the oxygen-free warehouses the big supermarkets use today. They had no preservatives or tin cans. When they caught an animal they had a feast, after which they might go days or even weeks without eating anything substantial.

It's not just our ancestors who fasted, various faiths and religions to this day still participate in different ceremonial fasts. Muslims celebrate Ramadan, the ninth month of the Islamic calendar, with a month-long fast known as Sawm. Christians participate in Lent and the Greek Orthodox Church asks that its followers fast for more than 180 days a year. Saint Nikolai Velimirović wrote, "Gluttony makes a man gloomy and fearful, but fasting makes him joyful and courageous. And, as gluttony calls forth greater and greater gluttony, so fasting stimulates greater and greater endurance. When a man realises the grace that comes through fasting, he desires to fast more and more. And the graces that come through fasting are countless".

What Happens To Our Metabolism When We Intermittently Fast?

Doesn't fasting mess with our metabolism? Doesn't it slow down our metabolic rate? Let me first explain metabolism and metabolic rate. Dictionary.com says, "In metabolism some substances are broken down to yield energy for vital processes while other substances, necessary for life, are synthesised". So metabolism is the breaking down of either our incoming food or our stored body fat to use as energy. But imagine what would have happened to our caveman ancestor if, on days when he couldn't catch anything, his metabolism slowed down. His energy levels would drop and his chances of catching his next meal would, just like his physique, get slimmer and slimmer. It would all be one huge downward spiral and before long he would starve and perish. When we fast our metabolism does not drop as many would have us believe, but in fact increases. The idea of 'don't skip breakfast because you need to kick-start your metabolism' is fiction, probably started by marketers for some hugely profitable cereal-producing company. According to Dr Michael VanDerschelden in his wonderfully researched book, *The Scientific Approach to Intermittent Fasting*, "Studies conducted right after a fasting period have shown a metabolic rate increase of 3.6–14% for up to 48 hours". He then goes on to say that our body does not see a slow down in metabolic rate for a period of three or four days after our last meal. Instead of slowing down our metabolic rate, our body releases the stress hormones adrenaline and noradrenaline, which provide us with energy as well as keeping the brain alert.

Dr Jason Fung in his book, *The Complete Guide to Fasting*, also arrives at the same conclusion: "Most people expect that a period of fasting will leave them feeling tired and drained of energy. However, the vast majority of people experience the exact opposite". He then goes on to say, "The increased adrenaline levels invigorate us and stimulate the metabolism". In what was music to our ears at Primal Cure, Dr VanDerschelden also writes, "Think what it must have been like for humans in the hunter-gatherer days. These desirable traits of mind enhancement and energy would allow them to effectively search for food and kill prey, increasing survival. With that said, after several days of not eating, these intelligent adaptations would do more harm than good. We would not want our body to sustain a high metabolism and keep burning fuel three or four days after eating for fear of starvation".

So, there you have it – fasting doesn't decrease our metabolic rate but actually increases it. Therefore, let's assume we normally consume 2500 calories a day spread across breakfast, lunch and dinner, but - if we fasted and ate them all in one meal we would start to lose weight because our metabolic rate would be marginally higher. Plus, what I experienced right from the very beginning with intermittent fasting is that we tend to eat way fewer calories in one meal than we would across three. Let's also remember that the only reason humans carry fat is to feed the body when there is no food available. So, if we are overweight or obese, doesn't it make sense to use some of our existing fat reserves to power our body? Many times throughout this book you will read the statement, 'that's what we are designed to do', and put simply our body was designed to go through periodical cycles of feast and famine. Don't fear intermittent fasting – embrace it.

Dr Dan Maggs

"I was never hungry in the mornings, but for many years I forced myself to eat breakfast because I thought it was the most important meal of the day. Would our Primal ancestors have eaten when they weren't hungry? I don't think so!"

Intermittent Fasting Prevents Numerous Diseases & Cures Others

The problem with eating little but often is that we constantly keep putting sugar back into our bloodstream. If we live constantly in feast mode, our liver and pancreas never get a break. As we read earlier, insulin is produced to carry poisonous sugar to our belly, bottom or thighs - and while it's active we simply cannot burn fat. But when we fast, insulin levels drop significantly and we turn into a fat-burning machine. The news gets better still. Our growth hormones (known as HGH) go through the roof when we fast. And as they are natural, they are far more powerful and beneficial than the synthetic ones that many athletes take to enhance performance.

What's more, our nervous system sends a little army of norepinephrines to our fat stores and they start breaking fat down into fatty acids that can be consumed as energy while we're fasting. It's kind of an either/or situation – either our body is focusing on creating insulin to deal with poisonous sugars or it is creating wonderfully beneficial HGH. They are kind of mutually exclusive. They really don't get on together and hate being in the same room. For those that don't fast, that's why getting a good long sleep is important, as it's about the only time they can produce HGH. A report by the American College of Cardiology stated that fasting triggered a 1,300% increase in HGH secretion for women and a whopping 2,000% increase for men.

In periods of fasting our body goes into a mode of repairing, rebuilding and renewing our cells – virtually all of them. Plus, one of the biggest advantages is that we don't keep spiking our insulin levels, and as a result there is a greatly reduced risk of becoming diabetic, getting cancer or suffering from heart conditions. There is also growing evidence that it enhances a number of different brain functions and helps to prevent both Alzheimer's and Parkinson's disease. But there's also one factor that was a huge part of making intermittent fasting part of my lifestyle, for now and forever – intermittent fasting has been scientifically proven to slow down the ageing process.

I think the most fascinating thing I read in Dr Michael VanDerschelden book *The Scientific Approach to Intermittent Fasting* was under the heading 'Top 10 Causes of Death' where he says, "Who would have thought that by doing an intervention like intermittent fasting, you could actually significantly go on to reduce your risk of the top two causes of death in the world, which are heart disease (cardiovascular disease) and cancer". Dr VanDerschelden then talks about how intermittent fasting can also prevent strokes (the fifth biggest killer) and of course we have already mentioned that it helps prevent Alzheimer's, which is the sixth largest cause of death. In addition, along with cutting out CARBS and other sugars, we know there is every chance we can avoid type 2 diabetes, which is the seventh biggest killer in the modern world.

There is another concept that I would like you to take to heart and it's called 'autophagy'. It is mentioned in many of the books I have researched, but one of the best and certainly simplest explanations I found was online, written by Nick English in July 2016: "It's a natural process called autophagy (literally 'self-eating'), and it's the body's system of cleaning house: Our cells create membranes that hunt out scraps of dead, diseased or worn-out cells; gobble them up; strip 'em for parts and use the resulting molecules for energy or to make new cell parts". Colin Champ, MD, a board-certified radiation oncologist, assistant professor at the University of Pittsburgh Medical Centre and author of *Misguided Medicine* has this to say: "Think of it as our body's innate recycling program. Autophagy makes us more efficient machines to get rid of faulty parts, stop cancerous growths and stop metabolic dysfunction like obesity and diabetes".

The good news is that there are three ways to get our body to perform autophagy (replacing our damaged cells with new ones), and they are completely aligned to the principles of Primal Cure:

1. Consume a diet high in quality fats and low in carbohydrates.
2. Embrace intermittent fasting.
3. Do high impact intensity training (you will read about Primal Cure's approach to exercise in the next chapter).

While autophagy is the process, the actual dustmen (or garbage collectors for those in the USA), are called lysosomes. They travel around the body constantly picking up the trash and performing a natural detox. But there is a small problem with lysosomes the older we get. They slow down and don't pick up the trash as efficiently as they did when we were younger. In our younger years lysosomes are very much our heroes. But in our older years they become irresponsible and play a pivotal role in the ageing process. The single best solution in order to get them to do their detoxing job properly is intermittent fasting.

Why is this? My theory goes something like this. If a caveman was sitting in his cave constantly feasting, having all of his food brought to him on a plate and not having to go out to hunt or gather, then nature would be misled into thinking that everything was wonderful in his body and therefore there would be no need to deploy a task force to make repairs. However, the reality of a caveman's life was very different. He was constantly going from feast to famine. When he was eating, nature sat back and let him enjoy the spoils of his hard work, but when there was no food available and he started to feel hungry, nature began to get concerned. His body asked, 'Why has he not caught anything today? To ensure he catches dinner tomorrow,

I better go and make sure I put everything into good working order'. The two main benefits of intermittent fasting are:

1. It gives the body a break from food, allowing it time to enter a self-repair mode.
2. It helps us to safely lose weight.

But If I Intermittently Fast Wont I Lose Muscle Mass?

People considering fasting may ask themselves, 'Okay, so it doesn't slow down our metabolism, it reduces our chance of getting numerous diseases and is even considered by many as a way of curing type 2 diabetes, but don't those who intermittently fast lose muscle?'. Not true! If our caveman started to lose muscle on days when he couldn't catch lunch, then he would never catch an animal again. If it was true, the human race would likely be extinct and you would not be reading this right now. After measuring my muscle mass after a 4-day fast, it had actually increased rather than decreased.

According to research, for our body to consume our muscles as a source of energy when intermittent fasting, we would have to have less than 4% of our body as fat. Even elite sports people are rarely below 8%, so we most likely have quite a long way to go before burning up any muscle!

In *The Scientific Approach to Intermittent Fasting*, Dr VanDerschelden suggests that those who lose weight by restricting the calories they consume (the calorie-counters among us) will find that approximately 25% of the loss is in fact muscle, but those who lose weight by intermittently fasting tend to only lose 10%. Now that is a huge difference. The data was taken from the Obesity Reviews journal, but it doesn't say whether those figures relate to people who regularly exercised or lived an inactive lifestyle. It has to be the latter, because I find that if I do half an hour in the gym while I am fasting, my muscle percentage at worst stays neutral but normally increases. I am convinced through monitoring many of my friends who intermittently fast, and from detailed analysis of my own body, that if we stay active while fasting we do not lose muscle at all, just heaps and heaps of unwanted and highly dangerous body fat.

Remember that fat doesn't really consume much energy, but muscles do. So, we want to keep strong and healthy muscles because that way we burn more energy and the body finds it harder to put on weight. Have you noticed how most people who go on one of the many different diets that are based on restricting calories actually put on more weight after they quit? That's because when they diet they lose muscle and when they stop dieting their reduced muscle, mass burns fewer calories. Let me make it very clear that constantly going on diets is counterproductive, and it is detrimental to our health too. As I stated in the introduction, Primal Cure is not a diet but a lifestyle. Because we don't have to count calories and instead work on understanding how different food types behave inside our body, it's simple to stick to and most importantly we get to eat lots of fantastic wholesome and tasty foods. Let's now look at the different ways of fasting. I recommend you read up on these and then just try whichever one you think fits in best with your daily routine, or just happens to peak your interest the most.

The 5:2 Diet

The 5:2 Diet by Michael Mosley and Mimi Spencer is a great read for those who are sceptical about intermittent fasting. I fully recommend you purchase the 5:2 book before you start as it gives you both lots of tips on how to integrate fasting into your life, and more importantly will provide the motivation to keep on the right track once you have started. It's the first book I read on intermittent fasting and as early as 20 pages in, I knew I had to make it part of my regular routine. On the 5:2 diet, we eat normally for five days a week, and we get to choose which two days we restrict our calorie intake to just 600 calories for males and 500 calories for females. As long as we don't overeat on the other five days, then we have reduced our calorie intake by approximately 3000 to 4000 calories per week, and therefore mathematically should lose approximately a pound in weight each week. However, the authors are also believers in food with a low glycemic index (GI) and high intensity training, so the likelihood is that if you follow the book closely, you will lose weight even faster.

The 1:1 Diet Or Alternate Day Fasting

The 1:1 or alternate day fasting is similar to the 5:2 diet, but we alternate our fasting day with a normal day. This doesn't work for me because of my lifestyle, but thousands of people swear by it. Of course, what is great about this technique is that if we restrict our food intake to around 500 calories a day on our fasting days and managed to maintain it for a year (which believe it or not is easier than you might think once you get into it), 180 days of 500 calories a day sees us consuming around 360,000 calories less in a year, which equates to around 45kg or 100lb (more than seven stone). If you haven't got seven stone to lose, then once you have your body fat where you want it to be you can either slightly overeat on your non-fasting days, or move to the 5:2 method or even just fast once a week. Dr Krista Varady and Bill Gottlieb have written a great book promoting the merits of this approach called *The Every Other Day Diet*.

The 18 Hour Fast Diet

The 18-hour fast diet is where you commit to only eating in a six-hour timeframe each day, so that you are regularly fasting for 18 hours every day. This is very similar to the approach I use and it has now become a lifestyle that I find extremely easy to adhere too. I never feel hungry, I never feel like I am missing out, I always feel energised and my brain seems to be able to focus on things with much better clarity.

The Three- Or Four-Day Fast

With so many benefits of fasting, we might want to occasionally think about doing an extended fast. While there are many articles written and research done on fasting periods in excess of several weeks and in some cases even months, I haven't yet researched them sufficiently to entertain trying it for myself. And I would never recommend anything to others that I hadn't experimented with on myself. What

I have tried and had wonderful experiences with are three- and four-day fasts. While they may sound difficult to do, they actually get easier and easier the further into the fast we get. What's quite amazing is how the body reacts on a three- or four-day total fast. By day three, rather than feeling tired and sluggish like we might expect, we feel amazing and the body reaches peak performance. Research by the American Society for Clinical Nutrition carried out a study on people participating in elongated fasts and discovered that their basal metabolic rate (BMR) was at its highest on day three. Isn't that incredible? While most people believe our metabolism slows down if we even skip just one meal, it's actually at a peak on the third day of a fast! In fact, the same research showed that day three was also the day when those on the trial were at their maximum exercise capacity. So much for needing a sports gel and a bottle of sugar-loaded energy drink to be at our physical best.

Imagine the repair the body can do in three or four days without food. We really do starve all of those free radicals, especially those that like to kick-start cancer. We also stop or at least dramatically slow down any inflammation, and we give our guts time to complete a full spring clean of our entire digestive tract. I personally try to do a three- or four-day fast at least once every month. Now and again I might enter an extended fast and end up having to attend an evening function on, say, day three and therefore only manage to complete two and three-quarter days, but even then I still feel fantastic. I fully recommend that once you have kicked the CARBS and experimented with either the 5:2, the alternate day fast or the 18-hour fast, that you pick a three or four day period where you know you have no dining commitments and give it a go. I promise you that you will feel wonderful. If in the unlikely, and I mean *really* unlikely, event that it makes you feel ill, then you can always stop.

So as not to deplete the body's store of vitamins and minerals, one thing you might want to consider during a 3 or 4 day fast, is to increase the number of supplements that you take.

Starting Out

Let's say we have lots of weight to lose. We might start on the alternate day fasting method, and as we near our desired goal switch to the 5:2 diet. Then when we are happy with where we have arrived we move to the 18-hour fast. Here we get all the health benefits of fasting and our body gets to enter its repair mode every single day, but we are able to maintain our desired weight. Remember I promised in the introduction of the book where I said that you wouldn't need to count calories? When it comes to fasting, for a short while you're going to need to. It's not that I lied in the beginning or that I forgot to mention this, it's just that it is going to take a few weeks into any of the above fasting programs for you to know what 500 or 600 calories looks like.

Even though we are restricting the calorie intake to 500 calories, we should of course try to consume plenty of nutrients and minerals. And don't do what I did when I first started to fast and allow some of your calories to come from wine! During fast days we shouldn't consume any alcohol, as we really want the body to fully maximise the benefit of its repairing mode.

Now if on your first attempt you feel giddy, experience a headache or you really dislike the rumble in the stomach, then you have two options:

1. Just push on. Remember that this is how our body is designed to eat and you will soon get used to it. Personally, I have come to love the hungry feeling, because it's my body's way of sending me a message to say, "all is well boss, I am in repair mode and things are taking shape down here". But I confess it can take a bit of getting used too.

2. Don't give up, but instead for a few weeks don't drop straight to 500 calories but slowly start decreasing them on your fast day. Maybe try 1200 calories for a few attempts, then when you have got used to it try 900 or 800.

But, whatever you do, no matter how hard you find it at first you must not give up. If you are on medication of any kind, then do check with your doctor before you try it. But try it you should, as it's crucial to our body to occasionally enter its natural repairing mode.

Fasting Conclusion

It's important to experiment a little and find an intermittent fasting regime that works for you. But don't even think of trying to fast until you are on a low CARB diet as it will be too difficult and unpleasant. Once you have moved over to the colourful side of life and ditched all the starchy, sugary white boring stuff, you will find intermittently fasting a breeze. One of the key things to try is to fit fasting into your life rather than your life around fasting. You don't need to do it in any type of rhythm. Because of social events and family holidays, you might find it harder in the summer months or at Christmas, but that's absolutely fine. When the time is right, just return to a method of fasting that suits your needs. I personally tend to mix it all up. Most weekdays ,if I am working, I don't eat anything all day and then just have an evening meal. At the weekends or on holiday, I might sit down and have a little breakfast with the kids. Then, once every month or so I will try to do a three- or four-day fast. I love them, I really do. By day three I feel on top of the world – full of energy, totally liberated and buzzing from consuming nothing but my own body fat.

Regardless of which approach you finally settle into, let me summarise some of the potential benefits you might experience by becoming part of the intermittent fasting generation:

- Improved memory
- Slowing the ageing process
- Better concentration
- Reduced inflammation
- Lower heart rate
- Less fatty liver
- Reduced blood pressure

- Increase fat burning
- Decreased leptin
- Increased insulin sensitivity
- Decreased risk of cancer

GO KETOGENIC GO GO

You have surely guessed by now that we believe that CARBS and other sugars are pretty much evil stuff. All wheat, grain, potatoes, rice, pasta etc gets turned into sugar in the body, then insulin comes to our rescue and caries the poisonous sugar off to our fat deposits and stores it as a future source of energy. However, the only time we can ever access this fat store is when there is virtually no insulin in our bloodstream. When insulin is limited and when we restrict the supply of new energy, we enter a state of what is known as ketosis. Here the body produces ketones (turning your fat into a usable energy source) to replace the sugar in our bloodstream. How do we get into a state of ketosis? Either we intermittently fast or our diet is very high in fat and very low in carbohydrates – preferably both!

Ketosis, Ketones, Ketogenic And Ketoacidosis... What Are The Differences?

- **Ketosis** – when we eat very few CARBS and a diet high in fat, eventually we turn our body from running on sugar to running on fat. An analogy would be like knowing that diesel engines aren't any good for the environment, therefore we modify our car so it can run on petrol (or gas as they say in America). Ketosis is a metabolic state where we are burning ketones for fuel, not glucose. And by the way it's a truly wonderful free ride when we eventually get there.
- **Ketones** – is the name of the fuel. Simplifying it a little, glucose (sugar) is one type of fuel and ketones (fat) is another.
- **Ketogenic Diet** – a ketogenic diet is one whereby we eat very small amounts of CARBS (almost exclusively green ones), moderate protein and lots of organic, healthy and delicious fats.
- **Ketoacidosis** – even though its name sounds similar, this has

nothing to do with any of the above. Ketoacidosis is a dangerous medical condition whereby there is a build-up of acid in the blood. It's a dangerous medical condition that mostly happens to people with type 1 diabetes who forget to take their insulin. The only reason I even mention it is that sometimes you will hear people saying that a ketogenic diet is dangerous. As they say, a little knowledge is often dangerous, and they are simply confusing two different things. Being in a ketosis metabolic state is what we were designed to do! Ketosis is Primal living at its best.

Where do ketones get produced? While insulin is created by the pancreas, ketones are produced by the liver. Just like a powerful motorbike that has been sat in the garage for too long, if we have been eating a diet high in carbohydrates and haven't intermittently fasted before, it might take a while to kick-start our ketone machine into order, but once it fires up we begin to feel like a completely different person. This period of firing up our ability to consume our own body fat as an energy source is known as the keto-adaptation period.

On a normal diet where we restrict calories, if we do manage to burn more than we consume then, while we might lose a little weight, we will most likely feel sluggish and irritable. If we are still eating CARBS but just fewer of them, our body will still be using the sugar as energy and only dipping into our fat store after its sugar supply becomes completely exhausted. I describe it as the body in a state of confusion – it doesn't know which way to turn. To our body, using CARBS for energy is as simple as opening up the breadbin in our kitchen. It requires minimal effort. The food supply might not be the cleanest or the healthiest, but it is easily accessed. But to use our own fat, it's like going down into the basement to open the freezer. The food here is definitely safer, but it's a pain to keep going downstairs to get it. What we need to do is to tell our brain that the breadbin is not going to be filled up again. We need to tell it to stop looking there for fuel and to go and fetch all of the food from the freezer downstairs and to put it in the fridge right next to the breadbin, which is going unfilled.

This conversion normally takes around two weeks of severely restricted CARB intake for the body to understand how to enter ketosis without any effort. It might take as long as six weeks if we have really damaged our metabolism through many years of CARB indulgence. The first days can leave us a little light on energy and we might end up missing a gym session or two, but it soon passes and before we know it we will have more energy than ever.

Once we have become keto-adaptive, rather than relying on the 2,000 to 2,500 maximum calories that our body can store in the form of glucose, depending on our weight we will instead have access to more than 40,000 to 100,000 calories sitting there switched on and waiting for us to deploy as required! I know which fuel tank I would rather be able to access. But remember, it takes a while for the body to know where to look and this is the only time on the Primal journey where patience is a virtue.

> **PRIMAL CURE FACT:**
> We can exercise as much as we like – we can run for miles or cycle for hours, but if we have sugar or insulin in our body we are not going to lose any weight. We can't burn fat in the presence of carbs, sugar, insulin or starch. Period!

UNDERSTANDING KETOSIS

Our body has two main sources of fuel: sugar/glucose produced from CARBS or burning fat through ketosis. Our body doesn't really differentiate between incoming fat or stored body fat, as it can produce ketones from either. Once we learn to switch on our ketosis metabolism, when we restrict incoming calories, losing weight becomes both a breeze and enjoyable.

Before we look at burning ketones, let's go back to what prevents us losing our fat. As we have discussed numerous times already (repetition helps things sink in so I am not going to apologise), when we eat CARBS our body converts them to sugar, and, as our body regards sugar as both fuel and poison, our pancreas creates insulin that takes the glucose and either helps us burn it if we need the energy immediately or dispatches it to our fat stores.

While insulin is active, even if we are on a long run or cycle ride, it prevents us from using our body fat as fuel. This is where I personally went wrong for so many years. I could never understand why I wasn't losing weight even when I was running three or four mornings a week. I just didn't realise it was the pizza the night before, or the early morning orange juice and cereal, that was secretly ganging up on me and sending their by-product insulin to render all my good intentions and painstaking efforts worthless.

So before we can even start burning our body fat and entering a state of ketosis, we must rid our body of as much sugar/CARBS/insulin as possible. Once we're rid of insulin, our body will turn to our fat stores for energy. Then, when we open the door of our fat store, our body releases energy in the form of ketones. Ketones are effectively an alternative fuel source to sugar/glucose. Not just energy to drive our vital organs, but as fuel for our muscles and brain too. In fact ketones are the fuel of preference for our brain, heart, liver and muscles, yet many individuals haven't been able to supply this rich energy source since they were infants consuming their mother's breast milk!

Once we open the door and enter our fat stores we are said to be in 'ketosis'. Until we enter ketosis it is impossible to lose body weight. For decades, as I stood on my bathroom scales after my early morning runs, the scales always showed that I had duly lost weight as a result of my hard hour slogging my guts out. But I was misinterpreting the results. Because I always had sugar/insulin in my body, it was preventing me entering ketosis and therefore all I had really lost was water and not fat. It is so important to understand this that I am going to repeat myself one more time.

During that long jog or cycle, we will be putting stress on our joints and limbs while not really gaining any benefit, and do more harm than good. Plus, as we will be burning lots of calories, we are sure to replace them with even more CARBS and other sugars as soon as we finish. Remember, just like nicotine makes a smoker want another cigarette as soon as it starts to exit the body, as insulin gets burnt it makes us crave more sugar and empty calories. I would like to blame the food corporations exclusively for this addiction. While it is true that in many cases, just like they do with cigarettes, manufacturers insert chemicals into food to make us crave them or even worse become addicted, Mother Nature had a hand in it too.

You see, at the end of the summer when she knew food was about to become scarce, she loaded her bushes and trees with sugar-rich fruit. To ensure that our caveman ancestors ate as much as they possibly could, stocking up their internal fat stores for the barren cold winter, she made it possible for us to consume carbs, store them quickly and then fool our brain to eat even more. She effectively shut down the creation of the 'I am full hormone' leptin, so our caveman took on board and stored as much calories as possible.

While today the vast majority of adults in the Western world never enter a state of ketosis, Primal man spent far more time in ketosis than out of it and if you were breastfed from birth you previously did too. In his brilliant book *Keto Clarity* – a book that if you really want to get a detailed understanding of how to enter ketosis I recommend you purchase – author Jimmy Moore explains that within 12 hours of being delivered into the world we enter a state of ketosis, with ketones from our mother's milk providing around a quarter of our total energy. What I also found fascinating in Jimmy Moore's book was that breast milk is rich in MCTs (medium-chain triglycerides – you will be reading a lot about these amazing fats later), which is what coconuts provide by the bucket-load. It is for this very same reason why much packaged baby milk contains either coconut oil or MCT oil.

It is too early in the book to go off on a tangent (again) and start talking about one of my favourite subjects, but for your health's sake please do everything possible from this point forward to fall in love with coconuts. They are simply one of nature's miracle foods and can actually accelerate the speed at which we enter the metabolic state of ketosis. So much so, that in order to bring forward the entry point into ketosis, many people take MCT supplements. I don't personally recommend them unless you are trying to get there for medical reasons. Instead just eat lots of coconut produce.

Because our Primal forefathers often went days without catching their food, and during the winter ate very sparsely indeed, they were constantly engaged in an intermittent fast orchestrated by nature. It's important to remember that when the supply of CARBS and protein is low, our body will run on fat. It doesn't distinguish from stored fat or free fat. Our stored fat, whether it is from our buttocks, love handles, waistline, results in exactly the same ketones as the free fat waiting to be stored. So our caveman ancestors didn't have to worry about balancing their food, the fact that their bellies were often empty meant that their ketosis metabolism kicked in automatically once any glucose in the body and liver had been consumed.

If we have a lot of weight to shed and really want to shift it, then one sure way to do so is to avoid as many CARBS as possible (even the good ones for a short while) and enter into a state of ketosis. If we can exercise as well and remain in ketosis for prolonged periods, then our weight should drop off. Warning: Don't drop the green carbs (broccoli, spinach, etc) for long as we need to eat healthy CARBS such as leafy green vegetables and low-sugar fruits. The only time we should drop them from our diet might be for just a few weeks while we teach our body how to enter ketosis.

So how do we become keto-adaptive? We need to get our daily CARB intake to below 50g and ideally these should come from complex CARBS such as leafy greens. Jeff S. Volek, PhD, RD, and Stephen D. Phinney, MD, PhD in their book *The Art and Science of Low Carbohydrate Performance* sum it up brilliantly: "When it comes to cereals, breads, pasta, potatoes, pastry, candy, juices or other carb-dense foods we'll say it once… just don't go there. Because all of these are like the nuclear option in suppressing ketones, we've started calling them 'carbage'". They have created this wonderful word 'carbage' by combining CARB and garbage, and I think it should be added to the English dictionary! Now you might wonder why I say low CARB, moderate protein and lots of quality organic fats. Why do we need to be careful of our protein intake? Aren't proteins the good guys? Yes, proteins are the good guys, and play a crucial role in our well-being. However, our body is really clever. It has the ability to turn protein into sugar. In the absence of CARBS, the body turns any excess protein into sugar and therefore while attempting to enter ketosis we need to be careful not to overdo the protein. If you remember back to Chapter 1, I said that while the body must intake protein and fats to survive, it can function happily forever without a single CARB. Now we are getting into the detail, let me explain that the body does occasionally need glucose to function. If it can't locate it when it's needed, through a process called gluconeogenesis, it synthesises it from proteins. This is really important to understand if we want to either enter ketosis or lose weight, or more commonly both! While protein is undoubtedly vital to our survival and a critical macronutrient for our body's self-repair mechanisms, when we consume too much of it, in the absence of CARBS our body will convert any excess into the same by-product of CARBS – sugar.

In *Keto Clarity*, author Jimmy Moore explains, "The liver normalises and maintains blood glucose levels in the body by creating glucose through gluconeogenesis. During those times when the body is not taking in any food (for instance, when we are sleeping), the liver goes to work on gluconeogenesis, using amino acids (the building blocks of protein), lactic acid and glycerol (a molecule that comes from fat) to create the sugar the body needs". What's really interesting to understand, especially for those like myself who love fasting, is that after the liver has used up all of the glucose it can store (stored glucose in the liver is known as glycogen), which is typically around 12 to 18 hours depending on the level of activity we are performing, gluconeogenesis kicks in and starts converting glycogen to fuel from other sources. Of course, what we really want to happen once all of our glycogen is spent is that the body stops searching for it and instead switches its fuel tank and starts metabolising ketones.

Although we don't count calories, while we are training our body to enter ketosis it's ideal to aim for around 20% of our calories from green CARBS and protein and 80% from healthy fats. But remember these are just guidelines and every single one of us is different. For example, because I have damaged my metabolism so badly in the past, I only have to look at CARBS to put on weight. Seriously, it seems I am that sensitive to processed CARBS I only have to sniff a pizza and my waistline bulges! And the same happens when I consume too much protein. I seem fine with 30g of protein during or immediately after a workout, but on days when I am not exercising I have to be just as strict about my protein intake as I am about CARBS.

> **As counting calories is not Primal, a simple summary for ketosis is – virtually no carbs, reduced protein and double our organic fat intake.**

So if we want to enter ketosis, it's all about maximising the amount of healthy fats we consume. But which fats I here you cry? We will learn about all of these little miracles of nature in detail later, but for now here is a snapshot of what can help us make up the 80% fat part of the diet:

- Organic grass-fed fatty meat (no need to trim the fat off)
- Oily fish
- Butter from organic grass-fed cows
- Extra virgin olive oil
- Coconut oil or coconut milk
- Coconut chunks
- Avocado or extra virgin avocado oil

Is Ketosis Healthy?
My wife's first impression was no, it's not! A side effect of being in ketosis is that one of the three different kinds of ketones, acetone, is

primarily detected in our breath. And boy does it sometimes smell very pungent! The first time I went into the blissful state of ketosis, my wife was so convinced that I had a stomach ulcer she pleaded with me to go to the doctor. However, I was feeling wonderful and healthy and knew that there was nothing wrong. It was only recently that I discovered that my initial bad breath was just the body learning how to burn its new clean fuel. If the same happens to you, then just chew on some fresh mint until it goes away.

I believe that bad breath for a few days is a small price to pay for something that can slow down the ageing process, reduces the risk of such horrible diseases as cancer (remember cancer needs glucose to fuel its growth) and improves virtually all cognitive functions, so much so that many specialists are recommending ketogenic diets for patients suffering with Alzheimer's. In addition it:

- Helps accelerate weight loss
- Improves the quality of sleep
- Benefits the skin and can eradicate acne
- Helps hormones better control appetite
- Lowers blood pressure
- Makes it far easier to intermittently fast
- Provides the body with a superior amount of energy
- Increases testosterone for a better sex drive
- Improves moods and fights depression
- Increases the good cholesterol HDL

How Do I Know If I Am Metabolising Ketones?

The first time will be fairly easy as you will probably get smelly breath! We can also purchase ketone strips, which when we pee on them will measure the level of acetoacetate ketones in our urine. They cost under £10 for 50 strips and they seem to work quite well when we are starting out and therefore provide excellent moral support, but as the body gets more use to being in ketosis tend to work less well over time. If you are happy to prick your finger to obtain a small blood sample, for around £30 you can purchase a ketone tester commonly used by diabetics. While it's a little less convenient, it's by far the most accurate as it measures on beta-hydroxybutyrate, which is the main source of ketones in the blood. You can also now purchase breath testers, but as of yet the reviews seem very mixed.

Dr Dan Maggs

"I lost nearly 5 stone (31kg) on a ketogenic diet. It works by allowing your body to access all the energy you have stored as fat. Aside from that, the feeling of clarity and energy you get when you brain is mainly running on ketones is incredible."

Chapter 3 Highlights

- Fasting doesn't decrease our metabolic rate but actually increases it.
- The best diet is one that mirrors our 'feast and famine' history and gives the body sufficient resting periods in which to heal itself.
- Primal Alignment: Our caveman ancestors didn't plan their famine and feasts, their food supply always dictated it.
- If possible, vary your fasting styles just like our Primal ancestors did. Without fridges or fast foods, the only eating routine they had was no routine.
- There is no such thing as losing body weight, we instead have to burn it. And we can only truly burn it when we have become keto-adaptive.
- Our body can only use one fuel source at a time, either glucose or ketones. Over time, on a very low CARB, medium protein and high fat diet, our brain acts Primally and turns to our fat deposits as its primary source of fuel.

04.
MOMMS
Exercise
Principles

In this chapter we discuss the basics of Primal exercise and how we are designed to benefit from short, intense bursts of physical activity. For too long endurance sports have caused havoc with our body, and in many instances been shown to not do us any good at all.

INTRODUCTION TO PRIMAL CURE ON FITNESS

"If I could give every individual the right amount of nourishment and exercise, not too little and not too much, we would have found the safest way to health."
Hippocrates

We need to stop spending so much time worrying about our chronological age and instead focus on our biological age. Our chronological age is just a number. I hate it when I hear someone claiming, "I'm too old to exercise". To my mind the term 'old' should be permanently replaced with 'older'. We're never old, we're only ever older. Maybe Jamaican Violet Brown who died in September 2017 or Italian Emma Morano who died in April of the same year – both of whom were 117 – might have earned the right to claim they were old, but for the rest of us we should just consider ourselves as older.

Unless someone suffers from a physical disability, the vast majority of the following advice is applicable to everyone, regardless of age.

In Chapter 2 we looked at the right type of foods we should be eating to live a long and healthy life. If you skipped any of it and jumped straight to this section, unless you are already lean and healthy, then can I politely request that you go back and read it in full? It's crucial for our well-being that we have a good understanding of what we should eat, and when to eat it, before we jump into exercise and other Primal Cure health principles.

From my own experience, a little knowledge of food is dangerous. By knowing only a small piece of the puzzle, I was overweight for 25 years, simply because I fell victim to advertising nonsense that I found on food packaging and in TV adverts. By not understanding the full picture, we are more likely to be easily persuaded by relatives, colleagues or friends who genuinely believe that they know better. Once you are happy that you have got a good understanding of food, then let's move on to the Primal Cure exercise methodology.

Dr Shan Hussain

"Exercise is proven beyond doubt to be beneficial in the prevention and treatment of so many conditions, including cardiovascular disease, diabetes, depression and even some cancers."

MAX OUT - MOVE MORE - SPRINT (MOMMS)

Let us now look at the two most important and most fundamental Primal Cure principles of all:

1. We must eat what we are designed to eat.
2. We must exercise in a manner that's as close to ancestral daily life as possible.

To capture in its entirety the Primal Cure approach to fitness, we are going to use an easily remembered acronym, MOMMS. It stands for 'Max Out – Move More – Sprint'. 'Max Out' refers to our approach to weight training, where we use a specific type of routine that pushes us 'to the max'. We then focus on moving more in our everyday life and eventually get to build a couple of extremely short sprints into our weekly routine. These three separate areas of fitness build muscles and at the same time increase our flexibility and help us feel younger for longer.

The principle behind the Primal Cure MOMMS approach is to emulate what our Primal ancestors did during daylight. It is about moving more, occasionally sprinting and lifting heavy rocks (in our case weights). It is not about laborious hours on a treadmill or exercise bike, nor is it about attending the latest craze in keep-fit classes. Caveman didn't jog for hours on end, nor did he stand outside his cave with all of his hunter friends and do an hour of floor exercises to the beat of a jungle drum.

What we desire is to be fit, but not at the expense of our health. What do I mean by that? While there are many overweight individuals that need to start eating and exercising Primally, there are some fit people that while they might look lean but are actually unhealthy. You may have come across the word 'TOFI' before, if you haven't it's an acronym for 'Thin Outside, Fat Inside' and refers to people who might slip nicely into skinny jeans, but have a lot of dangerous internal visceral fat around some very important organs. Then there are other athletic people that put their body through hell on the running track, which in the short term makes them look fit, but in the long term potentially leads to an onslaught of health problems.

Research carried out by Dr James O'Keefe at the Mid America Heart Institute at St Luke's Hospital in Kansas City suggests that people who exercise regularly live seven years longer than those who are physically inactive. No surprise there really. However, his latest research revealed something that will most likely astonish you and that is: 'Those individuals who participated in extreme endurance sports experienced significant heart damage'. More on this later.

Throughout this chapter, I will keep trying to highlight that MOMMS is the safest and most reliable way to achieve healthy longevity, and that the jogging fraternity and long-distance cyclists (and for many years I have worn both caps), are most likely causing themselves a lot of long-term damage.

Let me start by introducing you to a highly relevant scientific concept: Hormesis. It's a geeky word summarising the saying "a little of what doesn't kill you makes you stronger". An example of hormesis would be a vaccination, where we are injected with a small dose of the very thing the vaccination is trying to protect against. Stress is another example of hormesis. A small amount of stress is a good thing, while a large amount can kill you. Too much stress is linked to all sorts of horrible diseases, including cardiovascular and cancer. But a small amount of stress, as in the type caused by sprinting or by weightlifting, is a good thing. Sadly, we can't say the same about jogging long distances for hours on end, which can cause unhealthy damaging levels of stress.

> **Primal Cure exercise principles are geared around hormesis.**

MOVE MORE

Caveman didn't jump in a car and sit in a two-hour traffic jam on the way to an office, where he sat for seven hours before going home to slump in front of the TV. Put simply, in Great Britain we don't move enough.

Even 40 years ago, I can remember my mother carrying half a dozen heavy grocery bags in each hand, the handles cutting into her fingers, half a mile from the nearest shop. Today what do we do? So that we don't have to push the shopping trolley too far, we drive around the supermarket car park multiple times trying to find a space as close to the entrance as possible! It's terrible to think how inactive we have become.

If you are overweight or obese and just starting out with Primal Cure, then it is important to pay a little attention to that old saying, 'don't run before you can walk'. In fact, we don't want you to run at all, ever… well, unless a lion is chasing you. Looking at the three distinct areas of MOMMS – Max Out – Move More – Sprint – we are going to advise that you start moving more immediately, so depending on your current circumstances, potentially leave the weightlifting for a short while and only entertain sprinting when your weight is under control.

As Dr Spencer Nadolsky says in his book *The Fat Loss Prescription*, "All of the little movements you do in the course of a day fall under the blanket term of 'non-exercise activity thermogenesis, or NEAT'". When we get on to exercise (Max Out), and we mean real exercise where - 'without-pain-there-is-no-gain' type exercise - then that's a different principle that surprisingly doesn't take up much time at all. However, in our Move More phase, it's crucial for our health, especially if currently you live a very sedentary lifestyle, that you start to move about a lot more on your feet.

Get outdoors in the fresh air, walking, gardening, hiking, slow bike rides, skiing, rowing, it really doesn't matter what it is, but get moving. Get involved with a swimming class or bowls or anything that gets you moving, but not so much that you're out of breath. Now there is a good reason we don't want you out of breath, because we want to have a clear distinction between movement and exercise. Both are vital for our health, but both perform very different functions. I always tell my children to take the stairs and not the lift, but if this gets you out of breath, don't do it yet, as that would be exercise and until our weight starts to fall off, we want to concentrate on just getting moving.

> **PRIMAL FACT:**
> **Even 2000 years ago, Hippocrates - the father of western medicine - told us, "Walking is man's best medicine".**

If you live a few miles from work, try to walk there occasionally. If you live too far away, then park a mile or so from your destination and walk the last part. You will be amazed how you feel. Sir Richard Branson likes to get dropped off a mile or so from a meeting and walk. He will also often hold meetings with his directors while walking. Richard is patron of a charity my brother John and I started called The Colourful Life Foundation, and whenever we are with him it's really interesting to see how he never sits still for long, he is on his feet at every opportunity.

At the weekend, drive to a park or lake and take a stroll. There are dozens of health benefits from simply getting up and moving more. So find something you enjoy, maybe something a little different to the norm, and for your health's sake, get out and start moving.

Dr Shan Hussain

"One foot in front of the other. A study presented at the European society of Cardiology Congress in 2015, showed that 25 minutes of brisk walking a day could add up to seven years to your life and halve the risk of dying from a heart attack."

MAX OUT

While I truly believe that 80% of the way we look is shaped in the kitchen and only 10% in the gym, (with the other 10% being made up of combination of such things as sleep, stress and sunshine), I believe that, for numerous reasons, it is important to look after our muscles.

To understand the Max Out principle of Primal Cure, which is a modified version of HIIT – High Intensity Interval Training – we need to go back and look at the daily activities of our Primal ancestors. After a successful hunt, they would carry small animals across their shoulders, or drag heavier ones by their hooves - to get them back to their dwelling. While out gathering, without modern tools they would hack down trees and move heavy rocks looking for mushrooms and other fungi. None of these activities would take hours and hours, but our Primal ancestors must have been able to muster great strength when required. Therefore, our body is designed, and in fact programmed, to do the occasional bout of heavy lifting.

But before you rush out and start lifting heavy weights, let's invest some time in planning what our workout should look like; in business we call this the '5Ps Principle' – 'Prior Planning Prevents Poor Performance'. To start, we need to understand the concept of homeostasis. Every cell and system in our body relies on a stable environment to function. Homeostasis refers to the internal balance the body must maintain to ensure health. When we exercise, we break down our muscles (catabolic process) and then ask our body to rebuild them (anabolic process) stronger and bigger than before.

Unless we lift heavy things, our body no longer engages in any meaningful level of catabolism, but for our Primal ancestors the balance was perfect. They had to expend energy to catch and gather their food (catabolic) and then while feasting on their kill for several days their body had time to rebuild its muscles (anabolic). If the only exercise we currently do is opening the door to the grocery deliveryman, then our homeostasis is going to be well out of whack.

My good friend Angeline has been wonderful and dedicated a lot of time helping me edit this book. While working her way through this chapter, she came to see me because she was a little concerned. Let me explain. Angeline likes to keep in shape. She has two wonderful children and, as a TV presenter, both her fitness and body shape are very important to her.

Like many mums, Angeline treasures her gym sessions, and works hard to carve out the time in what is a very hectic schedule to ensure they happen. She loves to run for 30 minutes on a treadmill several times each week. However, she was upset to discover that jogging is more likely to have negative effects rather than beneficial, but even worse she really didn't want to lift weights because she didn't want to become muscular.

If you fall into the same category, and don't want to build visible muscles, don't fear MOMMS! If you download the Primal Cure app, you will find lots of exercises that you can do that won't build muscle in areas where you don't want them. For example, Angeline doesn't want visible biceps, but is more than happy to tighten up her triceps. The app has more than 10 exercises that isolate just the triceps. If you want to firm up your bottom, but not develop muscles in your legs, that's easily achieved too. My point is this – you need to develop muscles in order to:

1. Burn more calories.
2. Support your joints and bones.
3. Reduce the risk of injury.
4. Replicate the lifestyle of our Primal ancestors

However, if you don't want to look ripped, then you don't need to. For Angeline, by following the MOMMS philosophy, she still has her precious personal time in the gym, but now sprints intermittently within her four-kilometre walk on the running machine and lifts weights that target the parts of her body she wants to look firmer.

Weight Training Frequency

When I was in my teenage years, and competing at an international level in sailing, I only had to go to the gym once or at most twice a week to maintain a fit shape. But throughout my forties I was running several times a week and weight training in the gym at least three or four times a week, but the more I trained, the more I was progressively getting fatter.

So, what was the cause? It turns out that when we exercise too frequently, and when that exercise finishes without us maxing out, then our muscles may actually shrink (atrophy) rather than grow (hypertrophy). Ouch! All those half-assed hours in the gym and I was doing more harm than good. I would have been far better off just staying at home spending more time with my children.

The science behind the problems caused by my over-training goes something like this: When we exercise our muscles but don't completely deplete them of glycogen they actually can suffer atrophy. By leaving glycogen in the muscles each day while at the gym, it slowly begins to reduce the energy storage capacity in each cell in the muscle. This problem is encountered not just by the weightlifter that does not Max Out, but also by those that jog. To make matters worse, if during our gym session we do too many repetitions and sets, then the exercise becomes more aerobic (with oxygen), which can cause a build-up of dangerous free radicals.

In Ben Greenfield's book, *Beyond Training*, he quotes research conducted by the McMaster University (Ontario) and the Washington University School of Medicine in St Louis that, "The repair process appears to peak about twenty-four hours after a workout" and, "By about thirty-six hours post workout, the whole process is pretty much complete. So every time we beat up or tear down muscle fibres, especially with running and weight training, we're looking at approximately thirty-six hours of recovery before another high-quality session is doable or efficacious".

As I mentioned at the beginning of this book, we are all built differently. Our age, sex and current fitness level plays a big part in how quickly our muscles recover between sessions, and therefore what our recovery period should be. Plus, it also depends on whether we truly Max Out our muscles during training or just put them under duress. I know from personal experience that when I have completed a gym session where I have been truly in the zone, my body almost tells me not to train for at least a week. But then in other sessions, where I just couldn't motivate myself or push myself hard enough, I am itching to get another session in two or three days later.

Quality of sleep, diet, alcohol consumption, dehydration and even how stressed we are at work or home can also play a big part in determining how quickly our muscles recover from exercise. And remember that all movement and exercise is accumulative. If we weight train on a Monday and then take in a game of golf or a yoga class on Tuesday or Wednesday, we might find we are not feeling ready for the next gym session for an extra day or two. My personal approach is that as long as I do at least one weight training session a week and walk plenty of miles, then the rest of the time I just listen to my body.

Age also plays a part in training frequency. In our late thirties or early forties we start to lose muscles (known as sarcopenia). If we don't exercise we lose as much as 3 to 5% of muscle every decade. Sarcopenia increases the older we get, and by our seventies shifts into top gear. As we can't quite lift the same big weights as we once did, and as we tire a little earlier during gym sessions - therefore not truly Maxing Out - most weeks we ideally need to train at least two or three times. But once again, I can't emphasise enough that we are all built differently and that we should use the above as guidelines, while in the main listening to our body for when to hit the gym.

> **Visit PrimalCure.com where you will find over 100 different exercises with full descriptions, photos and videos.**

> **PRIMAL CURE EXERCISE FREQUENCY PRINCIPLE:**
> Recovery time between gym sessions is a crucial part of maintaining health, don't get into a routine of forcing sessions on yourself, instead listen to your body. While we are on it, never sacrifice a good night's sleep for an early gym session.

One last thought on exercising as we age – in reality we should see more 70-year-olds bench pressing in the gym than we do those in their twenties! Brad Schoenfeld in his book *Science and Development of Muscle Hypertrophy* says, "After age 40, the body loses progressively more muscle mass each year. Regular resistance training can reduce this loss. Although the elderly do have a diminished hypertrophic response, they can gain muscle mass; however, a greater weekly training dose appears necessary to maintain the gains".

As we get older, losing muscles not only reduces our strength, but also leads to a serious decline in metabolic function. And that's really important, because keeping our metabolic system healthy by maintaining our muscle mass helps slow down the ageing process, fuels the brain and helps protect us against obesity, cardiovascular disease and diabetes.

Method Of Exercise - Time Under Load

Okay, so now we understand how often to hit the gym, let's state something quite obvious – do everything you can to avoid injury. I say this because I constantly meet people who injure themselves training and spend as much time laid-up as they actually do in the gym. Certainly the older we get, as our recovery time gets longer and longer we really need to make avoiding injury a priority.

The Primal Cure preferred method of exercise, which is also one of the safest, isn't to swing huge weights using momentum, but to keep each repetition nice and strict, really focusing the mind on the muscles we want to work on. This might sound straightforward, but many people – including myself – are not very good at isolating muscles. Without the ability to isolate which muscle we want to work on, then the approach we are going to discuss will not prove as effective as it otherwise could be.

This might sound a little vain, but stand in front of a mirror and pose like a bodybuilder on stage. Try first without any weights to tense the muscle you intend to work on. This will send a signal to the brain and help focus its attention. Let's say we want to work your biceps. We should be able to tense them for about a minute and really feel a burning sensation without lifting any weights at all. If I am still struggling to connect brain and muscle (and this is going to sound even weirder), I tickle the muscle before starting the exercise.

The heightened awareness (known as kinesthesia – pronounced 'ken-es-teez-ya') from either or both of these methods increases our ability to focus on the muscle we want to exercise.

The Primal Cure Max Out method might sound a little strange to some readers at first, but I assure you that it works. Before you even lift your first weights, I am going to ask you to take some measurements. This way, you will be able to track your progression. While it is true that when it comes to eating, Primal Cure never counts calories, when it comes to exercise, we like to measure virtually everything. Rather than fill lots of pages with where and how to measure each muscle, you can find loads of useful photos and information at www.primalcure.com. You can also download the Primal Cure app to store all of your measurements. Once you have got all of your vital statistics noted, it's time to head off to the gym.

It's really beneficial in your first few sessions to either hire a personal trainer or go along with a good friend, but make sure whoever it is reads at least this section of the book. If you can't get some help, then download our Primal Cure app (it's totally free and really easy to use), or visit our website where we give you advice on more than 100 different exercises.

Using a watch or a clock, or better still our app, we are going to slowly and deliberately carry out each repetition (one complete motion of the exercise), whether it be a press-up or bicep curl, a pull-down or deadlift. The repetition should take between six and 20 seconds depending both on our preference and the actual exercise we are doing. Our aim is to keep going until we reach complete failure. This is where we just can't move the weight any further without cheating. Once we hit this point, we are not going to put the weight down, but continue to push to the max for at least 10 more seconds, even if the weight is not moving at all. While we are holding for these last seconds, in a phase of exercise called 'isometric training' or 'static contraction', we should in most exercises find our muscles twitching or whole parts of our body shaking. Don't panic, hang in there.

At this point, and this point only, do we class that we have reached Max Out. Unless we Max Out, we will still have spare glycogen in our muscles and not only will we limit our growth, we might actually make our muscles smaller! Before we give up, we should remind ourselves that this is the only shoulder press we are going to be doing for possibly an entire week and therefore we MUST Max Out.

Our ability to push to our true max, and the more microtrauma (damage) we can inflict on our muscles at a cellular level, combined with sufficient rest time, determines our success. Remember, weight training and sprinting are very different exercises to endurance jogging. They are polar opposites. Endurance sports are aerobic (with oxygen) and interval training is anaerobic (without oxygen). Effectively when we do short intense exercises (aka High Intensity Intermittent Training – HIIT), our muscles don't have time to take on board oxygen or fuel. Our body is forced to use an energy supply within our muscle cells called glycogen. When our muscles burn glycogen they produce lactic acid, which if I simplify it a little is what causes the burn we sometimes experience when weightlifting.

I want to explain a little further about what's happening inside our muscles as we exercise by using the analogy of a sponge. I can't claim its mine as it is mentioned in several books and it explains the process brilliantly. Each and every muscle in our body acts like a sponge. If we Max Out properly, we are effectively wringing out the sponge so that there is no water (or energy in our muscle's case) left inside. Once our glycogen has gone, our sponge will soak up everything it possibly can to replace it. Any sugars floating around the body will be quickly grabbed by our muscles before insulin has a chance to hand it over to our fat stores. What's more, we will be producing far less insulin as well, as our muscles will be hungry for any sugars and will temporarily make insulin semi-redundant. It's also why, when we eat straight after a training session, our muscles are said to grow. But be aware, this is not the same for aerobic exercises where the muscles aren't fully depleted.

Let's get back to Maxing Out. At that point, when the movement has stopped and you have held for roughly 10 seconds more, note down the time. For most exercises you are targeting the total time from starting to Max Out to be between 45 and 120 seconds. The total time is what we refer to as Time Under Load (TUL) or, as some people call it, Time Under Tension (TUT). If you didn't manage to last 45 seconds, then in your next session you must decrease the weight. If you managed to do more than 120 seconds, then in your next session you are going to add more weight. Remember my earlier point 'you can't manage what you can't measure'? What we are looking for over a period of a few months is to be able to slowly increase the weight and still last for between 45 to 120 seconds. Once you start to increase the heaviness, you will have proven to yourself beyond any doubt that you have become stronger.

Top 8 Primal Max Out Tips

1. Download the Primal Cure app. It will help you both measure your sessions (remember: 'You can't manage what you can't measure') and also motivate you to push just that little bit harder.
2. Remember that with some exercises, great things can be achieved even with very small weights or even static contraction exercises

(just holding the muscle tense without movement).

3. With Primal Max Out we achieve greater results by putting all of our effort into just one set per session. In other words, just performing the exercise once, where we truly Max Out yields better results than multiple sets where we didn't push ourselves as hard.

4. It's best to forbid ourselves from doing more than one set of the same workout, because if our body knows there is an option of a second set we might subconsciously find ourselves giving up too early in the first.

5. To ensure we Max Out, it is not possible to aim for a precise time or a nice round number of reps – we will fail when we fail.

6. Make sure we don't hold our breath and breathe out during the hardest part of each repetition.

7. Don't screw up the face – it doesn't help us lift anything and just makes us get wrinkles and lines!

8. We should remember that our sessions take up less than 1% of our week, but these short sessions are only effective if we are truly pushing our body hard.

Other Benefits Of Max Out Exercising

1. By lifting weights and Maxing Out, we increase our bone density and help increase our natural growth hormone.

2. We increase insulin sensitivity.

3. We become more metabolically efficient.

4. We limit inflammation, certainly when compared to endurance athletes.

5. When we Max Out Primally, we get both a hormonal rush and heaps of mental simulation that slows down the ageing process.

Let me now conclude this section on Primal Max Out with an extract taken from the summary of the research carried out by the Southampton Solent University with the aptly named title 'Resistance Training to Momentary Muscular Failure Improves Cardiovascular Fitness in Humans'.

"Resistance training performed to failure can induce acute and chronic physiological effects, which appear to be similar to aerobic endurance training. Which in turn produces similar enhancements in CV [cardiovascular] fitness ... We are optimistic and encouraged that this review will help to promote a paradigm shift in this area of training and research identifying a particular modality of exercise as being aerobic or CV constitutes a misnomer. The extent that any modality of exercise produces CV fitness adaptations appears to be dependent primarily upon the intensity of the exercise ... Indeed we are not the first to consider this false dichotomy between RT [resistance training, i.e. weight training] and aerobic training Phillips and Winnett have questioned the RT/aerobic dichotomy with regard to health outcomes. They too suggest that reconsideration of the value of RT is important. We hope that this review will encourage researchers and practitioners to consider the implications in the design and interpretation of future research as well as when prescribing exercise for the purpose of improving CV fitness. Thus in conclusion we contend that performance of RT to failure will produce significant improvement in CV fitness that occurs through physiological adaptations such as up-regulation of mitochondrial enzymes".

SPRINTING

If you remember back to Chapter 1, we discussed how we have only been at the top of the food chain for around 100,000 years. When predators chased our Primal ancestors, boy could they sprint. But can you ever imagine them going on a long jog? And of course, both the wheel and Lycra were a long way from being invented, so cycling was also off the Primal exercise agenda.

But shouldn't we include aerobic exercise like jogging or cycling in our exercise regime? No. In fact for the sake of your mid- to long-term health, you really shouldn't. Believe me when I say endurance training (ET) is actually unhealthy! But when we replace ET with SIT (Sprint Interval Training) we experience huge gains. Over the coming pages

I am going to explain why we should say goodbye to those laborious long runs and hardcore cycle rides, and instead master the art of sprinting.

Back in Chapter 1, we discussed the mitochondria, the powerhouse/battery of our cells. It turns out that they love sprinting so much that they start to procreate, creating a greater and greater power source. When our hunter-gatherer ancestors experienced a close call with predators snapping at their heels, during the ensuing good night's sleep, nature decided to provide the cells with more power for the next encounter. The good news of course is the more mitochondria organelles we have in each cell, the more fat and glucose we can burn. However, our mitochondria don't reproduce when we're jogging or cycling because the last thing the body wants to do while undergoing endurance activities is to create something that burns more fuel!

Before we make sprinting part of our weekly routine, it is really important to get our weight down first. We will do more harm than good if our body fat is above 25% and we start pounding the tarmac. Sprinting should be seen as pretty much the last thing on our list of lifestyle changes – in fact it's the Primal icing on the cake.

What are the benefits of sprinting and why should we do it? Let's face it, even if there was no scientific reason it's kind of obvious that we are designed to sprint - as if our Primal ancestors were not able to do so you wouldn't be around to read this book and I wouldn't be here to write it. Our species would not have lasted long if we could not sprint. As we have required the ability to sprint away from danger for more than 2 million years, you can bet your bottom dollar that nature has designed us to be good sprinters and to gain benefits from doing so.

In terms of return on investment, nothing gets close to sprint training. It burns fat while building muscle, increases the health of our heart and lungs, improves circulation and metabolism and provides us with better mental cognition. While long jogs and cycle rides rarely result in fat loss, sprinting is the king of fat burning. Even just sprinting for 10 to 20 seconds, three to six times a week, conducted over just one or two sessions can burn off heaps of fat. How is that possible? When we sprint properly, our muscles continue to burn up fat for days after the actual exercise. If you think sprinting only improves the muscles in our legs, think again. If we really want to find our six-pack, forget hundreds of sit-ups and ab-crunches – nothing beats flat-out sprinting.

Don't panic, when I say the word sprint, it doesn't normally mean on the road. You will most likely start with short sprints on an exercise bike in the gym or with a rowing machine, both of which are much safer for our body when we first start to sprint. However, once we have our body in shape and when we feel comfortable in giving it a go, then many people will naturally want to progress to sprinting on the road or track. Whether we are sitting on the bike or rower, or indeed running, the principles are all the same. Let's first look at the 'why' and then move to the 'how'.

When we sprint for short distances, it is done without the intake of much oxygen. It is therefore classed as an anaerobic exercise. This builds strength quickly, especially in our powerful, fast twitching muscle fibres. With muscle's fast explosion of instant requirements, the heart has to pump really hard to deliver blood, which in return helps to strengthen the heart. And a stronger heart is a heart more resilient to disease.

> **PRIMAL SPRINTING:**
> When we sprint, the body believes we are running for our lives and rewards us with extra mitochondria for our next dangerous encounter. This helps us burn calories faster and lose weight.

Sprinting is really challenging both physically and mentally. When we train with a friend, we will be able to measure our results in various ways. We might for example, take a marker pen and score our starting position on a kerb, and then using a stopwatch run flat-out for 10 seconds and mark where we finish. Then, after resting for four or five minutes, we try to beat that time. This mental challenge is great for the brain. The endorphins that are released act as a natural painkiller and provide us with a real feeling of well-being.

If you are looking to start sprinting for the first time, then visit our website for full details on how to sprint on foot, on a bike and on a rowing machine. Also download the Primal Cure app to record your sprints.

Return On Investment

As we say in business, when it comes to achieving a return on investment, very little in life beats sprinting. In return for less than two minutes of significant discomfort, in a week containing more than 10,000 minutes (less than 1/5000th of utter exhaustion) we received all of the following benefits from our flat-out sprints:

- Lose weight (post-sprint we will experience an increased metabolic rate for several days)
- Build core strength, not just in our legs but our abs and bottom too
- Increased growth hormones
- Growth in our heart and arteries (a true cardiovascular workout)
- Lowered blood pressure and blood sugar levels
- Lower levels of insulin
- Improved cognitive skills (yes, we become smarter)

> **PRIMAL CURE SPRINTING BELIEF:**
> **Each week achieve immense gains from just two**
> **minutes of intense pain.**

Personally I normally try to do two lots of sprints each week. Sometimes it's one run and one exercise bike, other weeks if the weather is not so good I might do one session on the bike and one on the rowing machine. I normally do them after I have finished a weight training session, but occasionally I'll do them on their own and use the rest of the time in the gym to improve my form or muscle kinesthesia (awareness). In total I normally do two or three sessions a week in the gym and never for more than one hour at a time (normally it's just 45 minutes). So my entire weight training and sprint sessions are on average just 10 hours per month. That's not a huge investment of time to ensure that the body is in good working order. If you don't want to go to a gym, you will probably need to spend around £200 to get a good exercise bike, a few dumbbells and some suspension cables and turn your garage or spare bedroom into your own fitness studio. It will most likely be the best financial outlay you will ever make.

One cautionary note on sprinting: while the legs are going to burn like crazy and our breathing becomes very loud and heavy through gritted teeth, we should not feel any pain or tightening of the chest. If we do, we should immediately stop and let somebody in the gym know and once we recover go and see a doctor.

Endurance Sports Aren't All That Healthy

As I mentioned in the introduction to this book, I was a regular jogger for many years. I had completed three full marathons and several half marathons and all in respectable times. But throughout the entire period I was overweight and constantly injuring myself.

It wasn't until I read a book with the head-turning title *Eat Bacon Don't Jog* by Grant Peterson, that I realised how totally unnecessary - and in fact harmful to my well-being - all those painful miles I had accumulated had been. Grant writes, "Your body responds to too much running by releasing cortisol, a stress hormone. Cortisol triggers a process called gluconeogenesis, in which your muscles (made up of protein) break down into glucose". Grant then goes on to dig the knife in deeper to the committed jogger who suffers pain in the belief they are doing themselves good by revealing, "Jogging doesn't build strength or fitness – it just trains muscles to tolerate more jogging, and in the real world that's close to useless".

In *Beyond Training*, America's top personal trainer, Ben Greenfield cites lots of research detailing the long-term dangers awaiting those who undertake too many endurance sessions. For example he writes, "The heart generally returns to normal within a week after completing a tough endurance workout or race. But for those who frequently compete in such events the results can be repetitive cardiac injury over days, months, even years". He goes on to describe a whole list of detrimental health conditions that can develop from undertaking endurance exercises, such as jogging and long-distance cycling.

"Jogging doesn't build strength or fitness – it just trains muscles to tolerate more jogging, and in the real world that's close to useless."
Grant Peterson
Author of *Eat Bacon Don't Jog*

Research carried out by the Public Library of Science (PLOS) in California during 2016 discovered, "Low cardiorespiratory [relating to the action of both heart and lungs] fitness is a strong independent risk factor for cardiovascular disease and all cause mortality. It has been known for decades that interval training involving brief hard efforts is a potent stimulus to improve cardiorespiratory fitness. Recent studies have shown that protocols involving as little as one minute of sprint interval training per session can be very effective in this regard". In the conclusion to their findings they state, "In summary, we report that a SIT [short interval training] protocol involving three minutes of intense intermittent exercise per week, within a total time commitment of 30 minutes, is as effective as 150 minutes per week of moderate-intensity continuous training for increasing insulin sensitivity, cardiorespiratory fitness and skeletal muscle mitochondrial content in previously inactive men. This investigation represents the longest comparison of SIT and MICT [moderate intense continuous training, aka jogging/cycling] to date and demonstrates the efficacy of brief, intense exercise to improve indices of cardiometabolic health". [For comprehension I added the explanation in brackets].

So what are the clever people at PLOS trying to tell us? Simply that jogging and cycling carries an increased risk of cardiovascular disease and other causes of death. Yet sprinting, if we are able to motivate ourselves to really push hard, achieves the same positive results, is safer and takes up a lot less time.

> **PRIMAL CURE SPRINTING BENEFITS SUMMARY:**
> **Sprinting achieves the same positive results as spending hours slogging our guts out endlessly jogging, but is not a catalyst of cardiovascular diseases.**

For many reading this section, you will find it hard to believe that cardio isn't necessarily healthy. Don't get me wrong, it's not quite as dangerous as living a life glued to the sofa, but it's not that much better either. It certainly took me a lot of convincing to hang up my running shoes. Even worse, it seemed that virtually every single Christmas present I got in 2014 was cycling gear. That year I had become obsessed with the sport and became a real MAMIL (Middle-aged Man in Lycra). My entire family bought me some brilliant stuff that year and my wife spent a fortune on electronics so I could measure my performances. Yet two months later, after reading so much about the dangers of cardio, I decided cycling or jogging would no longer play any part of my fitness regime.

Let me be very clear, this is one of the biggest u-turns of opinion in the fitness world. I am personally full of admiration for people who realise that the advice they have been giving is flawed and are subsequently brave enough to explain how they got it wrong. Far too many people in life, especially medical and health professionals, never seem to admit to errors in judgement and spend their lives defending their flawed principles. So with great pleasure, let me introduce Dr Kenneth Cooper who in 1968 became known as the Father of Aerobics (later creating The Cooper Institute for Aerobic Research) and who went on to sell more than 30 million fitness and health books worldwide. Reporting on the success of *Aerobics*, the book that rocketed Dr Cooper to fame, Texas Monthly quoted, "The book was revolutionary, shaking up the sedentary sixties. Before its release only

100,000 eccentrics called themselves joggers, but by late 1968, the nation's trails were overflowing, and now more than 34 million people run regularly … and Aerobics brought instant fame to the unassuming Cooper – here and around the world. To this day, Brazilians call aerobic workouts 'Coopering'".

But here is the game changer. In a recent interview with a reporter, Dr Cooper he reveals, "At the time, I knew scientific evidence had established that regular exercise was essential to good health and an effective life. But I erroneously assumed that more was better – that the longer you ran, cycled or swam, the healthier you would be". He shares statistics about thousands of his clients – many of whom were rich and famous and even included President George Bush. He talked at length about how many Olympians had prematurely died of cancer and heart disease and goes on to speak about the effects of free radicals in our cells. Dr Cooper concludes, "Too much exercise can kill you". Today, The Cooper Institute for Aerobic Research instead recommends a new approach to aerobics for cardiovascular fitness that centres around strength training, muscle mass and increasing our suppleness/flexibility. Yes you read that correctly - the father of modern jogging, now believes it is dangerous and instead we should lift weights!

> **PRIMAL THOUGHT:**
> **You only get so many heartbeats, don't use them up too quickly!**

If you are a committed cyclist or runner, I am not suggesting you have to give up completely, but you need to either slow down to the most leisurely pace possible, ideally below 60–70% of your heart rate maximum (so not really cardio at all), or use your equipment to perform extremely short sprints of less than 30 seconds duration.

Still Not Ready To Hang Up Your Jogging Shoes?
Of course, people undertake endurance sports for a variety of reasons. It might be to lose weight, to build muscle and to look good in front

of the mirror, to live healthier and longer or to appeal to a prospective partner. It might relax you or you might be one of the very few individuals who actually enjoy putting yourself through hell. I am sure there are a few other reasons as well, but let's look at each one of these in isolation and see how participating in endurance sports such as jogging and cycling aids or harms us in reaching our desired outcome.

"I jog because of the aerobic and cardiovascular benefits."

Have you ever stopped to wonder what the two words 'aerobic' and 'cardiovascular' really mean? Aerobic simply means 'with oxygen'. In other words aerobic exercises are those where you take in more oxygen than normal. Is that good for us? Over the past 40 years that's what we have been led to believe, and it's probably the main reason we see more and more joggers on our streets. However, the reality is that forcing more oxygen into our body, beyond just normal breathing, is actually hazardous. It is the fuel needed to set lose free radicals within our cells, leading to the inflammation that itself is the root cause of many of today's modern diseases. So too much aerobic exercise is by and large a negative and not a positive.

But what about the cardiovascular system, doesn't that need to be exercised? It turns out that jogging and cycling for long periods of time at medium intensity does very little for our well-being above that of just walking and talking! The only way to really put excessive load on our cardiovascular system is to put excessive load on our muscles – in other words sprinting and lifting heavy things.

"I jog/cycle to lose weight."

We might lose water spending hours jogging and therefore jump on the scales and look like the run did us good, but we're not really burning fat. Remember, there is no such thing as losing weight. We can't just lose weight, we have to burn off our body fat.

It might be possible under a few specific circumstances to burn a little fat while jogging, but we are just as likely to burn off muscle and as muscle requires more energy than fat, when we eventually hang up our running shoes as our knees or joints give way, our metabolic rate decreases as we now have less muscle to consume energy. If we give away our muscles too cheaply to the jogging gods, in addition to those which we naturally lose as we age, then we are setting ourselves up to gain weight later in life. Every step taken forward while jogging or cycling might potentially make a minuscule gain right now, but will actually result in a bigger backwards step later in life.

Plus there is another huge problem. My good friend Glenn Lehrer, who is regarded by many as the number one cutter of gemstones on our planet and who is also an accomplished crystallographer and philosopher, taught me that everything in life is about seeking the most stable state of harmony and balance. In our body the pursuit of harmony is known as homeostasis. If, while we exercise, we are getting most of our energy from CARBS or other sugars, the moment the exercise is complete homeostasis kicks in and notifies our brain that we are starving and that we must be fed. It's not our fault that we reach for the sugar-loaded sports drink or CARB-loaded energy bar. Don't beat yourself up about it or try to take full responsibility – our desire for more energy is squarely the fault of homeostasis.

And there is another reason why so many of us struggle to lose those extra pounds through jogging. It is because we would have to run some serious miles to burn off lots of weight. Just look at the maths: One pound of fat = 3,500 calories, or for the younger generation one kilogram = 7,700 calories. Let's assume we're a fast and fit runner and we have the ability to burn 750 calories an hour. It therefore takes us more than four and a half hours to burn off one pound of fat. That's approximately the time it took me to complete each marathon! Plus, this assumes that we didn't intake any sports drinks, gels or bars on our way around and that we didn't stuff our face as a reward for our effort once we crossed the finish line. But we do! We all do – right?

In his book, *The IF Diet*, Robert Skinner refers to our caveman ancestors and says, "Your brain evolved a safety mechanism. If it sensed that you'd been moving for a long time, steadily depleting your blood sugar – and not replacing it – something was wrong. Either food was in short supply or you were a useless hunter. This is what your brain senses during traditional exercise".

In the book *Primal Blueprint*, Mark Sisson says, "It's ironic that many in their 40s and 50s start engaging in marathon or triathlon training with hopes of improving health and delaying the ageing process when, quite often, it has the exact opposite effect".

"I am a jogger because I want to build muscle."
Sorry, but other than maybe a minimal size increase in a couple of muscles in our legs, we are going to lose muscle elsewhere. You just don't see muscled marathon runners, they tend to be thin and wiry. Plus, when we lose muscle mass we decrease our metabolic rate and get fatter in the long run (if you'll pardon the pun).

"I am a jogger because I want to live healthier and longer."
That's exactly why I did it for all those years too. But as mentioned above, we then consume more bad calories after we finish the jog or cycle and therefore we don't lose weight. And as we pile on the miles over repeated sessions, we begin to lose muscle mass, which we certainly need in later years to preserve our precious joints and to maintain our metabolic rate. The amount of damage you can also do to your knees and hips is huge. I eventually had to have my anterior cruciate ligament replaced in my right knee and my rehabilitation took almost 12 months. I am not alone – it is believed that more than 60% of runners get injured one or more times every year. And even if we don't, the constant pounding on our joints might cause a problem to manifest years down the road.

Research has revealed that those who jog for more than 30 minutes continuously, with a heart rate of more than 85% of their maximum, are likely to damage their immune system and trigger inflammation for periods of up to three days post-exercise. Even at 75% of our maximum heart rate, joggers will experience raised cortisol levels (stress hormone) and reduced levels of both testosterone and growth hormones. Incidentally, both sprinting and weight training or any other form of high intensity intermittent training (HIIT) actually increases both testosterone and growth hormones. These hormones are critical components of helping us to live more healthily and happily, and become leaner and fitter.

"I am an endurance jogger/cyclist because I love it."
First of all, make sure it is the endurance aspect that you love, and not the fact that you are just exercising. Why not try the Primal MOMMS method for a few weeks and see how it makes you feel? If, after trying the Primal approach to fitness, you are convinced that you still prefer the relentless jog or long-distance two-wheel slog, then my advice is this. Make sure that you only participate in endurance activities when your body is accustomed to burning your own fat.

We have talked about ketosis, but put simply when there is no sugar in your bloodstream to use as energy, then the body starts to burn its own fat and this is known as ketosis. In this state, when you finish your mammoth workout, rather than homeostasis telling your brain it's hungry and forcing you to consume as much energy as you have just exerted, it will simply satisfy your hunger by burning up your own fat.

THE CONCLUSION ON JOGGING

I don't want you to think that I am advising you to either hang up your running shoes, or drop off your bike at the local tip, and return to a life on the sofa. Nothing could be further from the truth! If you love jogging or cycling, then I recommend that you purchase a heart rate monitor and still go outdoors and jog or cycle, but so slowly that your heart rate is only mildly elevated between 55 to 70% of your maximum heart rate. Then, just two or three times throughout your journey, try to sprint flat-out for around 10 to 20 seconds. This way, your workout will better reflect the type of exertion the heart has been designed to support and will not place it under excessive stress.

Mixing up slow jogging, cycling and walking with the occasional sprint is going to feel really weird at first to all who, like me, have spent years pushing on through the pain barrier. It is so annoying to think that all the times where I berated and even hated myself for taking any respite during my runs, the breaks were actually beneficial to my long-term health. With the Primal way of slow cycling or jogging, leaving all the huffing and puffing to the wolf, the entire outing becomes more enjoyable, more sociable and much better for our long-term health.

Dr Dan Maggs

"I want to say one thing in defence of jogging. I'm a big fan of Parkrun, which are free, 5km timed runs that take place all around the world every Saturday morning. It is a fantastic thing to do with friends - and when exercise is also a social activity you're more likely to stick at it! You can walk it if you want, too! Plus at 5k, you're not in a state of cardiovascular exercise for long."

It's Just One Per Cent

With the exception of walking and moving more often, if we don't participate in un-Primal endurance sports, we can become extremely strong and fit by just spending around 1% of our life exercising. All our sprinting and gym sessions needn't consume more than 1% of our week. Or if we find it hard to picture this, it accumulates to one full day of exercise in the spring, summer, autumn and winter!

Yes – to both look and feel fit, we only cumulatively need to exercise for four days each year!

Chapter 4 Highlights

- Our hunter-gatherer ancestors didn't jump in a car and pop to the local store and wander around filling their basket with man-made processed foods, they walked and climbed in search of plants and then sprinted after animals.
- Primal Cure MOMMS approach to exercise: Max Out – Move More – Sprint.
- MOMMS could also be called 'The 6S Movement', Slow Steady Strolls, Short Strains and Sprints.
- Research suggests that just 25 minutes of brisk walking a day is associated with adding up to 7 years to your life and halving the risk of dying from a heart attack.
- Once we have our food figured out, are moving more and exercising, have sorted out our lifestyle, then and only then do we need to start sprinting.
- Don't participate in long cardio exercises as they can play havoc with our joints, damage our heart and wreck our metabolism.

05.
Primal
Lifestyle

Living Primally isn't all about diet and exercise – it's a lifestyle change. In this chapter we find out how simple things like the amount of sleep we get, and the stress we have to deal with, can be optimised to help us beat the sick statistics.

Now we are eating the right things, intermittently fasting and participating in the right type of exercise. Excellent! We're almost there. Let's also look at other areas where our Primal ancestors did things a little differently, and at some changes we might want to make to ensure we live as super healthily as possible.

SUNBATHING - SENSIBLE OR STUPID?

Have you ever wondered why the further we live from the equator the paler our skins become? One of the most important vitamins to maintain good health is vitamin D, and what is the best source of vitamin D? The sun. Through evolution, as tribes migrated further and further from the equator, their skin became paler, so they could absorb as much Vitamin D as possible from the diminishing sunrays, I find nature astoundingly resilient and, as a back-up plan to the fading of skin tones, the more north and south humans began to travel - receiving less and less benefit from the sun - it also provided an intense source of vitamin D in cold-water oily fish.

There is a huge trick we can play on our body by being outdoors more often. Once out in the sun, our Primally-designed body says, "Hey, spring must be around the corner, the days will be longer and I will catch or gather more food". As a result our metabolism gets a boost and we feel full of energy. In contrast, when we stay indoors and avoid the sun, hibernating on our sofas, the body predicts that winter must be coming – food will be become scarce - and therefore the body releases hormones that slow everything down. We feel lethargic, and as our metabolism becomes sluggish, we have neither the energy nor inclination to do anything remotely energetic. Isn't it remarkable that something as simple as being indoors or outdoors can have either a positive or negative spiralling effect on our well-being and energy levels?

Sadly, my mother refuses to come on many summer holidays with my wife, our children and me because she has been told by her doctors not to go out in the sun. She has missed out on so much over recent years, and even though many experts are now advising completely the opposite, it is proving difficult to get her to listen to recent research. Even when we explain that there is so much evidence that we are more likely to get cancer by avoiding the sun than going out in it, my mother just won't have it!

Of course, while going lobster red is dangerous for all of us, getting an all-over light suntan is extremely beneficial. Not only does it make us feel great, it increases our body's ability to create vitamin D, which is one of the most essential vitamins of all. Did caveman stay in his cave all day? Of course not, he was out and about trying to catch dinner. Did he smear factor 50 all over his body? Again, the point is our DNA expects us to be in the sun. Just as ancient hunter-gatherers would have done, we should shelter in the shade when it gets too hot, or after we have had enough exposure for our natural skin tone, but for those who avoid the sun altogether it's a huge health risk.

On 6th March 2017, *The Daily Telegraph* newspaper reported, "Experts have overturned decades of advice by urging people to go out in the midday sun without sunblock – because the dangers of missing out on vitamin D can outweigh the risk of cancer". It goes on to say, "The definitive statement by seven leading health groups and charities, including Cancer Research UK, the National Osteoporosis Society and Multiple Sclerosis Society, is designed to clarify conflicting messages. It concluded that surrendering your body to the sun for 10 minutes should take place at midday during the summer months because that is when the sun is strong enough to trigger the body into making vitamin D". The research was also supported by the British Association of Dermatologists, Diabetes UK, the National Heart Forum and the Primary Care Dermatology Society – that's a pretty comprehensive bunch of leading authorities.

The 10-minute exposure recommendation seems to be advice that is now appearing in lots of articles. The key seems to be short stints, as regular as we can. It also appears that the more of our body we can expose to the sun, the more our body will synthesise vitamin D. While we should avoid getting burnt and looking like a red-hot chilli pepper, as that's obviously not going to be good for our health, we should go out in the sun in short bursts as often as we can as it will aid the creation of a reserve of vitamin D.

How Much Vitamin D Do I Need?

The US government recommends that children should receive 200IUs a day, those of us aged between 50 and 70, 400IUs and once we are more than 70 years old, 600IUs. But what is an IU? It stands for International Unit and it is used to measure the weight of how much of a vitamin we should consume daily, so 1000IU = 1g. While the US government issue the above recommendations for vitamin D, many other specialists and nutritionists suggest we all benefit from substantially more. From all of the research I have read, it appears adults should aim to consume at least 1000IUs per day. But how long does it take us to generate 1g of vitamin D by being in the sun? It is believed that if we stay out for just a few minutes each day, revealing most of our body to the light, then we will easily set the body up to create 1000IUs. If we want to build up a reserve of vitamin D, then we should stay outside a little longer. However, to avoid burning, we shouldn't sit in the sun for more than 25–50% of the time that it would normally take us to turn a pinkish colour.

In 2002, scientists in Boston came to the conclusion that, "Small amounts of sunshine can greatly reduce the risk of breast, colon and prostate cancers". More recently, research released in March 2016 - after studying 29,518 women in Sweden over a 20-year period - suggested that those who avoided the sun were likely to die prematurely, with frighteningly similar statistics to those who smoked! They went on to say that, "Compared to the highest sun exposure group, life expectancy of avoiders of sun exposure was reduced by 0.6–2.1 years". Sunlight hitting the skin helps the body produce vitamin D, which in turn plays an important role in calcium metabolism, which in turn leads to healthier bones. The good news for those of us who live in the sun-deprived UK is that, as Vitamin

D is fat soluble, it can be stored in the body for fairly long periods of time. Unfortunately, as we get older our body becomes less efficient at converting sun exposure into vitamin D. My poor mother has been made so scared of going out in the sun by her doctor, that I just can't convince her that his thinking is outdated. At the precise period in her life when she needs to be going out in the sun for longer periods, and uncovering more of her body to the healing benefits of the sun, on the odd occasion that she does venture outdoors on a sunny day, she dresses more like a teenager wearing a onesie and a hoodie! Getting outdoors in the sun is not just about providing a much-needed boost to our vitamin D reserves. Exposure to sunlight tends to lift our mood and reduce stress. It's also good for reducing both blood pressure and acne!

On the 27th June 2016, *The Mirror* newspaper ran an article with the headline, 'Health benefits of sunbathing outweigh skin cancer risks'. The article goes on to say, "Sunbathing also reduces blood pressure, cuts the risk of heart attacks and is more likely to prolong life than shorten it. Sun worshippers worried by gloomy warnings [that] they risk getting skin cancer can start looking on the bright side. Sunbathing also reduces blood pressure, cuts the risk of heart attacks and is more likely to prolong life than shorten it, ground-breaking research has found". Dermatologist Dr Richard Weller, whose team conducted the study said, "We suspect that the benefits to heart health of sunlight will outweigh the risk of skin cancer". The same article goes further by stating, "The big discovery is that when skin is exposed to sunlight, a compound called nitric oxide is released in blood vessels that helps lower blood pressure". Living in the UK, with our infrequent bouts of sunshine, what we need to know is how long after we return from our holidays abroad can our body store vitamin D? According to a 2010 article published by Pediatric Nephrology, vitamin D can be stored in the fat tissue for approximately two months. It's important to note the same article reveals that, once we have been in the sun, we shouldn't go and immediately have a soapy shower, as it apparently can take half an hour or so for the skin to complete the cycle of synthesising vitamin D.

What about sunbeds – are they a valid way to obtain a suntan? It appears that as long as they effectively balance UVA and UVB rays in a similar proportion to the sun, and that they are fitted with modern low-pressure lamps, then they are no different to sitting out in the sun and similar precautions, such as how long we should be exposed, therefore apply. If it's an older machine that only produces UVA rays, then other than getting a tan there is little medical benefit. This is because we need UVB rays to stimulate vitamin D production. So should we use a sunbed? It's obviously more Primal to harness the sun's magic healing powers – not only is it free, it doesn't use expensive electricity, so therefore it's kinder to the planet. But if we don't have a chance to get out in the sun, then by all means use a sunbed, however remain respectful of its powers and don't go getting burnt, as it still holds true that overexposure can lead to skin cancer. You may also have heard some people say that they like to build a base tan on a sunbed before going on their annual holiday. There is some logic in this, as it is possible to build-up melanin levels in our skin that can provide a little bit of natural protection against burning. But please do it in moderation and in short bursts.

If you want to learn more about the benefits of being in the sun, let me recommend you read Dr Michael Holick's book, *The UV Advantage*, in which he states, "Lack of sunlight is associated with a host of conditions from colon, breast, prostate and ovarian cancer to heart disease, high blood pressure, type 1 diabetes, multiple sclerosis and depression". Dr Holick is an endocrinologist, and he has some very sensible advice on sun cream too. He believes that the higher the SPF, the less vitamin D gets through, and once we get to SPF 15 or above, the benefit of the sun is reduced by 99.9%. Dr Holick says that when he goes out in the sun, he does 10 minutes without sun cream and then puts it on to prevent overdoing it. Later in his book, he goes on to say that he believes the correct exposure to sunlight has an equal benefit on the health of our heart to that of exercise! Then, in a section under the heading 'In the Beginning', Dr Holick talks of how ancient man understood the benefit of sunlight. From studying paintings in caves, he suggests that we can assume that even Primal man understood the benefits of sun therapy.

Here's one final thought from Dr Holick, which fits with my belief that too many companies care more about their profit than they do people or the planet: "How did we reach a point in our history when sun became something to be feared instead of worshipped? Shunned instead of desired? The simple answer lies in the fact that there are many billions of dollars to be made in emphasising the only major medical downside of sun exposure (non-melanoma skin cancer) and not much money to be made in promoting the sun's many benefits".

American Dr William Grant believes, "An increase of sun exposure in the USA would result in 185,000 less cases of internal cancer". Compare that to the 1,200 people who sadly die of skin cancer, and I am sure you will draw the same conclusion as I have that sensible sunbathing is extremely beneficial for our health. However, let me repeat the sunburn warning. While we are after a light suntan, we don't want to burn. Remember, it takes approximately three or four hours after being in the sun for our sunburn to reveal itself. This is caused by extra blood flow to the burnt areas, and doesn't normally reach its peak for around 18 hours after overexposure. So please, whatever you do, don't sit in the sun until you burn, otherwise it is going to be extremely detrimental to your health. Put simply, suntans are good for health on so many levels, and can prevent multiple cancers, yet sunburn caused by overexposure can cause skin cancer.

Let me explain the approach I take for my family and myself. We try on most school holidays to take the kids somewhere warm, where we can top up their vitamin D levels. We ensure each day that they go outside in the morning and play or swim without sunscreen. Jack, Tom, and even our little two-year-old Louie, go a lovely light-brown shade, and for them 30 minutes exposure is absolutely fine without any protection. I believe the girls would start going red after about 40 minutes, so I get them to go under the shade after about 20. (These are only approximations as it depends how close to the equator we have ventured.) Once they have hit about 50% of the exposure that would normally make them turn slightly red, they go in the shade and chill out for about half an hour, allowing their bodies sufficient time to maximise the gift they have received from nature. Then we slap on the sunscreen, allow it to soak in for 10 minutes or so, and let them go back out and play. What's more, we always make sure the lotions are as organic as possible, and when the kids or my wife and I are at a level where a SPF factor 8 is sufficient, we no longer use sun lotion and instead use coconut oil. Believe it or not, the very same oil that we recommend we cook our food in is Mother Nature's SPF level 8!

Depending on what you have been taught, you might feel that letting our two-year-old son out in the sun without any protection is irresponsible. But it really isn't. Sadly, we see too many misinformed parents who, with only the child's best interest at heart, slap on sun protection before the kid has had any chance to take in sufficient sunrays to convert to vitamin D. As long as we soak up plenty of sunshine in the summer, it will almost see us through the early part of the winter - especially if we can top it up by eating plenty of oily fish. If we feel we are running low on vitamin D, we can always ask our doctor to test our blood specifically for vitamin D levels - if he or she feels we are running low, then there are plenty of vitamin D supplements on the market. It's also likely that, if we are running low, our kids are too and therefore the whole family could do with eating more oily fish or taking vitamin D supplements. Better still of course, jet off abroad with one of the low-cost airlines and boost your vitamin D levels through nature's natural source, sunshine.

If you still are not convinced about spending more time in the sun, then be sure to eat plenty of eggs, oily fish and consider taking a quality vitamin D supplement. Or get hold of Jeff T. Bowles book *Vitamin D3 Miracle*. If I haven't convinced you I am sure Jeff will. One of my favourite quotes from his brilliantly written self-published work is, "Since the early 1980s, when doctors started warning us about too much sun, obesity rates in adult humans and many other diseases (including asthma and autism) have skyrocketed!"

> **VITAMIN D TIP:**
> When it is sunny, go outside without sunscreen for up to 50%
> of the time that it would normally take you to turn slightly red.
> Then go under the shade, chill for half an hour and then slap
> on a natural mineral sunscreen.

The latest data from the Public Health England National Diet and
Nutrition Survey (2008 to 2012), shows that 23% of adults aged 19 to
64 years, 21% of adults aged 65 years and above and 22% of children
aged 11 to 18 years have low levels of vitamin D in their blood. Public
Health England advises that, "in spring and summer, the majority of
the population get enough vitamin D through sunlight on the skin
and a healthy, balanced diet. During autumn and winter, everyone will
need to rely on dietary sources of vitamin D. Since it is difficult for
people to meet the 10 microgram recommendation from consuming
foods naturally containing or fortified with vitamin D, people should
consider taking a daily supplement containing 10 micrograms of
vitamin D in autumn and winter". What I find very encouraging about
this article, is that it is one of the first times I have seen the British
government recommend the use of supplements. Let's hope this is a
change of tide to one of prevention rather than cure.

A GOOD NIGHT'S SLEEP

For someone who has run their own businesses for more than 25
years - burning the candle at both ends trying to setup and launch
numerous ventures - researching how much sleep we require has had
a profound effect on how I live my life. Those who know me well will
be astounded by what they read here.

There will always be periods in everyone's lives where - due to external
factors such as work, having young children or even party season -
getting a good night's sleep becomes a low priority. While the odd
day or two of not getting enough sleep shouldn't cause any long-term
health problems, sleep deprivation over a sustained period can be very

harmful. I personally found the views I am about to share with you very hard to swallow. For the past quarter of a century I have preached that the early bird catches the worm; that while you rest you rust; that I will sleep enough when I'm dead - and a number of other pithy one-liners that in the main suggest that life is just too short to sleep. What I have now discovered by reading several books and dozens of research papers is something very different indeed, and that leads us nicely to the Primal Cure sleep principle:

> **The theory that "life's too short to sleep" is incorrect, it should be restated as, "life is cut short without sleep".**

When I sailed across the Atlantic in my small boat in 2009, none of my family had sailed an ocean before, so I went six whole days and nights without more than the odd minute or two of sleep. I managed to survive, but if the sleep deprivation had gone on much longer it apparently would have killed me! Scientific studies on rats show that they can only last three weeks without sleep; and for those poor people who suffer from insomnia to the point where they cannot sleep at all, the body eventually shuts down completely after a few months.

It is really important that we don't confuse rest with sleep, as they are two very different things. While resting for a few hours on the sofa watching a movie might help us de-stress and unwind, it does not allow our body to go into repair mode. It does not allow the brain to process its learnings from the day or let our various hormones get themselves organised.

Dr Shan Hussain

"One of the most common complaints I hear from patients is, "I'm tired all the time." On occasion, there may be medical causes for this, but the vast majority of the time the solution is very simple: sleep more, and then review your energy intake and expenditure."

Our Circadian Clock

In September 2017, American scientists Jeffrey C Hall, Michael Rosbash and Michael W Young won a Nobel Prize (physiology or medicine) for their work on the internal clock of living organisms. Today, our internal biological timepiece is referred to as the circadian clock. We have already mentioned the stress hormone cortisol, and how it can wreak havoc in our body if it not controlled properly. It turns out that, if we don't get enough sleep at the right time of night, then as well as keeping ourselves awake we also rouse our cortisol monster. To explain why this happens we need to learn a little about our circadian clock.

Way before the British invented the grandfather clock and the Swiss perfected the wristwatch, Mother Nature beat them to it by creating the body's circadian (pronounced 'sir-kay-dian') clock. It doesn't need winding up or batteries, but keeps time primarily by the rising and setting of the sun, which activates a hormone in our body called melatonin.

Nature didn't create the circadian cycle (often referred to as the biological rhythm) exclusively for us humans, but for every living thing on the planet – from animals to fish, plants to microbes. Understanding the cycle is extremely important to our health, so much so that in the 1980s a whole new field of science was created to study it – chronobiology.

For those of us who live a distance from the equator, our body has to adapt to huge swings in the hours of sunlight that we receive throughout the different seasons. In the UK, during the darkest winter days, we get as little as eight hours of sunlight, but in the middle of the summer we receive a whopping 16. With our circadian clock being regulated by sunlight, it's a good thing that the change happens subtly, with sunrise and sunset changing by approximately just one minute each day.

Remember that what keeps our biological clock in sync is sunlight. The chart on the following page is based on the sun rising at 6.00am and then setting at 6.00pm, as it does mid-spring and autumn in the UK - and pretty much all year round near the equator. At other times of the year, as the hours of sunlight move backwards or forwards by only a minute each day, our circadian clock is able to fairly reliably reset itself. Problems arise when we travel abroad or work night shifts. Ironically, I am writing this section on a flight to India where the time difference is currently 4.5 hours ahead of the UK. Our body really struggles to adjust to instant big time changes and it can cause a variety of health problems.

However, it is possible to limit the damage by tricking our biological clock. This is what I did the past two days before boarding the plane. I got up earlier than I normally would and immediately went out into my garden with a cup of coffee. Both bright sunlight and caffeine stimulate the production of cortisol, and I effectively forced it to kick-start the cycle a little earlier. I also went to bed at 9.30pm and made sure it was completely dark in my bedroom. By being in bed an hour earlier than normal, I fooled my body clock into thinking it was later than it really was. As soon as I got on the plane at 8.00pm, I turned the brightness right down on my laptop screen and got ready to put on my earmuffs and eyeshades. I want my body's clock to think it's a lot later than it really is. Then for the next few days in India I have already set my meetings up so that they don't start too early, but go on until later than I would at home. I will stay up as late as I possibly can each evening, with every light in my hotel room turned up full until an hour before I want to sleep. This helps my body clock stay in tune with the time in the UK, where it is still daylight. Then in the morning I will sleep in later than I would back in the UK, tricking my body's clock to think it's earlier than it really is.

> **PRIMAL SLEEP:**
> When we sleep, our brain begins its magic show, collating, storing and making sense of what we learnt during the day.

Considering I am on an aeroplane as I write this, I just had a fairly decent night's sleep. Back home I am sure all of my kids are all still fast asleep, but until a few months ago this might not have been the case. Both of my two youngest daughters, Jessica and Lili - used to always sleep with their bedroom lights on. I tried everything to get them to sleep in the dark. I taught them about our biological clock and how, if they kept their lights on, or left their iPads and iPhones blinking all night how they wouldn't produce enough melanin - and without it they wouldn't get smarter at school. But it all went in one ear and out the other. Then I remembered a two-word phrase that everyone has heard. I reminded them that, as well as feeling healthy and improving their intelligence, if they turned off their lights they would become even more beautiful than they already were. I simply told them that it's called 'beauty sleep' for a very good reason, but it only becomes real beauty sleep when the room is totally dark. Any light in the room at all and the magic just doesn't happen!

Let's look at our 24-hour clock, starting at midnight, give or take 30 minutes:

- **00:00** To make sure we feel tired, melatonin production reaches its peak around midnight. The thyroid gets to work and tells the mitochondria in our cells to burn energy to keep our inactive body warm. This is how we lose weight when we sleep properly.
- **01:00** Melatonin slows down our brain activity so that we can process what we have learnt in the day and form long-term memories.
- **02:00** Our deepest sleep, where the body starts to enter repair mode.
- **04:00** We are at our most relaxed at this time, and both our neurological and immune systems are hard at work.
- **05:00** It takes five or six hours of sleep for our body to reach its lowest temperature, this is why it's nonsense to get less than seven hours sleep.
- **06:00** We get a surge of cortisol and blood pressure rises in an attempt to wake us, and the brain mobilises our muscles.

- **07:00** The body stops producing our sleep hormone melatonin and switches on our hunger hormone ghrelin.
- **08:00** Our bowels become active and if we ate the day before they stir action downstairs.
- **09:00** The height of testosterone secretion for the day.
- **13:00** The most alert we will be all day.
- **14:00** Height of co-ordination (so we could track animals after the midday sun).
- **15:00** Fastest reaction times (so that we could catch said animals).
- **17:00** Maximum muscle strength and cardiovascular efficiency (in case we didn't catch an animal the first time).
- **18:00** Highest blood pressure of the day. As long as we are on a low carb diet, in order to stop us eating too much, leptin will continue to rise until it's time for sleep. If for some reason it doesn't, then for goodness' sake don't eat CARBS, but try some coconut or avocado instead.
- **19:00** Peak of body temperature.
- **21:00** The body starts to produce melatonin to tell us we are tired and ready for sleep.
- **23:00** So that we are not going to the toilet all night, our gastrointestinal works start to go to sleep.

The saying 'beauty sleep' is based on the fact that, while we sleep, our skin regenerates itself up to eight times faster than when we are awake. We all want to look more beautiful, but let's look at what happens on a less superficial level.

While We Are Asleep

- The body goes into repair mode and increases our growth hormones
- The brain assembles the jigsaw puzzle of knowledge that we learnt during the day
- The brain takes the daily knowledge and stores it neatly into our mental filing cabinets, so that we can more easily retrieve and recall it in the future

- The liver doesn't have to deal with incoming food (it's difficult to eat when we are asleep) so gets to work detoxifying our body
- The body increases the production of testosterone

Without Sufficient Sleep

- Knowledge and memories from the day's activities become scrambled
- The body struggles to regulate our body temperature, and becomes particularly inefficient at dealing with extreme cold or heat
- The body creates an excess of cortisol, and we become easily stressed. Have you noticed how short-tempered we become after a poor night's sleep? It's not our fault that we become irritable and ratty, it's an excess of the hormone cortisol
- Our immune system begins to fail
- Insulin struggles to regulate blood sugar levels, and a lack of sleep over time can lead to type 2 diabetes
- Leptin and ghrelin hormones don't function properly, leading to overeating
- Our body can lose control of its fight with inflammation

For 26 years, I limited how much sleep I got because I thought it made me a better person, a smarter businessman, and because I believed it gave me more time to achieve things. Yet it turns out that, while I had a feeling of self-righteousness by getting out of bed at the crack of dawn, I was actually becoming a weakling by stopping my muscles from growing properly. I was becoming dumber by not allowing my brain to properly organise what it was learning, and I was killing my sex drive by not producing sufficient testosterone. Putting on my running shoes at 5.00am, feeling like the smarter martyr who was getting fitter than the rest of the population who were still in bed sleeping their life away, it was actually counterproductive - and rather than improving my overall health was actually impeding it. Many chronobiologists now believe that certain diseases are caused by continual disruption to rhythm of our circadian system.

How Much Sleep Do We Need?

There is no simple answer to this question as we are all different. The more active we are, the more sleep we potentially need. I also believe that it can vary a little from day to day. I personally sleep around seven to eight hours during weekdays, but get as much as 10 hours a night at the weekend. So what do experts recommend? The National Sleep Foundation of America recently assembled 18 leading scientists and researchers and gave them the task of bringing their official recommendations up to date. As of June 2017, this is their suggestion:

Age	Hours Needed	May Be Appropriate
Newborn - 3 months	14 to 17	11 to 19
4 months - 11 months	12 to 15	10 to 18
1 - 2 years	11 to 14	9 to 16
3 - 5 years old	10 to 13	8 to 14
6 - 13 years old	9 to 11	7 to 12
14 -17 years old	8 to 10	7 to 11
18 - 25 years old	7 to 9	6 to 11
26 - 64 years old	7 to 9	6 to 10
65 years +	7 to 8	5 to 9

While we also have similar guidelines in the UK, the US study is so well researched that I personally prefer their findings.

It might be true that politicians such as Margaret Thatcher got by on four hours sleep each night, just as Donald Trump also claims to only need four to five hours, but is that actually good for our health? The simple answer is no! Researchers at the University of California in San Francisco discovered that 3% of people have a gene that enables them to perform well on just six hours sleep per night. But for the other 97% of us, in order to live a healthy, happy and long life we need to follow the above recommendations.

Dr Dan Maggs

"You need as much sleep as you need! Don't try and cheat it else it will catch up with you eventually... somehow."

Chilling Out & Cat Naps

There is definitely a place for taking time to relax in the Primal Cure approach, but that does not mean we are endorsing the couch potato way of life. Without doubt we are living in the laziest, fattest and most sedentary era ever. Think about the progression. We used to hunt for food, then we had to walk to stores to carry home food, then we could travel to restaurants – and even this burnt some calories. But today we can simply go online and order any takeaway we desire.

In the UK there is even a food portal called Just Eat which can now deliver us almost any meal we desire. We then sit down, turn on our TV (or more commonly these days our computer or phone or tablet) and scoff down our food without even registering we're doing so. And remember 'scoffin' is only one letter away from 'coffin'!

But it would be naive to think that our Primal ancestors were on the go from sunrise to sunset. What we believe is that we should get around eight to nine hours of quality sleep each night. If we aren't able to do that during the dark hours, maybe because of work commitments or childcare, then we should try to make up our missing hours of sleep with a Spanish-like siesta in the afternoons, or if we are unable to doze off at that time of day then we should at least try and take our foot off the gas for a while.

Interestingly, on the isle of Ikaria, where there is a high percentage of centenarians, afternoon naps are commonplace. Plus, the Harvard School of Public Health reported that just napping for 30 minutes, at least 3 times a week, lowered coronary mortality. Now I normally discard this type of research, as it is not derived from a controlled randomised, interventional study, but in this case the conclusion feels logical and it's certainly backed up by the longevity of people in regions where naps and siestas are regarded normal.

AVOID STRESS & BE HAPPY

Stress-related diseases are one of the biggest killers in the Western world. From cancer to heart attacks, so many illnesses and early deaths can be attributed to it. While a little bit of stress, such as that from exercise, is good for us, prolonged exposure – whether it be conscious or subconscious – is really bad for our health. One of the best pieces of advice I have ever been given is to try everything possible to never waste time worrying about events that have happened, or those that we can't change. Instead, only invest time deliberating about things that we can influence.

Our family have always made 'creating happiness' a central belief in the companies that we have built. Our holding company is even called the Bennett Health & Happiness Group, and BHH Publishing - an abbreviation for Bennett Health & Happiness Publishing Ltd -brings this book to you. With this in mind, I have spent years trying to uncover what makes people truly happy, and have come up with five recurring traits of happy people:

1. They don't worry much and therefore aren't stressed.
2. They have a close circle of friends or family and therefore a sense of belonging.
3. They challenge themselves frequently.
4. They have a purpose in life.
5. They have a high level of tolerance.

PRIMAL CURE HEALTH PRINCIPLE: :
Try to be happier by reducing stress in your life, and just take everything and everyone less seriously. If you can't change something, don't waste precious time thinking about it.

Dr Shan Hussain

"As a doctor, I regard stress as any physical, mental or emotional factor that causes strain or tension on the body or mind. Mental or emotional stress often results from adverse situations, such as family conflicts, worries about work, or health issues, but it's important to remember that stress is highly individual. What's highly stressful for one person may be regarded as normal for another. Whenever a patient tells me they feel ill or mentally exhausted or depressed from stress, I take it seriously, even if the stress they describe doesn't seem that stressful. After all, I believe physical, mental, or social stress may well be the fundamental basis of most, if not all, disease."

Minimise Worry

Let's start with what Regina Brett, the author of *45 Lessons Life Taught Me*, says: "Don't take yourself too seriously. No one else does". Relax a little, and try not to take everything to heart. If you can't change something or it has already happened, just whistle or hum to yourself Bobby McFerrin's 1988 song 'Don't Worry, Be Happy'. Adopt the more laid-back approach of the African tribes in Kenya and Tanzania, who in real life really do use the phrase from The Lion King, 'Hakuna matata' – the Swahili saying for 'no worries'.

If you hate your boss because he or she is unreasonable, have a chat with them to try to help them see the error of their ways - and if nothing changes try to get them fired! I know this might sound like strange advice from someone who employs hundreds of managers, but bad managers are bad for both business and health. While work should be both hard and challenging, it should also be enjoyable and rewarding. I teach our managers that they have a duty to create a working environment where team members don't have to leave 'pleasure to be in their leisure'. Work must make you happy. If you hate your job, then leave and find something else that you enjoy. Life is too short to be stuck in a job you don't like. And never stay in a job just because the pay is good. Cash only buys possessions, not happiness.

Family, Friends, Colleagues & Dogs

In the first edition of Primal Cure I told a story about Ikaria. Here is a snippet that highlights the importance of social interaction. On a small mountainous Greek island, just a stone's throw from the Turkish coast, lives a small community of people who, when its comes to living healthily into old age, are breaking all sorts of records. Most evenings you find elders wandering into their neighbours' homes and sharing freshly prepared meals and several glasses of locally-produced wine. Here they don't send parents into care homes, they remain together in strong family units. Their sense of community seems all but lost on the rest of the Westernised world. Interestingly, The World Health Organisation defines health as "a state of complete physical, mental and social well-being and not merely the absence of disease or infirmity".

There is a brilliant book written by Dan Buettner called *The Blue Zones*. Dan travels the world to regions with the highest concentration of centenarians (those that have lived to over 100 years), to discover the truth about living longer. One of the key similarities across all regions was a strong family bond, where people of old age still put their loved ones first.

Dr Shan Hussain

"High-quality social interaction on a regular basis with your immediate peers is helpful for reducing and managing stress. In other words, make an effort to get together with your friends and family when you can. If your social circle is small, have you thought about getting a dog? A recent study in Sweden showed that dog owners were 23 percent less likely to die of cardiovascular disease, and they also experienced a 20 percent lower risk of mortality from all causes. The authors were unable to explain this link, but it was felt the additional physical activity and emotional connection between dogs and owners played the most critical roles."

Challenges

A challenge is something that stretches us physically or mentally. It might not give us pleasure at the time – it might be delayed until the activity has passed, such as the feeling of relaxation and achievement after a hard gym session or learning to play an instrument or speak a foreign language. Not only do these activities prevent stress, they also keep the brain functioning well.

Have Fun

We have a saying in our business: we never take ourselves too seriously, just our customers and our products. I insist that all managers who work with me make having fun part of the culture within their team. After all, life's just too short not to enjoy yourself.

While having fun at work is important and helps alleviate stress, it's even more crucial that life outside of the office is as enjoyable and fun as possible. Going to the cinema, laughing with friends, reading a book, watching a sunset with a loved one, playing catch with your dog, are all associated with numerous health benefits. How so? I hear you ask? Well having fun helps to reduce the levels of the stress hormone 'cortisol', while at the same time increasing levels of serotonin (kind of a happiness neurotransmitter). It boosts energy, helps us get a better night sleep and may even help improve memory!

Dr Shan Hussain

"A recent Norwegian study showed that women with a good sense of humour had 48 percent lower mortality rates, but the authors were unable to find a similar link for men. However, they did notice that men with a good sense of humour were less likely to die from infectious disease, and concluded that "a sense of humour is a health-protecting cognitive coping resource"."

Purpose

In addition to setting ourselves challenges, to be truly happy it's important to believe that our actions are making a contribution to something that we consider to be worthwhile.

It's been proven in several pieces of research that people who win huge amounts on the lottery usually become unhappy people. Why is this? Whilst everyone will have different opinions on what makes us happy, I am convinced that truly happy people are those who have few worries, people who enjoy sharing experiences with friends and family, but most importantly have a sense of purpose in their life. Lottery winners tend to have lots of worries - they worry about losing what they have quickly gained. They often become isolated from friends and have fewer challenges and less purpose in their lives! My advice is not to do the lottery, if you were to win it could ruin your life and whilst you are sitting there waiting to win, you are not engaged in actions that will fulfil your purpose and enhance your self-worth.

Tolerance

In both our personal and work lives, the strongest relationships are the ones that give and take. There has to be an element of tolerance in life, because without it we are likely to become very stressed indeed. Leading on from tolerance is the ability to rationalise. I recently walked passed two elderly ladies sitting on a bench, admiring the views across the river in Dartmouth, and heard one say to the other, "how do you always look so happy, I never see you depressed", the lady smiled at her friend and said, "I am always able to rationalise things". From this I took it that she had a "let it be" attitude, or as the French call say laissez faire.

Virginia Satir who was an American author and therapist, known especially for her approach to family therapy, famously said, "Life is not what it's supposed to be. It's what it is. The way you cope with it is what makes the difference".

Switch Off The TV & Read A Book

I am going to hand you over to Dr Shan for this topic.

Dr Shan Hussain

"Common sense tells us that too much TV is bad for our health. But is this really true, and how much is too much? Aside from working and sleeping, watching TV is the most commonly reported daily activity in many developed countries. A large 40 year meta-analysis in 2011 confirmed that prolonged TV viewing is associated with increased risk of type 2 diabetes, cardiovascular disease and all-cause mortality. The association was linear and strongest among people watching TV for over three hours per day.

But reading books, well that's a whole different matter. According to a 12-year study performed at Yale University and published in Social Science And Medicine, book readers experienced a 20 percent reduction in mortality compared to non-book readers. Reading for only 30 minutes each day helped people live an average of 23 months longer compared with non-book readers, regardless of gender, wealth, education or health."

Eating Rubbish Leaves Us Stressed

Primal though: Good food equals great mood!

You will read throughout this book various ways to avoid stress and other brain-related disorders by eating the right food. The main culprits of course, are CARBS and other sugars, which become deadly poisons that stress out the body when over-consumed. For now, let's keep it as simple as possible - out of all the courses we eat, which are the most laden with sugar and most damaging to our health? Desserts of course! And if we write desserts backwards what does it spell? STRESSED. Enough said!

FLAT FEET - STRAIGHT BACK

Primal man didn't wear high heels or platform shoes. When he needed an elevation to view his prey he climbed a tree. Constantly wearing high heels can cause all sorts of problems for our body. It's kind of obvious really, that the more time we can spend without shoes on, the better it must be for our posture and our body. And even for us gents, constantly wearing a half-inch heel shoe is not natural for the body either. That said, this is one of the smaller principles, and if wearing heels makes you feel more confident and less stressed, then continue to do so. However, whenever we find ourselves alone we should try to go barefoot as often as possible.

There is also another reason for ditching the shoes and socks, and that is because it can reduce the chances of getting fungus under our toenails. My two big toes were a real mess, and have been for many years. However, taking a leaf out of my own book, I have made a real effort to remain barefooted for as long as possible in the past two years and I frequently wear open-toe sandals in my office. The results have been fantastic. I think the combination of exposing my toes to fresh air - and also getting my vitamin D levels boosted - have both contributed to my nails returning to full health. I guess it shouldn't come as a surprise because, if you think about it logically, fungi grows in dark damp places - and that's exactly what my feet were experiencing while covered by socks and shoes.

When it comes to sitting down, put simply we do too much of it! And what's worse is that we're not actually very good at it. Recent research has suggested that those of us who work in offices now spend more time sitting than those who are retired! On the NHS website it says, "Studies have linked excessive sitting with being overweight and obese, type 2 diabetes, some types of cancer and early death. Sitting for long periods is thought to slow the metabolism, which affects the body's ability to regulate blood sugar, blood pressure and break down body fat".

The Guardian newspaper ran an article in 2014 suggesting that, "We spend half our lives sitting down – and studies show it increases our risk of dying from practically any disease you can think of. But there is something we can do about it – we can simply stand up. Research in the British Journal of Sports Medicine shows that reducing sitting time increases the length of your telomeres". What are telomeres? They turn out be a cap that sits at the end of each DNA strand that helps protect our chromosomes from fraying. Picture them like the little plastic tips (called 'aglets') that stop our shoelaces from fraying. If we spend too much time sitting then we apparently damage our telomeres, preventing our cells from doing their job properly.

In January 2017, *The Daily Telegraph*'s website stated, "Elderly people who spend most of their time sitting down age significantly quicker than more active contemporaries, according to new research. A study of 1,500 pensioners found those who kept to a sedentary position for 10 hours or more a day and who did less than 40 minutes moderate physical activity had the body of people eight years older".

You would think that, because we practice the art of sitting for so many hours each day, we must be pretty good at it - but as you have just read, we're not. In fact we're rubbish at it! We slouch, round the shoulders, and put all sorts of stress in the wrong areas. It must be something that we slowly develop, because I have noticed that my two-year-old son Louie sits with a perfectly straight back. I am certainly no physiotherapist, so I won't go into chapter and verse about how we should sit properly, other than recommend that when you get five minutes, you go to Google and type in 'how to sit properly' or 'good posture' and you will find lots of articles.

ALCOHOL

This is the hardest principle for me to write about, as I do like a drink. So here I am going to start by quoting an old proverb, 'do as I say, not as I do'. That said, if you like the odd drink you will be pleased to hear that I am not going to suggest you stop completely. Remember, this book is about happiness as much as it is about health - and if the occasional drink makes us happy, then we should go ahead and have one. If a glass of wine helps us unwind after a hard day at work, our overall health will probably benefit from having a drink rather than going out of our way to avoid it. But we are talking about only one or two glasses. We aren't talking about drowning our sorrows, we're talking about a little relaxation. If we feel the need to get drunk to be happy, then it's important to seek help in getting to the root cause of our unhappiness.

Let's take a look at units. While we don't count calories when we live Primally, we really do need to count our alcohol units. Firstly, where the British government got that '21 units a week for men and 14 for women' is a complete mystery. Only last week I read they are now saying men should only drink 14 units. Plus, in many books I have read about our gut, the common recommendation to keep our healthy bacteria in good working order is to suggest no more than one unit of alcohol per day.

But here is my take on booze. First of all, we all know you can set fire to brandy, if you didn't then you have never lit a Christmas pudding! If something can catch fire it must be a really good fuel. Forget calorie counting, if something can easily ignite then the body must use it as a fuel. 'So what', you might be asking. If we are eating and drinking too, it seems to make sense that the body is going to choose to burn the fuel that's easiest to burn first, i.e. the alcohol, before it even thinks of burning up that evening meal we just ate.

Virtually every time I step on my bathroom scales in the morning after consuming more than two units of alcohol the night before, I find that my weight has increased. During almost three years of charting my daily weight, almost every time where I have consumed more than two units of alcohol the night before, my weight is higher the next morning- even if I exercised and ate very Primally.

At the end of the day, alcohol is full of empty calories – a whopping seven of them per gram. But it's not just the calories that are a problem, alcohol seems to disrupt our blood sugar control, makes our muscles less likely to take in the energy and instead deposits it all in our fat stores. The Drinkaware website sums it up very well, "While we can store nutrients, protein, carbohydrates and fat in our bodies, we can't store alcohol. So our system wants to get rid of it, and doing so takes priority. All of the other processes that should be taking place (including absorbing nutrients and burning fat) are interrupted". One of the biggest sacrifices the body makes while dealing with too much alcohol is it fails to metabolise vitamin B. Among other things this can lead to depression, lack of concentration and damage to several cognitive functions.

I heard Olympic diver Tom Daley being interviewed on the Chris Evans radio show some time ago, and he said something along the lines of a glass of wine has the same calories as a donut - and if he was going to have to chose one, he would rather have a donut! This made perfect sense to me. I had been eating strictly Primal that week, but the night before hearing Tom, for no apparent reason, I had three glasses of wine. That's the equivalent of three donuts and on hearing what he had to say, I finally got the message.

> **THE ALCOHOL DILEMMA:**
> Undoubtedly a small amount of alcohol is good for us, but there is little margin for error, as over consumption is very unhealthy.

Now, if we like the occasional drink, then all the research I have ever read points to our best bet being red wine. Tannins are a chemical found in the skin of the grape that helps protect it from bugs, and they are excellent antioxidants and in sensible quantity may help prevent cellular damage that leads to cancer. Also resveratrol found in red grapes further adds to its healing benefits, although recent researchers have suggested that we would need to consume way too much wine for the benefit of resveratrol to be meaningful.

One final thought on alcohol, but this time it's aimed just at us men. Did you know when we consume lots of booze, our body converts the male sex hormone testosterone into the female hormone oestrogen? Yes gents, the more we drink the more feminine we become. Now that might explain a lot of the man boobs that we see in pubs!

> ### Wine Hangovers
> Imagine the scenario: you own a winery and are asked to supply a huge supermarket halfway around the world. They are happy to purchase large volumes from you, but aren't prepared to pay too much per bottle. So the cheapest solution is not to bottle your wine at your vineyard, but to pour it into a vast container the size of a small swimming pool and put it on a ship. But there is a problem, what happens if on the ocean your huge vat becomes contaminated? The solution is you stuff the container full of your precious wine with chemicals! Ever woken up with a sore head after a wedding or office party, but are sure you didn't drink too much? Chances are it was an assortment of nasty chemicals that you consumed. Therefore, always purchase wine where the label includes the message 'bottled at source'.

TURN OFF THE HEAT

When my son-in-law Jake and I decided to walk to the North Pole (you can watch the documentary on YouTube, it's called 'The Last Degree North Pole'), we were advised that, due to the extreme low temperatures, we would need to consume 9,000 calories each day of our week-long adventure. As it turns out, our clothing was so good that we only burnt 6,000 calories per day. But that's still a whooping 3,400 more than we would normally expend. What was really interesting was that, while we were walking and pulling our sledges, we took off our thick overcoats and even at -40°C we walked wearing very thin jackets. The core of our bodies stayed warm the whole time we were moving, but not our feet and hands – they needed covering up at all times. When it was time to go to the toilet, we had to bare our man bits and bottoms to the elements. The amazing thing is they never became overly cold, but when wiping our bottom required going from three layers of gloves to just two so that we could grip the toilet paper, our hands ached with intense pain. The point is this: when we are in cold conditions our body consumes a colossal amount of energy to keep us warm.

I once read that we actually burn more calories per hour standing in a cold sea on a British summer holiday than we do jogging for the same amount of time. Wow! Don't run a marathon, but get into surfing! Apparently, when we are shivering we burn around 100 calories every 15 minutes. But as someone who has spent a lot of his life in and on the water, let me stress that we must not take it to the extreme or we might get hypothermia, which can of course be fatal. If we get too cold and can't keep heating our entire body, then it focuses on our core and horrible things begin to happen to our arms and legs. I witnessed this first-hand when the doctor we took with us on our North Pole expedition got a small amount of damp into his gloves, and suffered terrible frostbite.

What about cold showers? I used to love them dearly and took them daily as they really woke me up, but these days I only have the guts to do them after a workout in the gym. But if you can, wow – what a great start to the day you are going to have. Actress Katherine Hepburn was said to have taken a cold bath or shower every day and swore by its benefits. So how does taking a cold shower contribute to our health? It makes us breathe deeply as we gasp so that we take in more oxygen. This leads to an increase in heart rate, releasing a rush of blood and energy throughout the body – that's why we should do it in the morning and not at bedtime.

Cold water is also great for our hair and skin too. It makes our hair shiny, stronger and generally healthier. It also closes our pores, which is why we should always use cold water after a shave. According to Dr Joseph Mercola, a natural health expert, "It can lower blood pressure, clear blocked arteries and improve our immune system".

In 2016, my brother and I, along with Sir Richard Branson, his daughter Holly and son Sam, plus a group of other crazy cyclists, cycled the entire length of Italy. To tell the truth, I only did part of the three weeks as I had some other commitments - and as you have already read I don't believe endurance sports to be healthy. At the end of each day's ride, which was around 130–195km (80–120 miles), waiting for us on the finishing line was a kiddie's paddling pool full of ice-cold water. Why? Because it dramatically reduces muscle pain.

It's absolutely brilliant at preventing the delayed onset of muscle soreness (known as the DOMS for short) that we often get 24–48 hours after a heavy gym session. The reason this happens is a little bit of complex biology, but in a nutshell cold temperatures activate a hormone called adiponectin, which quickly pushes glucose into muscles, resulting in an anabolic (building up) effect. This surge of energy into the muscles greatly enhances recovery.

On a technical level, taking a cold shower, exposure to cold temperatures, cold-water swimming or cold baths, is referred to as cold thermogenesis (CT) and many elite athletes embed it into their weekly training. CT can:

- Help cure or reduce stress, and as we have already read stress is possibly the biggest cause of heart attacks
- Increase the levels of our immune system
- Increase metabolism
- Activate adiponectin hormones, which increase consumption of glucose and breaks down fatty acids

Chapter 5 Highlights

- Health benefits of SENSIBLE sunbathing outweigh skin cancer risks.
- When it is sunny, go outside without sunscreen for up to 50% of the time that it would normally take you to turn slightly red. Then go under the shade, chill for half an hour and then slap on a mineral based, broad spectrum sunscreen.
- Aim for 7 to 9 hours sleep daily, if necessary take afternoon naps.
- Undoubtedly a small amount of alcohol is good for us, but there is little margin for error, as overconsumption is very unhealthy.
- Avoid toxic wines. Always purchase those where the label clearly says, 'Bottled at Source', or for French wines, 'Mis en Bouteille au Château'.
- Is it a coincidence that the increase in environmental toxicity levels is tracked almost identically by the rise in the cases of cancer? Now I appreciate correlation does not directly prove causation, but surely we should at least treat it as a cause for concern!
- Read the ingredients of all products you put on your skin and if you would not be happy to eat it, then don't apply or spritz it!

06.
Primal Environment

It's time to retreat back to our cave. In this chapter we look at how toxins are affecting our health and how to best avoid them.

AVOID MURDER BY TOXIN

In 2006, ex-Russian spy Alexander Litvinenko was killed in London, when apparently someone slipped polonium-210 – a radioactive substance – into his cup of tea. Then, in February 2017, the estranged older brother of North Korean leader, Kim Jong Nam, was attacked at Kuala Lumpur Airport. Two women wiped a highly toxic nerve agent called VX on his face, and he died within just 30 minutes.

Why mention these two high-profile cases? Just to highlight, without any uncertainty, that toxins can kill. Do I honestly believe that toxins kill more people than they are held responsible for? Yes, without a doubt. Pretty much the only toxins our Primal ancestors were exposed too were the odd poisonous mushroom or venomous bite. But fast-forward to today and we are exposed to a mass of toxins. These can be in the form of:

1. What we eat and drink
2. What we inhale
3. What we apply to the skin
4. Electromagnetic fields

Toxins In What We Eat And Drink

There is not much to cover here that we haven't already mentioned. If we are avoiding packaged food and only buying organic produce, then we are doing pretty much everything we possibly can do to be safe. On the odd occasion, when we unknowingly digest something that might be slightly toxic, as long as it's in a small dose then our clever gut and liver will likely be able to deal with it.

> **PRIMAL CURE PRINCIPLE:**
> To avoid consuming potentially deadly toxins, eat organically, avoid packaged food and don't consume anything where you don't recognise the words on the label.

As well as being very careful about our food choices, we should be equally careful in how we store and cook our foods. For example, don't store any food in plastic, unless you are 100% sure that they don't contain bisphenol A (BPAs). This is especially crucial if you are going to microwave your food. Also, avoid using Teflon-coated pans if they are scratched or chipped as they can potentially leak dangerous chemicals into food. Another metal that should be avoided for cooking is aluminium. There have been several studies where they have found a link between the regular use of cooking in aluminium and Alzheimer's. Food grade stainless steel is always the best choice for your health, as well as the longevity of your cooking utensils. When food burns it also becomes toxic, but we will cover this subject later when we discuss cancer.

Toxins In What We Inhale

Don't smoke, period. Hold your breath momentarily as you race past the smokers huddled together outside the airport or office. When it comes to traffic fumes, try to avoid busy roads and instead learn to walk along the quieter back streets. We should be really careful in city centres, especially where there are lots of traffic jams: the densely packed buildings and skyscrapers lock in the fumes, creating what some are now calling urban canyons.

A recent report compiled on behalf of the EU by the University of the West of England listed some very interesting findings. To measure air pollution, they fitted car drivers, cyclists and pedestrians with a carbon monoxide monitors. On studying their research, what I found most interesting was that, on open roads, the level of pollution falls off quite quickly the further we are from traffic. For example, cyclists at 2.5 metres from the middle of the road were on average exposed to 0.5 toxic parts per million, while pedestrians at six metres from the middle of the road were exposed to 0.1 toxic parts per million. So, when we can't avoid going into highly congested cities or towns, it's important to try to get as far away from traffic as possible.

Toxins In What We Apply To The Skin

Have you ever wondered what is in the shampoos and shower gels that we lather all over our body? Have you ever stopped and thought about how that antiperspirant stops us sweating all day? Do you know what's in the creams and makeup that we apply to our skin?

In Canada, some people decided to find out the answer to these questions. You can read the full report at www.environmentaldefence. ca by searching for 'heavy metal hazards'. They trawled through the handbags of six ladies and conducted tests on items including foundations, concealers, powders, blushes, mascaras, eyeliners, eye shadows, lipsticks and glosses. In total, they tested 49 different products, and the results were alarming. All 49 contained nickel, all but two contained lead, half contained cadmium and 10 contained the poison arsenic. And, before you start to think that Canadians use inferior cosmetics, nearly all of the products were brand names that you would recognise and most women in the UK use regularly.

One of the people who had their makeup scrutinised was Erin Charter. On hearing the findings she said, "The product that I spend the most money on, because I believed it was better for me, ended up being the worst out of everything tested! I'd like to have some indication of these ingredients on the label, so I could make informed choices. Or, better still, I'd like there to be rules to protect me from these chemicals so I don't need to worry so much".

While there are numerous white papers and continual scientific debates as to what constitutes 'safe' levels of heavy metal exposure, I find it hard to comprehend how anyone could ever tell. How is it possible to truly measure what is the safe level of covering your body in known poisons over a sustained period of many years? Imagine going to one of the many uncontacted tribes in Peru or Indonesia and saying, "Hey, would you like to make yourself look more attractive by putting on modern makeup? But before you do, we have to warn you that they contain at least nine different elements that are known to be poisonous". What do you think they would say? Would it be, "Hey, that sounds like a good idea, let's stop using the natural herbs and colourings that we have used for generations and go for your scary cocktail of prettily labelled toxins?"

Is it really that bad to put poisonous things on our skin and to spray them in our hair and under our arms? Think back to Chapter 1 where we discussed how, when the small intestine has done its job, it sends blood to the liver for a safety check before it is then allowed to be pumped around the body. The problem with what we put on our skin is that, without a safety check, it is free to be absorbed directly into the bloodstream. Am I really implying that we would therefore be safer swallowing our shampoo, deodorant and makeup than we are applying it to the skin? Yes I am. If we were to swallow them, our inbuilt safety mechanism would kick in and we would normally vomit. If we did somehow manage to swallow them, then our liver would give the thumbs down and send them to our back door for a quick and timely departure.

> **PRIMAL CURE PRINCIPLE:**
> **Read the ingredients of all products you put on your skin and if you would not be happy to eat it, then don't apply or spray it!**

Think about it this way: for 2 million years we have had to build a defence mechanism for poisonous things that we might consume. Every single month, our Primal ancestors had a varied diet of hundreds of different plants and bugs. This diversified diet meant that they would occasionally eat a berry, a mushroom or plant that was not healthy for them. Therefore, through evolution, Mother Nature has built in a fairly robust safety mechanism against things that we might accidentally consume.

But, as we have only been smearing our body in poisonous creams, makeup and cleansing products for just over a 100 years, nature hasn't yet had chance to evolve and create a natural defence mechanism. When I told my wife this, her immediate reaction was that I was wrong. She reminded me of how our daughter Lili had come out in a huge rash after having her face painted and how our sister-in-law Paula's eyes had become swollen from a reaction to sun cream. Of course, as always, my wife was right. However, these were reactions to highly concentrated poisons in just one application. The body was smart enough to detect this and react immediately, therefore alerting them not to use those products again. But what I am talking about here isn't huge concentrations of poisonous things in just one application, but a lifelong drip-feed of them into our systems.

Think about it another way. We know that toxins attack the immune system. We also know that underactive thyroids are related to the immune system, and it is a fact that this condition is much more prevalent in females. Why is this the case? Could it be because females apply far more products on the skin than males? In her insightful book, *Hashimoto's Protocol*, Dr Izabella Wentz makes a very similar point, "When we swallow a substance, our gut and liver process it first before it goes into the circulation system. When you apply substances through the skin, the substances skip the gatekeepers of the digestive tract and liver". In an article in The Huffington Post titled, 'Why Your Makeup is More Harmful than You Think,' it says, "When it comes to antiperspirant, you may want to consider going for the less potent, natural options. When you shave your armpits, you're scrapping off a layer of skin – and then you apply the carcinogenic-filled deodorant right onto the vulnerable area right near your lymph nodes. Yikes!"

It's not just the creams, makeup and sprays that can cause us harm, but the clothes that we wear too. We should try to avoid synthetic material, instead dressing in clothes made from natural fibres. While we are talking about clothes... There was a recent news clip on the BBC, where the fire brigade conducted an experiment to show the dangers of using skin creams containing paraffin. They set alight six identical ladies tops, one that hadn't been worn and the rest that had been worn for different periods of time. Amongst the points they were trying to highlight, it was frightening to see how quickly the clothes caught fire if they had been in contact with skin creams containing paraffin (of which sadly there are many on the market), even if the clothes had been washed. The conclusion was that tragically 44 women in Britain have died since 2010 due the paraffin in their clothes catching fire. Now while that is very frightening, what is more concerning to those of us living in "Sick Britain", is the toxic effects that same paraffin might be having on the health of our bodies.

Embracing The Coconut And Avoid Toxic-Hygiene

We have already talked about the huge health benefits of coconut oil and, in Chapter 9, we will look at other ways to make the coconut a staple in our diet. But here, under general health principles, I would like to discuss several other ways in which coconuts can help us avoid toxic substances and thereby improve our health and well-being. As well as being the only superfood that we should consider for our skin, hair, teeth, I highlight it here in an attempt to try and get everyone to start thinking about natural, non-toxic and non-poisonous solutions to personal hygiene.

Teeth & Gums

If we swirl coconut oil around our mouth for five to 10 minutes, not only do our teeth become whiter, we will be providing our entire mouth with a full detox. Known as oil pulling, you can create your own pulls or there are several brands available in health stores and online. As there are no added chemicals or other nasties, coconut pulling is extremely healthy and an additional benefit it makes our breath smell great too. No wonder so many celebrities, including the lovely Gwyneth Paltrow, are said to be now pulling with coconut.

By simply mixing it with baking soda, you can even use coconut as a toothpaste. If we miss the minty taste of chemical-laden commercial products, then we can always add a little bit of mint to it. It's really easy to make, and if you need a guide you can always visit our website.

Coconut & Our Skin

In the gemstone world, experts often liken the outer layers of a pearl to that of a woman's skin. If skin looks youthful and translucent it is sometimes described as pearlescent. When we are young, the fat in our skin has the ability to hold plenty of water, but as we age our fat breaks down and our skin dries out. To avoid wrinkling, it's important to keep skin moist. Obviously water is not the answer, as it doesn't penetrate the surface of the skin – if it did, we would never get out of the bath! The Primal answer to a pearlescent vibrant skin is, of course, the application of quality organic oils. Coconut is the king of all oils, and pretty much the only oil that has a medium-chain fatty acid (MCFA). Applying coconut oil directly to the skin helps maintain a youthful look. Don't just take my word for it. When Nicole Scherzinger was asked what was the one skin product she couldn't live without, she didn't name one of the beauty products that she was an ambassador for, but coconut oil! If you suffer from acne or spots, one of the best solutions is to apply a cream or lotion containing lauric acid. This has rich antibacterial, antiviral and antifungal properties and roughly half of the oil found in coconut is lauric acid, so it is great for applying to spots too.

If you arrive at a stage in your life where you are using coconut oils for virtually everything, and feel the need to take a short break, then another fantastic natural oil for our skin is shea butter. This is obtained from the nut of the shea tree. It is a complex triglyceride fat derived from stearic acid and oleic acid, widely used in the cosmetics industry as a moisturiser. It's also edible and can be used to cook with. But as always, make sure it is unrefined, organic and free from additives.

Coconut As An Organic Shampoo

For healthy hair, it's important to keep our entire body hydrated, so drinking plenty of water is extremely important. For a full, bouncy and shiny head of hair, coconut oil is simply the best Primal shampoo you will ever use. In fact, without realising it you probably inadvertently use a little already!

Many brands of shampoo and skin products blend coconut oils into their formulas, the only problem is, to make their product feel and foam like regular shampoos, they often blend it with chemicals that are toxic and potentially very dangerous to our health. According to leading nutritionist Dr Josh Axe, "It is the protein loss in hair that leads to dryness and breakage. The lauric acid has a low molecular weight, and is able to actually penetrate the hair shaft, nourishing the hair with vitamins, minerals and the medium-chain fatty acids".

If you suffer from dandruff, it's brilliant for the scalp too. You can now buy organic coconut shampoos from health stores, online or you can make your own at home for a fraction of the price. Visit www. primalcure.com for various shampoo recipes.

TOXINS IN ELECTROMAGNETIC FIELDS (EMF)

While not a toxin as described above, I couldn't leave out the dangers we face from putting our mobile phones to our ears too frequently. As a parent, I am concerned – or should I say frightened – by the fact that current claims that low frequency electromagnetic field exposure are safe is based on very little conclusive research. The World Health Organisation (WHO) currently state on their website, "The electromagnetic fields produced by mobile phones are classified by the International Agency for Research on Cancer as possibly carcinogenic to humans". Does that sound frightening? It does to me. Especially when you consider how big and powerful the telecommunication giants are, I doubt we will find out the truth for several more decades.

WHO's website goes on to say, "The power (and hence the radiofrequency exposure to a user) falls off rapidly with increasing distance from the handset. A person using a mobile phone 30–40cm away from their body – for example when text messaging, accessing the Internet or using a 'hands-free' device – will therefore have a much lower exposure to radiofrequency fields than someone holding the handset against their head. In addition to using hands-free devices, which keep mobile phones away from the head and body during phone calls, exposure is also reduced by limiting the number and length of calls. Using the phone in areas of good reception also decreases exposure as it allows the phone to transmit at reduced power".

My advice is go hands-free or don't use your mobile phone at all. However, it's not just your phone that produces a toxic electromagnetic field. The modern kitchen and bedroom are hotspots too. In the kitchen the microwave is the most harmful. While the food is fine once cooked, don't stand too close to it while it is cooking. Other appliances such as washing machines and blenders also generate an EMF, but they are far weaker. In the bedroom, try not to over use your hairdryer and let your hair dry naturally where possible, just as our Primal ancestors once did.

> Now I am not trying to scare anyone, but with Cancer Research UK now predicting that one in two people in the UK will get cancer at some time during their life, we simply need to do everything possible to protect ourselves.

PRIMAL DETOX

Every now and again, I believe there are huge gains to be made by undertaking a week-long detox. In the modern world, our immune system, which is controlled by our gut, really benefits from a deep clean. I have now done nine of these over the past two years and in April this year I felt so amazing at the end of my week-long cleanse, that I extended it to 19 days.

While detoxing has become something of a cult over recent years, I believe the type of detox most people actually take part in reaches nowhere near its full potential. You see, to really cleanse the body it's not just our food we need to clean up, but our environment too. For me, a true detox should consist of:

- Only consuming clean organic foods.
- Eating just the Top 20 Superfoods that you will read about later.
- All meals to include cruciferous vegetables whose glucosinolates supercharge detoxification.

- Eating foods high in sulphur, such as eggs, onions, garlic and chicken.
- Take curcumin supplements to aid detoxification.
- Consuming plenty of vitamin C as it helps flush toxins out of the body.
- Undertaking several fast days during the detox period.
- Consuming supplements to replace missing vitamins and nutrients.
- Not using a mobile phone or if we have to, ensuring its either on speaker mode or use headphones.
- Only drinking water that is filtered.
- Completely avoiding BPAs and plastic bottles.
- Avoiding antiperspirants, perfumes or aftershaves.
- Avoiding toxic shampoos or toothpaste.
- Wearing underwear made only of natural fibres.
- Drinking lots of green tea, which contains catechins that aids detoxification.

Flushing Toxins By Sweating

It's important to stop poisoning ourselves with unhealthy sprays, creams and shampoos, but we can also use our skin to clear toxins. One of the best ways to get our skin working for us is by sweating. When we sweat, our body naturally detoxes from the inside out.

As Primal Cure is not big on long jogs and epic bicycle rides - both activities where you would definitely sweat a lot - we need to look for alternative ways to detoxify. This is where taking a regular sauna can help. If you can't get to your local sauna, then when you do your gym routine try turning up the heat. If your gym owner won't let you do that, then put on lots of layers during your workout. It is really important that, on a regular basis, we find a way to sweat out our toxins. On a biological level, when we sweat it helps remove bacteria from our epidermal layer of skin, and increases the rate at which dead skin cells are replaced.

Chapter 6 Highlights

- Scientific research now suggests that up to 90% of all known illnesses can be traced back to an unhealthy gut.
- There are several things we must do to protect our microbiome: the most important is to avoid CARBS and other sugars and to eat a diet rich in fermented foods and fibre.
- To develop the right balance between the gut's two most important bacteria, firmicutes and bacteroidetes, we need to reduce our intake of CARBS and other sugars and increase the amount of fibre in our diet.
- When it comes to our health, happiness and longevity, our gut is responsible for far more than we may ever know. We must be mindful to ensure we give it the true care and respect it deserves.

07.
Gut Feeling: Taking Care Of Our Microbiome

In this chapter we look at how the British diet causes havoc with the natural flora and fauna of our gut and what we can do to fix it.

Hippocrates taught us that, 'All diseases begin in the gut'. As I believe this to be so true, I am not going to apologise for already quoting this twice. I know there is a lot to comprehend in this book, so if I was asked to draw your attention to just one statistic, it is the following:

> **PRIMAL CURE FACT:**
> Scientific research now suggests that up to 90% of all known illnesses can be traced back to an unhealthy gut.

Wow! Doesn't that suggest we need to knuckle down and learn a little more about this extremely complex organ? Grab a black coffee or a cup of green tea and let's begin…

Our bodies are not just single living individuals, but thriving ecosystems comprised of 100 trillion microscopic creatures living and working in and on us. As we discovered in Chapter 1, we are less likely to inherit diseases or illnesses that runs in our family than we probably fear, and one of the reasons for this is that only 10% of our cells contain any human DNA! The other 90% is made up of bacteria, fungi and microflora, all of which can't pass on anything genetically.

In *10% Human: How Your Body's Microbes Hold the Key to Health and Happiness*, author Dr Alanna Collen writes, "Over your lifetime, you will play host to bugs the equivalent weight of five African elephants. Your skin is crawling with them. There are more on your fingertip than there are people in Britain". Our 100 trillion microbes can be divided into more than 10,000 different species. This array of vastly different creatures living on and in our body are collectively referred to as our microbiome. As Dr Martin J. Blaser explains in *Missing Microbes*, "In ecology, biome refers to the set of plants and animals in a community such as a jungle, forest or coral reef. An enormous diversity of species, large and small, interact to form complex webs of mutual support. When a keystone species disappears or goes extinct the ecology suffers. It can even collapse".

A lot of today's research into the human body and how it functions is now focusing on the importance of our microbiome. While these tiny creatures exist all over our body, inside and out, it is primarily their accumulation in our gut that has the biggest impact on our health. Getting the varieties of microbes in our gut balanced is now believed by cutting-edge science to have positive effects on all aspects of our health. From weight control to a healthy heart, food metabolism to a good memory, these creatures need to be respected and controlled.

They say a picture paints a thousand words, and when I am trying to create an image of what's happening in my gut - where many creatures are so tiny you wouldn't even see them under a normal microscope - I close my eyes and visualise ants! Just like ants working in a cohort to perform tasks beyond our imagination, the bacterial army in our gut affect not just our health, but also our mood, emotions and behaviour. In *10% Human*, Dr Collen writes, "Imagine, for example, one strain of bacterium that feeds on a particular compound found in our food. If we eat that food, thus feeding these bacteria, and they are able to 'reward' us with a dose of happiness through the chemicals they produce, so much better for them. The chemicals they produce in us could cause us to crave the food they feed on, and even to remember where we found it".

It will come as no surprise to you that one of the best ways to get our microbiome under control is to follow the principles laid out in Primal Cure – avoiding CARBS and other sugars, eating protein, fibre and lots of berries and nuts. If possible, we should try to avoid taking any antibiotics and, if we do take a course, then make sure we immediately rebuild our microbiome by taking a quality course of probiotics.

Back in 2009, my wife and I were in India visiting one of our gemstone cutting factories, and in the evening we went out for a meal in one of the most popular restaurants in the city of Jaipur. When the waiter served me chicken, my wife commented that it didn't look properly cooked, but I told her that I thought it was just the colour of the spices making it look pink. The next morning on the flight home, I practically didn't leave the tiny toilet cubical. I had the worse diarrhoea and stomach cramps I have ever experienced. Little did I know at the time, but for the next five months I could never be more than 30 seconds from a toilet!

Our guts are a bit like a coral reef. While coral reefs can be devastated by a rapid rise in sea temperature, the colonies living in our microbiome can be eradicated by either a strong virus or antibiotics, and of course sometimes both. Just like the physical coral is still intact after bleaching, our intestines remain in place too, but they become barren. For months, maybe years afterwards, the gut's environment rests on a knife-edge. While some species are completely wiped out, one strand (firmicutes) seems to feed on disaster - and either avoid being exterminated, or are very quick to regroup after a big environmental event.

Firmicutes are the bacteria that make us fat by rinsing every last calorie out of the food we eat. While firmicutes survive, overall diversity is greatly reduced, and some species never return. This imbalance is known as dysbiosis (sometimes referred to as dysbacteriosis). While antibiotics and major infections can cause complete wipeouts, medicines, poor diets and mild illnesses can all knock our microbiome ecosystem off balance.

So, could it be that the dodgy chicken I ate in 2009 affected my microbiome and has contributed to me struggling to lose weight over recent years? I can't say for definite that this is the case, but this was the same year that, even though I was constantly on the toilet, my weight started to balloon!

> **PRIMAL CURE ON RECONSTRUCTING OUR MICROBIOME:** There are several things we must do, but the most important thing is to avoid CARBS and other sugars and to eat a diet rich in fermented foods and fibre.

How important is the state of our microbiome? In truth, we don't fully know yet. After all, with 100 trillion microscopic creatures in our body across 10,000 different species, it is an area of science that we will probably never fully understand. But logic suggests that, as the bacteria in our gut aid the break down of toxins, help in the creation of vitamins and are ultimately responsible for our immune system, then we should do everything we can to nurture them and keep them on our side. And talking of our immune system, did you know that 80% of it is located in our gut? What's your gut reaction to that fact? Hopefully it is to start taking better care of it!

With such a diverse range of tasks and skills, many scientists regard the gut as the second most complex engine in our body, only surpassed by the brain. It is now believed that a lot of the feelings that we can't always easily explain, such as depression, anxiety and stress, are driven from the gut and not from the brain. It is becoming increasingly evident that there is a connection between gut health and mental illness.

Many medical journals go as far as claiming that the gut is, in fact, our second brain. Think back to the small intestine, with its sensors the size of a tennis court. Compare it to all of our other sensors, such as our eyes, nose, ears and touch. It is vastly larger. It monitors way more than all of our other sensors put together, but we never give it credit or apportion blame for our feelings. Science is now discovering that we absolutely should. The 'gut feeling' is something we should not ignore any longer. In her book *Gut*, with the apt subtitle, 'The inside story of our body's most under-rated organ' author Giulia Enders says, "Cooperation between the gut and the brain begins very early in life. Together, they are responsible for a large proportion of our emotional world when we are babies".

Where Did Our Bacteria Originate?

First things first, this planet that we inhabit is really their domain and not ours. Earth formed some 4.5 billion years ago and, while us humans have only inhabited it for less than one thousandth of that time, it's been the home to single-celled bacteria for some 3.8 billion years! As you will read over the next few pages, we would be wise to view Earth as their planet and not ours.

Bacteria, plankton and single-celled organisms are far more shatterproof than us fragile humans. They can withstand temperatures so low that we would freeze to death in seconds. They can thrive, and indeed multiply, in temperatures so high that our skin would melt instantly. They have survived our planet's hostile environment through toxic periods, caused by mass volcanic activities and colliding tectonic plates, that would wipe us out in a heartbeat. Compared to us Homo sapiens, some species of bacteria are virtually indestructible. They were the first living life form on planet Earth and, in my mind, will ultimately be the last. To picture how long they have been on Earth, if you imagine a 24-hour clock, bacteria have thrived on our planet for the 24 hours - and us humans have only cohabited with them for the last two seconds!

In *The Diet Myth*, author Tim Spector writes, "These microbes are the true and permanent inhabitants on Earth; we humans are just passing through". I love this quote because it really makes me think hard about how important it is that we create harmony between our body and our microbiome.

Dr Martin J. Blaser says in *Missing Microbes*, "If you were to gather them all up, not only would they outnumber all the mice, whales, humans, birds, insects, worms and trees combined – indeed all of the visible life forms we are familiar with on Earth – they would outweigh them as well … Without microbes, we could not eat or breathe. Without us, nearly all microbes would be just fine". Whether we realise it or not, the bacteria in and on our body has played a huge part in the evolution of our species, and how we look after them and treat them today is very different to the way we have partnered with them since our evolution as a species. For more than 2 million years, we did nothing out of the norm to upset our bacteria. Every aspect of human life, until the agricultural revolution some 12,000 years ago, saw us living in harmony with our microscopic inhabitants. Our bacteria cells felt safe and unchallenged. After all, they greatly out-numbered the cells in the humans they became attached to. But fast-forward to today, and they are at constant war with a barrage of unhealthy, highly engineered and chemically enhanced foods that they are as estranged to, as we humans are too.

Here is another fantastic quote from *The Diet Myth*, "Over millions of years we have evolved together with microbes for mutual survival, yet recently this fine-tuning and selection has gone wrong".

What Role Do Bacteria Play In Our Body?

It's important to point out that not everyone will agree with what comes next, but what you will read is both highly researched and backed by lots of up-to-date independent data.

Whenever you participate in an activity, say a game of football, golf, tennis or a netball match, there is always a result. Put simply, the activity leads to a conclusion. Similarly, the bacteria in our microbiome participates in a whole host of activities, which in turn eventually lead to a whole host of different results.

Let's look at just some of the activities the bacteria in our body's microbiome play a part in: detoxification, inflammation, the functions of our immune system, neurotransmitter production, nutrient absorption, the synthesis of vitamins, the control of many hormones and how we utilise or store our macronutrients. Those activities in which our bacteria play an attacking role may lead to the following conditions (to name but a few): ADHD, Alzheimer's, asthma, autism, cancer, depression, diabetes, gum disease, high blood pressure, multiple sclerosis, obesity and Parkinson's disease.

To highlight how important our microbiome is to our health and well-being, let me start by asking you another question. The bacteria inhabiting our body are microscopic little things, containing just one cell each. If you could remove them all in one go and place them on your bathroom scales, what weight would you predict they would be? How about if I told you the bacteria in our body weighs about the same as our brain? I hope that shocked you, because it certainly caused me a mild panic.

Why Do Microbiomes Collapse?

Before I scare you half to death with what I am about to say, even if our microbiome is currently completely shot, broken beyond what you might believe repairable, I am pleased to announce that it is a graceful ecosystem, and with the right nurturing and conditioning we can return our intestines back to the positive working bacterial environment that nature designed. As Dr David Perlmutter reminds us, "Thankfully, the gut's microbiotic community is wonderfully receptive to rehabilitation".

It is now believed that, while in the womb, we don't have any bacteria in our body. But as we travel through the birth canal, a female organ rich with friendly bacteria, our skin acts like a magnet attracting billions of wonderful bacteria to climb on board. Those born by C-section never benefit from this microbiotic kick-start. What's more, most caesarean births (and according to recent research over a third of births now include major surgery) are conducted simultaneously with a course of antibiotics. As their name suggests, antibiotics are 'anti' our body's 'biotics', aka our bacteria. Sadly, they are not all that good at isolating and attacking just the bad bacteria, but often cause complete genocide, mass-murdering the good bacteria too. If you were born by C-section with antibiotics, and then didn't benefit from bacterial-rich breast milk, then your microbiome really did get off to a poor start (even though, of course, this was neither you nor your mother's fault).

There is also mounting evidence that people in built-up cities experience more immune diseases than those living rurally. Why is that? Because those of us living in built-up environments are living in a clinical, overly sterilised bubble. Our kids no longer bring muddy boots into the house, and at the first sight of a bit of muck, antibacterial wipes are whipped out! My daughter Lili screams at me every time I leave the toilet, "Wash your hands daddy!" The whole world seems obsessed with cleanliness, when the reality is that we are mass-murdering our friendly bacteria. As I am writing this sentence, Lili is sitting next to me on the sofa, still insisting that I need to wash my hands - and while she might be right when it comes to toilet visits, there are many other instances where we would be better off just being a little bit grubby!

Many scientists now believe that our obsession with hand sanitisers and bacterial wipes is not only killing off the bad bacteria, but the good bacteria too. Dr David Perlmutter in Brain Maker says, "There's immense value in being un-hygienic. Astonishingly new studies show a relationship between our increasingly sterile living environments and incidence of chronic illness, from heart disease and autoimmune disorders to cancer and dementia".

> **PRIMAL CURE COMPLAINT TO GOVERNMENTS:**
> Sadly, as of yet there is little publicity about how protecting our microbiome is as crucial for our health and longevity as preserving our rainforests, oceans and corals are to the survival of our planet.

How To Recolonise Our Microbiome

Later we will discuss fermented foods, and discover which are rich in positive bacteria. After being missing in action from supermarket shelves for decades, these probiotics foods - which were the norm - are mounting a resurgence. Regularly eating fermented foods (probiotics) such as yoghurts, kefir, sauerkraut and certain pickles will undoubtedly help rebuild most lacklustre immune systems.

Getting the gut back in good working order is actually a two-step process. We need to eat foods that are rich in healthy bacteria, as well as foods that the bacteria themselves like to feed on. These are known as prebiotics, and they are insoluble fibrous foods that cannot be absorbed or broken down by the gut, and as a result they remain there long enough to feed and fertilise our legions of healthy bacteria. While we can take prebiotics as a supplement, artichokes, raw garlic, chicory, onions (raw or cooked), raw asparagus and raw leeks are all natural sources.

Another way to take care of our microbiome is to regularly put our body into a ketogenic metabolic state. Research has shown that this increases the healthy variety of bacteria known as bacteroidetes and decreases the undesirable firmicutes. Let's remind ourselves what this means. Among other things, firmicutes are able to extract the most energy out of food, effectively stripping out maximum calories and leading to us putting on weight, getting fatter and eventually obese. Being ketogenic is effectively a spiral of upward health benefits. Our body not only consumes its own fat for fuel, but also removes the bacteria that over-extracts calories from food too.

> **PRIMAL CURE MICROBE MANTRA:**
> A ketogenic diet is a positively healthy double dose of
> goodness, where in collaboration we burn our own body fat
> as our primary fuel source and the good bacteria redirect
> any excessive incoming energy straight to the exit!

The Bacteria That Makes Us Fat And That Which Keeps Us Lean

I mentioned earlier that it's all too easy to criticise fat and obese people for overindulgence and being too lazy to exercise. It's a natural conclusion for those unaware of the effects of our bacteria. But knowledge is power, and I am hopeful that these next few sentences will help you understand one of the hidden secrets of why some people eat rubbish food and almost instantly get fat, while others seem to be naturally fat-defiant without any real effort. You see, even though there are thousands of different bacteria in our gut, much of it is killed off in the Western human, leaving just two to dominate the entire digestive system. I have mentioned them a few times already, their names are firmicutes and bacteroidetes. It is believed that, together, they might account for more than three-quarters of the bacteria in our body - the combined weight of their armed forces being in excess of 0.9kg (2lbs)! If we want to lose weight, we need to work out how to reduce the volume of firmicutes in our gut. These clever creatures are superefficient at extracting maximum calories from the food that we eat. Bacteroidetes just aren't as qualified at unbundling energy.

Remember the saying 'we are what we eat' or when it comes to meat, 'we are what we eat – eats'? In our gut, our bacteria are forced to eat what we eat. Different bacteria thrive and survive on different foods. This is one of the key reasons why we all have very different ecosystems. Is your diet encouraging the right bacteria? Is it providing a safe harbour for firmicutes? If it is, then you're most likely overweight. But don't take it the wrong way, because getting our weight down might be as simple as working out how to balance our microbiome. Once we have balanced our firmicutes and bacteroidetes, the next thing is to encourage as wide a variety of gut bacteria as possible. In *Brain Maker*, Dr David Perlmutter writes, "It's now firmly established that the gut community of lean people resembles a rainforest filled with many species and that of obese people is much less diverse".

> **PRIMAL CURE HEALTHY GUT GUIDANCE:**
> **Eat as many organic vegetables and fermented foods as possible, and take a quality probiotic supplement.**

At the University of Gothenburg in Sweden, Professor Fredrik Bäckhed, an award-winning expert in cellular microbiology, has performed numerous clinical studies with mice to uncover more about the critical role that microbes play in our gut. In 2004, he took a selection of skinny mice that were all born by C-section, and who had lived in a sterile environment to ensure that they didn't have any bacteria in their guts, and began his experiment. He took bacteria from the caecum (the pouch located between the small and large intestine) of normal mice and placed it in the fur of the sterile mice. So, as they licked their fur, the microbes started to arrive in their guts. Within weeks, even without changing their diets, these mice - which had been lean for their entire life - became fat. Seriously fat. Within

just weeks, on average they put on 60% more body weight.
The professor then reduced the amount of food the mice were eating
and they still put on weight. So without doubt, when it comes to mice,
certain varieties of microbes make them put on weight. You might
now question if there is any relevance to what goes on in the stomach
of a mouse and that of us humans, but let me just remind you that
while the vessel might be different, i.e. mouse vs human, the crew is
exactly the same! Certain microbes are able to extract more energy
out of food than the body can on its own. Whether they reside in mice
or humans, a microbe is a microbe. If they are experts at extracting
energy from food then they will perform their tasks regardless of their
host.

So, if we are fat or obese, the fault might not lie in just our food
choices, but the state of our microbiome. In fact, the microbiome can
also affect how good our body is at producing the hormone leptin,
which informs us when our stomachs are full and therefore when we
should stop eating. If we have damaged our body's ability to produce
sufficient leptin, and we have too many microbes that are experts in
extracting energy, then we could lay the blame of every excess pound
of body weight at their door!

> **POSSIBLE CAUSE OF OBESITY:**
> Bacterial damage to leptin production and an increase of gut
> bacterial varieties that specialise in extracting maximum calories
> from food could be the root cause of some cases of obesity.

In *10% Human*, Alanna Collen describes another mice experiment,
this time carried out by microbiologist Ruth Ley in America, where
she studied the DNA of a variety of supersized mice that are known
as ob/ob (their name appropriately derived from their obesity). These
mice are almost round in shape, and, because they just won't stop
eating, they are three times heavier than normal mice. Alanna writes,
"Although they appear to be a completely different species of mouse,
they actually have just a single mutation in their DNA that makes
them eat non-stop and become profoundly fat. That mutation is in

the gene that makes leptin, a hormone which dampens the appetite of both men and mice if they have a decent supply of stored fat".

Hang on a minute, if it's as simple as the satiety hormone leptin controlling our hunger, why can't we take leptin tablets or have leptin injections? Sadly, it's not so much a lack of the ability to produce leptin, but also the brain becoming insensitive to it. Just as type 2 diabetes can occur when cells stop accepting insulin (insulin resistance) due a long period of overwhelming abundance, the brain ignores the cries of leptin to stop eating if it has sustained periods where we have over-eaten when we were already full. To the brain, leptin's performance is viewed as a cry wolf scenario.

Dr Dan Maggs

"Watch this space! This is such an exciting area of medical research and we're only just starting to learn how important our microbiome is. Subscribe to our YouTube Channel where we'll be interviewing experts over the coming years as this area of research develops."

MORE GUT FACTS
Serotonin

If you take antidepressant tablets, their role is to simulate the brain's happiness neurotransmitter serotonin. However, some scientists suggest that as much as 90% of serotonin is not, as you might assume, created in the brain, but in our intestines. When we feel depressed, my recommendation would be not just to pop a pill and create temporary relief, but to spend time figuring out how to get our gut in order. Did you know that serotonin is synthesised from tryptophan, and foods rich in tryptophan include eggs, cheese, pineapple, salmon, turkey, nuts and seeds?

Stress

I know I have already covered the negative effect to our health caused by stress, and some of what I am about to say you have already read, but it's so important to our well-being that it's worth repeating. Stress plays havoc with our microbiome. It can send our bacteria into a frenzy. Short sharp moments of stress, such as what we experience during sprinting and weightlifting, don't set alarms bells off in our internal bacterial network. But persistent stress – caused by endurance sports and horrible bosses, for example – does. Our microbiome sees prolonged stress as a potential threat to the body, and summons the support of both steroids and adrenaline. Together, this mighty taskforce summons the help of a built-in safety device called inflammation. However, nature invented inflammation to protect injured joints, to isolate snakebites and other such dangers. Summoning inflammation when it's not really needed can lead to a whole host of diseases, from cancer to Alzheimer's, from MS to depression. It is therefore important to avoid stress at all costs.

If we don't avoid stress, the Guy Fawkes in our microbiome is going to start setting fire to many of our internal systems, leading to mass-inflammation. If we have a lot of healthy fire-fighting bacteria protecting our corner, then we should be okay at dealing with short exposure to stress. But if they have already left the building due to our diet or sedentary lifestyle, we could be in for big trouble. It's for this reason that many people who suffer from stress also suffer from a myriad of gut-related illnesses. For those that have never got to the root cause of their irritable bowel syndrome, reducing stress levels and rebuilding the health of their microbiome may resolve the issue.

GALT

The immune system has been mentioned several times throughout this book. It is effectively the body's inbuilt self-defence system, which is activated when potential trouble arises. Highlighting the importance of our gut, the Gut Associated Lymphatic Tissue (GALT) represents approximately three-quarters of our entire immune system. Why does the immune system deploy the vast majority of its army in our gut? Because this is where our body needs its defence bolstered in order to stop the enemy breaching the delicate lining of our intestinal wall, which is only one cell thick. Yes, the only thing that stands between all of the nasty stuff that we swallow, that keeps harmful ingredients inside our gut, is just one cell wide. When the bad guys penetrate the immune system's defensive line, it is referred to as a leaky gut.

Fructose

When our Primal ancestors came across a fruit tree, they would likely feast on 'nature's candy' until they were completely bloated or sick. Is it by design or by coincidence that fruit ripens at the very end of the summer, just before the nights close in and hunting and gathering becomes both intermittent and less rewarding? If by design maybe nature's intention was, "At the beginning of autumn, I will create a food type, full of nutrients and a heap of energy, and design the human species to eat copious amounts of it, building up a reserve of energy to see them throughout the winter months". If this hypothesis is correct, then in Chapter 1 where I mention our species was not designed to be fat, maybe I should add this one caveat, 'we were designed to be fat only at the end of summer'.

To encourage the body to keep eating the fruit, nature needed a way to bypass the 'I am full' hormone, leptin. The solution was to treat fructose slightly different to all other sugars, and not to produce insulin in the same way. Instead of calling on the pancreas to do the work, nature instead handed the job of storing fructose to the liver. As the liver also synthesises the hormone leptin to inform the brain that we are full, it has to give it a break while it is busy dealing with incoming fructose. As a result, humans keep eating and eating it without any signal of satiety. Why mention fructose in this gut-related chapter? Because, while small doses of fructose from fruit are not an issue, especially if it is locally grown and in season, high fructose corn syrup (HFCS), consumed en masse in packaged foods and sauces, ruins our healthy flora and fauna and colonises an army of deadly bacteria. In a recent report, the average American now eats 27kg (60lbs) of HFCS every year. This is simply way too much for the body to absorb, so lots of it ends up fermenting in our guts for long periods, resulting in many varieties of our microbes being poisoned by it.

IBS

Irritable Bowel Syndrome is rife, with around 10% of the adult population suffering from it, and two out of three people affected by it are female. This common disorder affects the large intestine and causes, among other things cramping, abdominal pain, gas, bloating, diarrhoea and constipation. While it tends to be used as a catch-all diagnosis when doctors can't pinpoint the exact cause of a patient's discomfort, I believe that, for most sufferers, the cause is an imbalanced microbiome. However, with thousands of varieties of microbes in our gut, where should sufferers turn for a solution? I am a big believer in the Pareto Principle, named after the Italian engineer, sociologist and economist Vilfredo Pareto (1848–1923), where 80% of an effect comes from 20% of the causes (also known as the 'law of the vital few'). Therefore, with firmicutes and bacteroidetes occupying around three-quarters of our gut bacteria by volume, weighing in at about 0.9kg (2lbs), more than three times heavier than the human heart, I am confident to recommend to IBS sufferers that they try two things – firstly commit to a diet that creates an environment that firmicutes do not like, and secondly, do everything possible to reduce stress in their life.

Dr Dan Maggs

"We must ensure that the good bacteria in our guts outnumbers the bad (collectively known as pathogenic bacteria)."

Obesity

Like I just stated, I have to be careful not to oversimplify something that is regarded as a complex matter. In all walks of life, I often feel sorry for professionals where too much knowledge can cloud their vision, and make it difficult to accept a simple solution. In business, I always ask my team to stand back from the coalface and search for a simple solution. Could obesity in the main be caused by a negative microbiome?

I have already mentioned the brilliant research carried out by Professor Ruth Ley. In another experiment she evaluated the balance of firmicutes and bacteroidetes in both lean and obese mice, and then repeated the experiment across lean and obese humans. The result: obese mice and obese humans have a higher number of firmicutes than bacteroidetes. Lean mice and humans have higher number of bacteroidetes than firmicutes.

> **PRIMAL CURE ON OBESITY:**
> **Once we have cut out the CARBS and other sugars and then began intermittent fasting, the next thing to sort out is the balance of bacteria in our guts.**

Akkermansia Muciniphila

I need to introduce another bacteria, a microbe that my personal trainer Sam recently referred to as 'the slimmer's bacterial friend'. Akkermansia muciniphila can constitute as much as 5% of the bacterial colony in lean people, but can be completely absent in those who are obese. In May 2013, researchers at the Belgium University of Louvain concluded that this bacteria possessed an amazing ability to promote weight loss in humans.

How do we encourage akkermansia muciniphila to reside in our guts? We need to eat foods rich in oligofructose, which include onions, bananas, artichokes, garlic and chicory. Interestingly, these foods are also known to be prebiotic, and there are plenty of articles online that suggest oligofructose suppresses hunger and promotes fullness. I find these articles interesting because we arrive at the same result from two different perspectives. Through scientific research we learn that akkermansia muciniphila helps us lose weight, and reading articles on the internet we discover what food types individuals have found beneficial in losing weight. Here, both science and anecdotal experiences are pointing to the same variety of bacteria – 'the slimmer's bacterial friend' is akkermansia muciniphila.

MICROBIOME CONCLUSION

Us living in Great Britain, where antibiotics and antibacterial wipes are the norm, where packaged food is stripped of nutrients, are in danger of developing a microbiome depleted of so many species of microbes that the human body was designed upon. To restore the very foundation on which nature created the human body, we all need to take steps to rebuild and then maintain our microbiome.

Chapter 7 Highlights

- It will come as no surprise to you that one of the best ways to get our microbiome under control is to follow the principles laid out in Primal Cure.
- With such a diverse range of tasks and skills, many scientists regard the gut as the second most complex engine in our body, only surpassed by the brain.
- Over millions of years we have evolved together with microbes for mutual survival, yet recently this fine-tuning and selection has gone wrong.
- Eat as many organic vegetables and fermented foods as possible, and take a quality probiotic supplement.
- There are 100 trillion microscopic creatures living on and in our body.
- Three-quarters of the weight of our faeces is bacteria.
- There are more than 10,000 different species in the human microbiome.
- Our faeces is made up of more than 4,000 species.
- Individual bacteria cells live from a few days to a few weeks.
- Around 90% of illnesses can be traced back to the gut.
- We are 90% bacteria, fungi and microflora and only 10% human.
- 80% of our immune system is located in our gut.
- Microbes have thrived on our planet for more than 3.8 billion years.
- Firmicutes make us fat.
- As much as 90% of serotonin is created in the gut.
- Our guts contain about 1.5kg (3.3lbs) of bacteria.

08.
Vitamins, Minerals, Herbs, Supplements & Medicine

This chapter explores the essentials needed for good health and how they can be obtained either from our diet or supplements. Plus, we take a look at the limitations of modern medicine and why we shouldn't rely on drugs to fix us.

Did our Primal ancestors take supplements? Of course not. So, staying true to the Primal Cure principles of healthy living, we ideally wouldn't want to recommend them. However, even when we buy everything organic, eat very few processed foods, avoid the deadly CARBS, even when we are completely abstaining from added sugars and as best as we can avoiding toxins, our health is still at a slight disadvantage to our Primal ancestors. You see, they ate hundreds of different plants, bugs, insects and animals and, as the seasons changed, so too did their food options. Their diet was far more diverse than what we eat today. Their soils were not full of toxins and chemically produced pesticides and they were not breathing in pollutants.

Ideally, just as our Primal ancestors did, we want to get all of our nutrients from our food and not have to worry about the state of our microbiome. However, while our body has yet to evolve to be in sync with the world around us, so much has changed in Great Britain in terms of our food and our environment, that a life without supplements leaves many individuals lacking in various areas.

With so much of the nutritional value in our food being suppressed, we would have to eat copious amounts of some items just to satisfy our basic requirements. Even with some organic foods, the soil has been so badly depleted over the years, they aren't able to soak up as much nutrients through their roots as they have done historically.

> **PRIMAL CURE PRINCIPLE:**
> Eat as much organic and nutritionally loaded food as possible and then supplement to meet any dietary shortfalls.

INTRODUCTION TO VITAMINS AND MINERALS

As we already know, the vast majority of the food we eat is made up of three main macronutrients: CARBS, fats and protein. In terms of weight, the three headline acts make up more than 90%. You will know by now that, when we want to get our weight under control, the balance of these three ingredients is essential, and that after digestion our body converts all CARBS into sugar, most proteins into amino acids and fats into fatty acids.

On top of our fuel, it's also necessary to top up our engine with certain things that are going to make it run smoothly, efficiently and for as long as possible. You might see these as the oils in our engine or the additives they add to premium unleaded fuels. As BP say on their website about their finest fuel, 'A formulation designed to bust the dirt in your engine and restore performance'. Welcome to vitamins and minerals, the premium fuels for our body.

> **PRIMAL FACT:**
> **Vitamins are organic compounds made by plants, animals and us humans. In other words, vitamins are derived from living things. Minerals are inorganic, occurring naturally in water and soil.**

Let us first get a basic understanding of vitamins. Vitamins form in all living things from cows to humans, from grapes to broccoli. While not every organic compound found in plants and animals are essential in our diet, some are. When our body's health is negatively affected by a deficiency in an organic compound it is then labelled as a vitamin.

> **PRIMAL VITAMIN THOUGHT:**
> **All vitamins are considered essential for a healthy life and it's ironic that there are 13 of them. Maybe it's unlucky to miss by just one!.**

The 13 vitamins that are essential for the human body fall into two categories: either they are fat-soluble or water-soluble. Fat-soluble vitamins are A, D, E and K. I remember these with a mnemonic – 'A Drunken Elephant Kills'. Those that are soluble in water are all the B vitamins and vitamin C. These are easier to remember if you picture a stuttering news reporter struggling to announce their employer – 'BBBBC'. But why is it good to remember which are which? The answer is because, as A, D, E and K aren't soluble in water, the body is very good at storing these vitamins and therefore worrying about our precise daily consumption isn't necessary. For example, experts once measured sailors in a submarine and found that after 10 weeks below the ocean, their vitamin D level fell by 50%. However, vitamin C and all of the B vitamins dissolve in water, making them harder for our body to retain, and for this reason we should try to ensure that we consume them in our daily diet or through the use of supplements.

Vitamins, just like minerals, don't just work in isolation, but in partnerships too. Some vitamins need the presence of others to perform certain tasks, while others partner with minerals to get their job done. For example, we all know that calcium is good for our bones, but our body needs sufficient levels of vitamin D in order for our skeleton to make full use of it.

GOVERNMENT GUIDELINES FOR VITAMINS

Alongside all vitamins and minerals mentioned on the following pages you will find the official daily recommended amount that we should consume. But before you get brainwashed by governmental data, let me start by saying that all these guidelines are founded on the basis of deficiency. Set by a panel of EU nutritional experts, the recommended Nutritional Reference Values (NRVs) are said to represent the required intake levels of all vitamins and a selection of minerals to help prevent deficiencies in the vast majority of healthy people in Europe. But let me give an example of how you have to take them with a pinch of salt; how on earth can the minimum level of vitamin D be the same for someone who works outdoors in the south of Italy as an office worker in Great Britain?

> **UNDERSTANDING NRV AMOUNTS:**
> Mg = 1/1,000th of a gram (one thousandth of a gram)
> µg = 1/1,000,000 of a gram (one millionth of a gram)

When it comes to vitamins and minerals we should always consider the recommended Nutritional Reference Values (NRVs) like we do a minimum wage, it's kind of a safety net, an entry point, not necessarily the amount anyone would really desire. And as I have pointed out several times, we are all very different. We eat different diets, are different ages, experience different stresses and lifestyles. We all have different microbiomes and even everyday our own nutritional requirements will vary a little. The key thing to remember is this; almost all chronic illnesses are a result of a nutritional deficiency. Whether it be a short-term deficiency or one that has built up overtime, it is crucial for our well-being to understand that the key to our own health, happiness and longevity lies in fueling our body with sufficient nutrients, especially vitamins and minerals.

Let me introduce you to a new word and one that if more people knew it, would certainly halt our nation's decline into ill health. "Orthomolecular" medicine. The phrase was first coined in 1968 by American biochemist Linus Pauling and refers to an approach to health that involves not the use of drugs, but a focus on nutrition or as one Orthomolecular practitioner Dr Carl C. Pfeiffer says, "For every drug that benefits a patient, there is a natural substance that can achieve the same effect". And, whilst Cure might be in the title of this book, prevention by ensuring our bodies are properly fuelled with sufficient vitamins and minerals, is what we 100% recommend.

> **PRIMAL CURE BELIEF:**
> **The European Union NRVs are assembled around**
> **avoiding deficiency, not ultimate health.**

FAT-SOLUBLE VITAMINS
Vitamin A *(NRV 800 µg)*
Plays an important role in maintaining healthy vision (especially improving our sight in low light), neurological functions and our immune system, and helps maintain healthy bones.

It's found in lots of vegetables, especially kale, spinach and broccoli, and eggs are rich in it too. But one of the best sources is carrot. Yes, it's scientifically proven that carrots really do help us see in the dark.

Vitamin D *(NRV 5 μg)*

Plays a vital role in calcium absorption in our bones, helping to fend off osteoporosis. By boosting the immune system, amongst other things, vitamin D helps the body to defend against cancer and Alzheimer's. Getting plenty of sunlight is a great way for the body to synthesise vitamin D.

When it comes to food, we can find rich sources of vitamin D in oily fish such as tuna, mackerel and salmon, plus dairy products and eggs, are all useful secondary sources. Plus, most multi-vitamin tablets also contain a sufficient quantity.

When you think about how much vitamin D you personally need, try and compare your lifestyle to that of the caveman. How much time do you spend outdoors compared to the caveman leaving his cave?

Vitamin E *(NRV 12 Mg)*

A powerful antioxidant and plays a vital role in the body's fight against free radicals. Among many other things, vitamin E helps protect against Alzheimer's and high blood pressure. Our Superfood list is full of natural sources, the best being sunflower seeds, almonds and hazelnuts, and just one portion can surpass our daily needs. If you are not big on nuts and seeds, then a secondary source is greens such as broccoli and spinach and one the biggest superfruits of all – avocado.

Vitamin K *(NRV 75 μg)*

Plays a leading role in keeping our bones healthy. If we cut ourselves, the blood clotting self-defence mechanism that kicks in is courtesy of vitamin K. It also fights against cancer, and maintains a healthy heart. There are actually two types of vitamin K, simply called K1 and K2. K1 is found in vegetables such as kale; it is also one of the best sources with just half a cup providing more than 100% of our recommended daily intake. We also get vitamin K1 from broccoli, cabbage, spring onions and spinach. K2 is found in diary products, and a healthy microbiome will also synthesise K2.

WATER SOLUBLE VITAMINS
Vitamin C (NRV 80 Mg)

A powerful antioxidant with numerous health benefits including curtailing high blood pressure, protecting against gallbladder infections, and defending against both strokes and certain cancers. It's also great for keeping wrinkly skin at bay, as well as colds and the flu too. The only problem is that the body can neither create nor store it. Therefore, we must consume plenty of vitamin C on a daily basis.

The best source is the Indian fruit guava, where consuming just one provides six times the daily-recommended amount. The trouble is, in the UK it's hard to get hold of it anything other than a juice. Alternatively, a cup of blackcurrants or raw red peppers will provide three times our daily requirement, with a kiwi or a cup of raw green peppers doubling what we need. An orange, a cup of strawberries, a portion of broccoli, kale or Brussels sprouts will also suffice. Or a cupful of grapefruit or pineapple chunks would do nicely too.

All of the following either surpass or come very close to providing us with our daily requirement of vitamin C:

- 1 yellow bell pepper (5 x NRV)
- 1 red bell pepper (3 x NRV)
- 1 green bell pepper (2 x NRV)
- 1 kiwi
- 1 cup of broccoli
- 1 cup Brussels sprouts
- 1 cup of green peas
- 1 cup of cauliflower
- 1 orange
- 1 grapefruit
- 2 large tomatoes
- 2 cups of blackberries
- 2 cups of raspberries
- 5 large strawberries

However, there is a word of warning. I actually believe the daily recommendation for vitamins, especially vitamin C, is way understated for most people. While the recommendation is between 65–90mg per day, I personally feel that we need closer to 2,000mg (2 grams).

You will find a great speech by Dr Thomas Levy on YouTube, where he claims Vitamin C is the very best antioxidant of all. Also, in his bestselling book *Stop America's Number 1 Killer*, he claims that atherosclerosis (the build-up of plaque in the arteries) is preventable and even sometimes reversible through high dose vitamin C and that it is the lack of vitamin C that causes it. Put simply, Dr Thomas Levy believes the number one cause of heart disease is a lack of vitamin C.

Vitamin B

Vitamin Bs can be a little confusing as there are eight of them, but there is no B4, B8, B10 or B11. It's all to do with when they were discovered, and how some vitamins that were once thought to be one vitamin later turned out to be several different types. To avoid confusion, many in the scientific and medical community prefer to use names for B vitamins instead of numbers.

Vitamin B1 - Thiamine *(NRV 1.1 Mg)*

Boosts the immune system, and is believed to be great for cognitive functions, reducing both stress and memory loss. In January 2017, *The Independent* newspaper ran an article with the headline, "A diet rich in thiamine can reduce your risk of getting Alzheimer's disease, but some groups, such as the elderly, aren't getting enough". Levels of vitamin B1 are often deficient in individuals who consume too much alcohol, as it blocks its absorption. Vegetables, meat, fish, seeds and nuts are all good sources of thiamine.

Vitamin B2 - Riboflavin *(NRV 1.4 Mg)*

Like several other B vitamins, B2 works alongside other coenzymes to help us extract nutrients from protein and carbohydrates. It is yet another vitamin that acts as a powerful antioxidant, and as we age it can prevent cracks from appearing around the mouth and nose, as well as counteract depression and sore throats. Food rich in B2 include meats and poultry (especially organs such as chicken liver), seaweed, shellfish, cheese, yogurt, eggs and green vegetables such as broccoli and spinach, as well as nuts and seeds.

Vitamin B3 - Niacin *(NRV 16 Mg)*

B3 is one of the most powerful vitamins of all and plays a role in over 500 different reactions in the human body. It helps to maintain a healthy cardiovascular system, as well as balancing blood cholesterol levels. As we age, it helps with cognitive functions and joint mobility, as well as preventing the skin from drying out. The best sources are chicken, beef, lamb and fishes such as tuna, sardines and salmon.

There is a great book called *Niacin: The Real Story*, where the authors talk about using large doses of niacin to cure a whole range of children's learning and behavioural disorders. It's a must read for anyone with a family member suffering from ADHD, after all Dr Lendon H Smith believes that, "ADHD is not a disease; it is a nutritional deficiency".

Niacin was almost worshipped by the founder of Alcoholics Anonymous (AA) Bill Wilson, who used mega doses (orthomolecular medicine) to cure many of his patients of their addiction.

Vitamin B5 - Pantothenic Acid *(NRV 6 Mg)*

Plays an important role in extracting valuable nutrients from food, and a critical role in maintaining the health of our nervous system. As the vitamin is found in lots of fresh foods, its name is derived from Greek – 'pantos' meaning 'everywhere'. However, it is easily lost during processing, so if we eat only packaged foods, beware. Avocado, sunflower seeds, beef, duck, chicken (especially its organs), salmon, mushrooms, eggs, kale, broccoli and yogurt are all rich sources of pantothenic acid.

Vitamin B6 - Pyridoxine *(NRV 1.4 Mg)*

Instrumental in producing the happiness neurotransmitter serotonin. It plays an important role in removing excessive homocystine (a form of amino acid) from our blood after eating meat. Some researchers therefore suggest it is as important to monitor our pyridoxine levels as it is cholesterol. Just like vitamin B1, individuals that consume too much alcohol can often suffer from pyridoxine deficiency. Good sources include vegetables such as carrots, spinach, meat and poultry (especially turkey and organs such as liver), fish, milk, cheese, nuts and seeds, avocado and eggs.

Vitamin B7 - Biotin *(NRV 50 µg)*

Often referred to as the beauty vitamin, as it thickens hair, nails and beautifies skin. So much so, you are likely to find biotin added to many beauty products in your bathroom cabinet. There are, in fact, eight different types of biotin, but only one is natural with all seven others being synthesised. Don't believe any company who tells you that the synthetics are just as good.

Marketeers who talk of vitamin H (for hair) or vitamin 8 are normally referring to synthetic versions of biotin. Vitamin B7 works as a coenzyme with other vitamin Bs to metabolise all three macronutrients. Sources include liver from both meat and poultry, eggs, salmon, nuts, cheese, avocado and berries.

Vitamin B9 - Folate *(NRV 200 µg)*

Plays a leading role in producing and repairing damaged cells, as well as supporting nerve and immune functions. It is said to prevent both cancer and cognitive decline. Some experts say that, in sufficient quantities, it delays or even prevents the onset of grey hair... I wish I had known this a few years ago, so I could have avoided my silver highlights! People who consume too much alcohol are often deficient in vitamin B9. Liver, vegetables such as spinach, asparagus, broccoli, Brussels sprouts and fruits (especially mango, avocado and oranges) are rich in folate.

Vitamin B12 - Cobalamin *(NRV 2.5 µg)*

Plays a major role in creating new red blood cells (preventing anaemia), and maintaining the nervous system. It also helps vitamin B6 in controlling homocystine, and is said to influence many parts of our health including energy levels, mood, digestion and cognitive functions. It's a unique vitamin that contains a mineral, and it's also the only one that's not found in plants. The best source for vitamin B12 is to get our gut in order and have bacteria produce it for us, but food sources include liver from cows and chickens, fish such as salmon, mackerel, sardines, tuna and trout, plus dairy products such as yogurt and milk.

B12 also highlights another flaw in the subject of NRVs, because as we age, our bodies get less efficient at processing this vitamin, resulting in the need for a higher daily intake.

VITAMIN SUMMARY

I don't expect you to memorise any of the above, and to be quite frank it would be pretty much a waste of time if you did. But if you scan back through them, you will notice how so many food types appear time after time. This is one of the ways that we designed our Superfood list. For example, look how many different vitamins olives, green vegetables, offal, avocados, nuts and seeds contain. Compare these to fast foods and packaged foods and the difference is chalk and cheese!

Also, fresh fruits and vegetables are often richer in vitamins than those that are approaching their sell-by dates, and the more raw, uncooked vegetables we can eat the better. When it comes to cooking them, those that are quickly stir-fried or briefly steamed will often retain more vitamins and healthy nutrients than those that are cooked slowly, or overheated. And for frozen foods, as they are often packed and frozen very quickly after picking, they can in some instances provide a richer source than those found in the fruit and vegetable aisle in the supermarket.

Dr Dan Maggs

"Avoid crap foods void of nutrition and live longer and happier with natural foods full of vitamins and minerals."

MARVELLOUS MINERALS

If we were playing the 20-question game, where the first question is animal, vegetable or mineral, virtually everything you will ever eat will fall into the first two categories. Minerals are not naturally found in animals or plants, and only climb on-board the food we consume through water and soil. The soil of our Primal ancestors, food was rich in minerals, and their water was quite simply mineral water. With the Earth's crust historically providing such a rich layer of diverse minerals, plants absorbed them en masse through their roots, in turn themselves becoming part plant, part mineral. Then, when animals ate the mineral-loaded plants, they too became part mineral.

Being so incredibly clever, nature decided that if plants and animals were constantly consuming minerals, and then in due course so were us humans, it made sense to put them to good use and incorporate them in a multitude of bodily tasks and functions. Over millennia, these minerals have literally become integral to our well-being, but sadly, like all good things, they have pretty much come to an end. Over recent generations we have damaged our soil so badly that plants no longer find abundant minerals to absorb, therefore animals lack them in their diet, and as we humans are 'what we eat - eats', we too have become very lacking in minerals.

As the definition of a minerals is 'a solid, naturally occurring inorganic substance', another way we might want to picture them in our diet is as a foundation. In the same way that houses are always built on a solid foundation, so our diet should be too. See minerals as building blocks for the body. They help construct healthy bones and teeth. They participate in producing muscles, skin, hair and blood, and are an essential tool in the metabolic process.

Depending on what definition we apply to nutrients, there are between 40 to 70 of them that are essential to our health and that we must ingest frequently. But, as over the past few generations we have completely ruined our soil with chemicals and pesticides, very little is available to be absorbed by today's plants. This is another reason why more than ever, we need to get a diverse healthy diet. Let's say one vegetable contains 10 minerals that the body needs, that leaves some 30 to 60 that are missing. The answer is to eat a wide and varied diet of natural organic food, just as our Primal ancestors did and to also take a quality multi-vitamin and mineral tablet.

Just like we separate vitamins into two separate groups – water-soluble or fat-soluble – we are going to do the same with minerals. Some we need in big measures, normally milligrams (mg), as these are the building blocks on which some bodily functions are cemented, while others we only need tiny trace elements.

Calcium *(NRV 800 Mg)*
Helps build strong bones and healthy teeth. In fact, our skeleton and teeth contain about 1.5kg (3lbs) of calcium, and for this reason we need to make sure we keep our levels regularly topped up. It is also used by our nerve cells to communicate with one another, and for keeping our muscles nice and flexible. It's believed that calcium helps us to fight off certain cancers, in particular colon cancer. And for those looking to shed a little weight, calcium is a definite fat buster. You will notice in the chart that the US recommendation suggests that we consume more calcium while we are young, when our bones are growing. While there are several cases to be made against milk, it certainly packs a punch when it comes to calcium, with one pint of whole milk containing around 85% of the NHS's recommend daily intake.

Our mothers were correct that milk is a rich source of calcium, but so too are other dairy products such as yogurt and cheese. Leafy greens such as broccoli and cabbage (but for once we can't rely on spinach)

also contain it, as well as some nuts and seeds and small fish such as
sardines, pilchards and white bait when we consume the bones.

> **PRIMAL SUNSHINE REMINDER:**
> Remember back to the section on sunbathing, for the body to
> properly absorb calcium we need vitamin D. Therefore it's pointless
> getting our kids to drink a daily pint of organic whole milk, only to
> then let them sit indoors playing computer games.

Phosphorus *(NRV 700 Mg)*

Has very similar properties to calcium, and is used by the body to
build and maintain healthy bones and teeth. Phosphorus is also a
messenger between cells, carrying vital information from one to
another about our DNA. If we don't have sufficient phosphorus in our
system, we might become somebody totally different! Okay, that might
be a bit far-fetched, but hopefully you get the message. Phosphorus
also prevents our body from becoming too acidic or alkaline (it
balances our pH levels). Red meat, dairy produce, fish, poultry, nuts
and seeds are rich in phosphorus and therefore it is rare for someone
to become deficient.

Magnesium *(NRV 375 Mg)*

One of the most important minerals, essential for our well-being,
and is required by more than 300 biochemical reactions in the body.
Magnesium plays a leading role in regulating our body temperature,
detoxification, formation and maintenance of healthy bones, blood
glucose control, regulation of blood pressure and much more.
Researchers in America found that approximately 75% of people
tested were deficient in magnesium, and this is a real health issue.
Being deficient in a mineral that is critical for us to function properly
can lead to an onslaught of illnesses, especially as we age. In her
bestselling book *The Magnesium Miracle*, author Dr Carolyn Dean
quotes 56 conditions that are associated with magnesium deficiency,
including acid reflux, Alzheimer's disease, angina, anxiety and panic

attacks, arthritis, asthma, blood clots, bowel disease, depression, diabetes, heart diseases, hypertension, indigestion, inflammation, insomnia, kidney stones, migraines, osteoporosis, Parkinson's disease, tooth decay and more. I believe so much in the curing powers of magnesium that I am going to dive into a little more detail.

Magnesium May Reverse Osteoporosis
Numerous research studies have concluded that calcium supplemented with magnesium improves bone mineral density. So much so that many women in the USA who are susceptible to the disease take magnesium supplements as a preservative measure.

Magnesium As A Treatment For Diabetes
Magnesium aids in the metabolism of CARBS which helps control blood glucose levels.

Magnesium Treats Headaches And Migraines
For those who suffer from frequent headaches or migraines, increasing your intake of magnesium might prove more effective in the long term than taking painkillers.

Taking Magnesium Before Bedtime
Can help you get a good night's sleep and can even help those suffering from insomnia.

Magnesium Prevents Cardiovascular Diseases
Magnesium has been demonstrated to lower the risk of coronary heart disease.

Now that you are aware of how beneficial magnesium can be, take a look at the NRV recommendations by the EU. As you can see these are quite high, but in my opinion still very conservative. Let's look at the types of food that we can find magnesium in, and how much we would need to consume.

Magnesium Rich Foods	Milligrams (mg) per serving	Percentage of NRV
Almonds, dry roasted, 28g (1oz)	80	20%
Spinach, boiled, ½ cup	78	20%
Cashews, dry roasted, 28g (1oz)	74	19%
Peanuts, oil roasted, ¼ cup	63	16%
Black beans, cooked, ½ cup	60	15%
Edamame, shelled, cooked, ½ cup	50	13%
Peanut butter, smooth, 2 tbsp	49	12%
Avocado, cubed, 1 cup	44	11%
Potato, baked with skin, 99g (3.5oz)	43	11%
Rice, brown, cooked, ½ cup	42	11%
Yogurt, plain, low fat, 227g (8oz)	42	11%

As you can see, it's pretty difficult to consume enough magnesium through food alone. I will cover this in more detail later.

Iron (NRV 14 Mg)
Works alongside the two proteins, haemoglobin and myoglobin, which transport oxygen via the blood to our cells. The human body finds it easier to absorb iron from animals than it does from plants. Liver, meat, nuts, seeds, eggs and leafy greens such as watercress and curly kale are all rich in iron.

Zinc (NRV 10 Mg)
Plays a role in creating new cells, hormones and enzymes. It also aids the metabolism of all three macronutrients. It's a vital mineral, and our body is better at absorbing it from meat and shellfish than from plants. That said, leafy greens are a reasonable secondary source.

Fluoride (NRV 3.5 Mg)
Not to be confused with fluorine, which is poisonous. A small amount

of fluoride is good for our teeth, and possibly our bones too. It's commonly found in toothpaste and in drinking water, and you can always top your level up with avocado and strawberries. We don't require much of it, and as a result the NHS don't detail any daily recommendations for our consumption, however in America they do.

TRACE MINERALS

Let's now turn our attention to some of the trace minerals that we should ensure are in our diet. While the doses we need are minimal, they are just as vital to our well-being as they are to making emeralds green and rubies red! Again, in the chart I have listed them from left to right in descending order of the amount we should consume.

Manganese (NRV 2 Mg)

Helps both create and activate several enzymes, and therefore most of it resides in our glands - with a smaller amount located in our bones. Tea is a rich source of manganese, as well as nuts, seeds, offal and some green vegetables such as peas and runner beans.

Copper (NRV 1,000 µg)

Used in the production of both white and red blood cells, and acts as a trigger to release iron to form haemoglobin - the protein that carries oxygen in blood cells. Copper also reduces free radicals, and can help defend the body against certain infections. Offal, nuts, tea and coffee, dark chocolate, most green vegetables and shellfish all contain copper. As we only need a small trace amount, Primal diets are rich enough not to overly concern ourselves with it.

Iodine (NRV 150 µg)

Contributes to the creation of thyroid hormones. It also helps rebuild and repair bones, as well as supporting a healthy nervous system. Good sources include fish, shellfish and seaweed. Iodine used to also be found in vegetables, but sadly today most soil is depleted. Not that I am promoting non-organic milk, but if you were ever tempted by it then you would also receive iodine, zinc and selenium from it. But please don't drink it! Instead get these three minerals elsewhere.

Selenium *(NRV 55 µg)*

Prevents damage to cells and tissue, and helps the immune system work properly. Researchers have also suggested that it helps prevent cancer and other diseases including heart failure. Sources include nuts (especially Brazil nuts), meat (especially organs), fish and eggs. In some countries, you can get selenium from vegetables, but in the UK our soil is now so poor that this is no longer likely.

Molybdenum *(NRV 50 µg)*

Pronounced 'molib-dunum', it helps create and then activate some enzymes. Sources include green vegetables like broccoli and spinach, cauliflower, nuts and seeds, beans, legumes and yoghurt.

Chromium *(NRV 40 µg)*

Influences how insulin behaves in the body, affecting the amount of energy we absorb from food. Good sources include meat, green vegetables (especially broccoli), nuts and seeds and various spices.

THE SIX ELECTROLYTES

While it might sound like a band name, electrolytes are a group of nutrients that produce an electrically conducting solution when dissolved in our body. In harmony, they perform many vital tasks in our body. Nutritionist and Primal living expert Nate Morrow says, "Your body is a complex and carefully-balanced superhighway of cells, tissues and fluids that, almost every second, directs an incomprehensible array of electrical impulses. This is only possible because those cells, tissues and fluids thrive in a homeostatic [a condition of balance or equilibrium] environment where they conduct electricity well enough to carry the signals to their intended destinations. The key to maintaining this conductive superhighway lies with our friend the electrolyte".

The name electrolyte is derived from the fact that they effectively carry an electrical current around our body. They regulate our heartbeat, enabling our muscles to properly contract in order for us to move. Electrolytes are essential for all of our cells and organs, and maintaining a healthy balance of them is critical. The core six electrolytes are sodium, potassium and chloride, plus calcium, phosphorus and magnesium, which we have just discussed.

Balancing our electrolytes can greatly improve our health, but be aware that if they are way out of balance they can actually kill us. What throws our electrolytes off balance? Dehydration, especially as a result of illness or excessive exercise without fluid intake, is the biggest cause. When we have diarrhoea or are sweating profusely, it's crucial that we up our intake of both water and electrolytes. Other causes of electrolyte imbalances include excessive urinating (caused by various infections), drinking too much alcohol or, believe it or not, even drinking too much water, poor diets and over-exercising.

As we age, we become more susceptible to both dehydration and overhydration, and therefore more prone to abnormal electrolyte levels. This is largely because our kidneys do not work as efficiently as when we were younger. Electrolyte imbalances can cause irregular heartbeats, twitching and muscle spasms, changes in blood pressure, confusion, seizures, numbness, headaches, fever, trouble sleeping, anxiety, weakness and fatigue, joint pain and dizziness, plus various nervous system disorders.

So how do we keep our electrolytes in balance? As we have already discussed, we would be wise to ensure we consume appropriate amounts of calcium, phosphorus and magnesium. In addition, we must consider the level of sodium, chloride and potassium that is in our diet.

Sodium, Chloride & Potassium

Salt that we sprinkle on our food is made of sodium chloride. Most people who eat packaged food and fast food will likely have too much sodium and chloride in their diet, and therefore their electrolyte balance might be compromised. The NHS report that the average British citizen eats double their daily recommendation. When we live Primally, our healthy diet and exercise routine might mean that we occasionally need to add a little to our food to top up our intake. The governmental daily-recommended amount for sodium is 1,600mg (1.6g) and for chloride it is 2,500mg (2.5g). If you add the two together it equates to about 4g of salt.

Potassium is found in various foods, and while it is recommended that we consume 3,500mg per day (3.5g), it's normally quite easy to do when we are eating Primally. Fruit (especially bananas), vegetables such as broccoli, parsnips and Brussels sprouts, nuts and seeds, beef, chicken, turkey and fish are all good sources.

HERBS & SPICES

Herbs and spices have been used for centuries as medicines in cultures from Asia to the Native Americans, from Southern Europe to the Aztecs. While, for thousands of years, herbal practitioners had no idea why or how herbs worked, they became extremely successful at identifying the right herb for the right aliment through trial and error. More than 2,000 years ago, to reduce fevers and inflammation in his patients, Hippocrates used to offer bark from the willow tree, and instruct sufferers to chew on it. Then in 1897, the German pharmaceutical company, Bayer, developed a branded tablet called Aspirin from the very same bark. In fact, most pioneering Western pharmaceutical companies created their pills by extracting nutrients from herbs. Even today, more than 100 well-known pills, medicines and tablets still base their remedies on plant extracts. While Aspirin no longer comes from willow bark (it's now synthetic), codeine and morphine are still made from opium poppy seeds.

Today, the industrialisation of both isolating and then mechanically extracting micronutrients from herbs and spices happens en masse.

However, it is so commercialised that it's hard to believe that anything other than very little of nature's remedies reside in the final product. At Primal Cure, we passionately believe that the balance of nutrients and the power of the remedy is far better when consumed the way nature intended. Today, I believe, we are so brainwashed by pharmaceutical propaganda and misinformed doctors that we are more likely to pop a pill containing extracts from a herb than actually consume the fresh herb or spice as intended and supplied by Mother Nature.

But let's return to herbs and spices as a prevention rather than a cure. What I love about using them in my cooking is that they add flavour to just about anything. And flavour is really important. As we start living Primally, there will undoubtedly be the odd occasion when we are going to miss our fast food or sugar-rich snacks. While it is okay now and again to fall off the wagon and have whatever we want (remember we are not promoting a diet but a lifestyle change), ideally the more times we can stay true to what we were designed to eat, the healthier we will ultimately be. I recommend you experiment with as many herbs and spices as you can get your hands on. Even better still, get out in the garden and grow your own. There is no more a satisfying meal than one where we know the flavour was created in our own backyard.

Plus, when we are trying to encourage our family and friends into a Primal way of living, tantalising their taste buds with herbs and spices makes it easy in helping them convert to our healthier lifestyle. And for those that you know who pop too many over-the-counter pills, as you read through the following pages you will be able to amass enough knowledge to be able to advise them to close the door on their medical cabinet, and instead plant their way back to good health.

PRIMAL HERBS:
The stronger the aroma and the more pungent the taste, the denser are both their nutrients and curing properties.

Let's look in detail at three truly supernatural herbs – ginger, turmeric and cacao – and then list other magically healthy herbs and spices.

Ginger

This miracle root vegetable is brilliant for curing sickness and digestive problems. In 2008, when I crossed the Atlantic with my family in a small sailing boat, we didn't know about the natural stomach-calming effect of ginger and instead relied on a barrage of tablets to prevent seasickness. The effectiveness of those man-made pills was very questionable indeed. But today, when feeling a bit sickly, whether it be travel sickness or anything else, the entire family opens the fridge and pulls out fresh ginger. While my eldest son and I love the strong taste and are happy just to chew on a small chunk, my younger children prefer to put ginger in the blender with a load of berries and yogurt.

A study carried out at the University of Georgia found that taking ginger supplements after exercise greatly reduced muscle soreness. Ginger is also known to reduce pain far more effectively than many pain killers, and is especially efficient at reducing discomfort during the menstrual cycle.

> ### ▶ Did You Know?
>
> Even more beneficial to our health than ginger's rapid action for sickness and pain is its ability to prevent inflammation. It contains a host of anti-inflammatory and antioxidants such as gingerols, capsaicin, caffeic acid, curcumin and salicylate. Ginger is also a rich source of vitamin B6, vitamin C, potassium, magnesium, phosphorus and folate. The BBC's website bbcgoodfood.com suggests, "The many curative properties of ginger are widely researched. Used on the skin it can stimulate the circulation and soothe burns. As a diaphoretic it encourages perspiration, so it can be used in feverish conditions such as influenza or colds".

Tumeric

Turmeric is one of the most powerful natural medicines we can add to our food. Just as fatty fish offers the finest source of Omega 3 and yellow bell peppers are the ultimate provider of vitamin C, turmeric is the richest source of the antioxidant substance curcumin. It's so beneficial for our health that I have written a far bigger article on it under supplements. I personally love to cook lots of dishes with this heaven-sent spice, but at the same time I still take a daily supplement to make sure I am not missing out on the goodness that it packs. After all, the spice is said to reduce the risk of prostate and skin cancer, brain tumours, leukemia, multiple sclerosis and depression. It's a natural painkiller that, for aches and pains in certain parts of the body, is said to be as effective as ibuprofen. And while I am a big believer that most research is misleading, as correlation rarely proves causation, I do believe turmeric is part of the reason why in India, where it is consumed by millions, Alzheimer's and Parkinson's is extremely uncommon.

Cacao

Keep a jar of raw unroasted cacao (pronounced 'ca-cow') powder in your Primal pantry and, whenever you need to make some sweet desserts for friends, you will be able to fool them that your chocolate-looking dish is no different to the regular sugar-infused milk chocolate they consume. But of course there is a difference - a huge difference.

Cacao powder is produced by cold-pressing unroasted cocoa beans from the cacao tree. Unlike regular cocoa powder, which is roasted at high temperatures, by keeping the temperature cool the process preserves living enzymes. The rawest of all chocolates, cacao contains more than 250 different nutritional ingredients, making it possibly the best source of antioxidants from plants on the planet! Rich in polyphenols, it even has more than a dozen times more antioxidants than the superfruit blueberries. No wonder the Aztecs used cocoa beans as a currency.

> **Always check that what you buy is raw and organic. You can normally tell as it has a slightly lighter colour than roasted cocoa.**

You may have noticed how most herbs have similar health benefits. That's great news because, unless we are looking for a specific cure or remedy, then all we need to remember is it that the more we can indulge in organic herbs, especially those that are home-grown, the more Primal we will be living and therefore the healthier we are likely to become.

SUPPLEMENTS

There are numerous different approaches to supplementing our food intake with vitamins and extracts. Some experts recommend taking loads and loads of pills, while there are others that don't believe in supplements at all. As you might expect, I don't believe that one approach fits all. For example, if you regularly go on holiday and also eat lots of oily fish, nuts and seeds, then there might be no need to take vitamin D tablets. However, if you rarely reveal your body to the sun, and don't receive sufficient amounts of vitamin D in your diet, then you most definitely would be wise to take it in the form of a supplement. And Public Health England have recently recommended us Brits take a Vitamin D supplement throughout the autumn and winter months, as we can pretty much guarantee living in this beautiful country unfortunately means we won't be getting enough vitamin D levels. Another example would be if someone eats chicken and eggs straight after a workout, then there would be little need for an additional protein shake.

When it comes to vitamins, other than water-soluble vitamin C and all of the Bs, as long as say over a 10-day period we ingest roughly 10 times the recommended daily amount, then the aggregation will be fine. Sunbathing is a great example. A one-week holiday in the sun with careful exposure can help our body accumulate enough vitamin D for several months.

> **PRIMAL CURE SUPPLEMENT PRINCIPLE:**
> **Eat foods rich in nutrients and fill any nutritional or vitamin**
> **shortfalls with reputable supplements.**

Everyone is different, so when it comes to supplements, without knowing you personally, it's difficult for me to recommend exactly which ones you should make part of your daily life. If you have both the time and the cash, you can go and have your blood and even your poo profiled. But, for most people just making an educated guess about what is right will be enough to help booster your well-being and longevity. And remember, what we are talking about here is not drugs, nor medication, but nutrition.

But aren't supplements dangerous, especially if I take too many? Interestingly, the American Association of Poisonous Control Centre, an organisation that monitors the causes of death each year in the USA, state that over the last 35 years of keeping records, there have been just 13 allegations that vitamins were a cause of death, yet not one of them was ever substantiated. Furthermore, Canadian biochemist Abram Hoffer, said flatly, "Nobody dies from vitamins". Contrast that with prescribed drugs, which many experts believe to now be the third largest cause of death after cancer and heart disease. I am not for one minute belittling prescribed medication, because in many instances they prolong life, I am just trying to highlight as powerfully as possible, that vitamins and minerals are simply good nutrition, but just in a different form. Let me summarise the use of supplements with three thoughts.

1. "For every drug that benefits a patient, there is a natural substance that can achieve the same effect". **Dr Carl C Peeiffer.** Whilst I don't believe this is always the case post diagnosis, I do believe that nearly all westernised illnesses are caused in the main by poor nutrition.
2. Nutritional based medicine (Orthomolecular medicine –meaning normal) is non-toxic whereas pharmaceutical medicine in the

main tends to be toxic (toxi-molecular).

3. Even though natural, herbal, nutritional medicine has been
    around since antiquity, as you can't patent a vitamin or a mineral,
    huge corporations don't get behind them.

Supplements Taken By The Author

For all the adults in my family and to all my friends, I always
recommend that they take the following five as a base; a multivitamin,
omega 3, turmeric, magnesium and a strong probiotic. To me even
without analysing their current diet, these are a no-brainer. To provide
you with a further example of what supplements you might want
to take, I will now explain both what I personally take and the logic
behind my selection. Some might not be necessary for you and there
might many others that you as an individual would benefit from
taking. But hopefully it will show you my thought process and act as a
catalyst to help you plan your supplementation. I religiously take nine
daily supplements:

1. Omega 3
2. Turmeric
3. Magnesium
4. Probiotics
5. Coenzyme Q10
6. Combined multi-mineral and multi-vitamin tablet
7. Vitamin C (2g)
8. Glucomannan & Inulin (SlimShotz)
9. Psyllium husk

Omega 3

Our caveman ancestor had a diet rich in Omega 3. He loved eating
whole animals, especially Omega 3-rich brains! He didn't face
the problem of factory manufactured beef, sourced from corn-
fed antibiotic-injected cattle, with its resulting Omega 3:6 balance
artificially adjusted from a healthy 1:1 ration to a noxious 1:7 ratio.

If every night you eat oily fish such as salmon, mackerel, anchovies and sardines and then consume a pack of walnuts as your daily snack, then you might be one of the exceptional few who don't need to take Omega 3 supplements. If you're not a fishy person, then taking Omega 3 will almost definitely improve your health. I personally eat loads of oily fish and love nuts, but still take an organic cold-water sourced Omega 3 capsules every morning. For me, Omega 3 is a must-have supplement.

If you don't want to take a supplement derived from fish, then flaxseed oil makes a perfectly good substitute.

▶ Scientific Stuff

There are three different types of Omega 3 (which is not related to the fact it is called Omega 3). They are alpha-linolenic acid (ALA), eicosapentaenoic acid (EPA) and docosahexaenoic acid (DHA). ALA is primarily sourced from plants, such as seeds and nuts. When animals such as cows, fish and us humans consume ALA, we convert some of it into EPA and DHA. Oily fish like salmon convert it best. EPA and DHA are the two types of Omega 3 fatty acids that are the most superior for our health. While the human body can convert a certain amount of ALA into EPA and DHA, it's not super-efficient at doing so. It is for this reason, even though we might consume enough Omega 3 by eating plenty of nuts and seeds, that we still need our oily fish or algae supplements to directly deliver EPA and DHA.

But why is it so important for our health? Omega 3, particularly those rich in docosahexaenoic acid (DHA), is quite simply food for the brain. In fact, one of the key components in the brain is docosahexaenoic acid, and for those of us who were breastfed, our mother's milk was loaded with it. It's not just about prevention either, in some instances Omega 3 can cure certain brain disorders! But surely this can't be true, because aren't we

> supposed to be stuck with the same brain cells throughout our entire life? Recent scientific research has turned this belief on its head. It now appears that we can grow new brain cells on a daily basis through a process known as neurogenesis. The area where neurogenesis is most effective is the hippocampus. This is the area of the brain that is responsible for storing long-term memories and learning new things. Therefore Omega 3 could make us even smarter than we already are!

I could list dozens and dozens of other amazing health benefits we receive from taking a quality Omega 3 supplement daily, but I would just be diluting this one very important advantage: It is an essential fuel for an active brain.

When it comes to selecting the right Omega 3 supplement, it's time to become a quality fanatic. While most softgel Omega 3 capsules on the market today are 1,000mg (1 gram), the concentration of the good stuff, EPA and DHA, can sometimes be woefully low. It always pays to check the labels when buying supplements. With Omega 3, there is also a danger of the supplement originating from highly toxic fish, full of mercury and other potentially harmful metals.

Turmeric/Curcumin

From the same family as ginger, turmeric is a brilliant anti-inflammatory herb that can either be consumed as a supplement, or used to spice up your food. While tablets and supplement manufacturers often claim their products are 10 to 100 times more potent than you would put in your homemade curry, if you are not a big fan of taking too many supplements, then heaping it on your chicken or beef is still very beneficial.

Supplements are made up of a compound found in turmeric called curcumin and not turmeric itself. There are more than 5,000 medical articles and pieces of research online, many claiming turmeric to be the most powerful herb on the planet. The benefits of turmeric could fill an entire book (many books actually – Amazon alone has 301 books with Turmeric in their title). Let's look at some of the main benefits of this incredible herb:

- Reduces chronic joint pain
- Reduces the pain of arthritis
- Can boost low energy levels
- If you mix with raw honey you can create a facemask to treat acne
- It can slow and even prevent blood clotting (for those that suffer side effects from Ibuprofen, curcumin is a godsend)
- In 2009, Auburn University of Alabama published a report that explored how taking turmeric supplements can help reverse type 2 diabetes
- It is a powerful anti-inflammatory and a very strong antioxidant
- It helps decrease memory loss
- Medical studies have demonstrated that it helps to prevent certain cancers

Magnesium

I personally love nuts, seeds, spinach, avocado and many other foods that are rich in magnesium and I consume them regularly. That said, I still don't feel that I regularly eat the 500 to 600mg that I believe I need. Why am I saying 500 to 600mg if the recommended daily allowance for my age, as suggested in the earlier chart, indicates 420mg? The more active we are, and the more we exercise, the quicker we deplete our mineral stores. With magnesium's benefits to health being so vast, I take a supplement every day. For those who don't like taking them, you can always buy bath salts rich in magnesium and, in addition to all of the other long-term benefits, your muscles will become relaxed, especially after exercising.

As magnesium helps us get a better night's sleep, it's the one supplement I like to consume just before I go to bed. To ensure I don't forget to take it, I store it in my bathroom next to my toothbrush, and not in the kitchen.

You can get magnesium tablets on their own or combined with other minerals and vitamins (especially calcium, vitamin D and vitamin K). Because I have had kidney stones in the past, I am conscious that I must not overdo my calcium intake. So I have two different magnesium choices in my bathroom. If, during the day, I have had either cheese or a probiotic yogurt, then I take my evening magnesium on its own. If, however, I haven't eaten foods rich in calcium during the day, then I take a combined magnesium and calcium supplement.

If you are unsure of whether you are getting enough magnesium, calcium and zinc in your diet, consider that, in 2005, The American Journal of Clinical Nutrition stated that 73.3% of Americans were not meeting the daily RDA of zinc, 65.1% were deficient in calcium and 61.6% were not consuming enough magnesium.

Probiotics

Once you have started eating fermented foods in your weekly routine, if you feel the need to take a probiotic supplement, then in his book *Brain Maker*, author Dr David Perlmutter suggests that it's advisable to purchase probiotics that contain the following helpful bacteria: Lactobacillus plantarum, Lactobacillus acidophilus, Lactobacillus brevis, Bifidobacterium lactis and Bifidobacterium longum.

Some brands claim their products contain thousands of different bacteria, but my concern with these is that the more they contain, the smaller the dose of each one. Aim for brands that contain 10 to 20 different strands, and if they contain all five recommended by Dr David Perlmutter, all the better. Make sure you don't wash these down with unfiltered tap water, or there is every chance that the chlorine in the water will kill off the helpful bacteria before they arrive in the gut!

Coenzyme Q10

This is the preferred food source for our mitochondria and our heart too. Our Primal ancestors ingested lots of it when they consumed entire animals, as coenzyme Q10 is found primarily in the heart, kidneys and liver. Smaller doses can be found in sardines, mackerel and peanuts and even smaller amounts in vegetables such as spinach, cauliflower and broccoli.

Our body naturally creates a certain amount of coenzyme and for this reason it is not considered a vitamin. However, we get less and less efficient at producing it as we age, and therefore can't provide our hearts and cells with the amount they need to stay healthy.

Therefore, if you're not a big organ/offal eater, and you are more than 40 years of age, you might need to consume this in the form of a supplement. There is no NRV for coenzyme Q10, and I guess this is because it's difficult to identify how much of it our body produces naturally. Dr Jonny Bowden, in his book *The Most Effective Natural Cures on Earth*, suggests that once we pass the age of 40, we should consume at least 60 to 100mg daily. And for those with a family history of heart disease, or those with high blood pressure or high cholesterol, he recommends taking between 100 and 300mg daily.

The US National Library of Medicine suggests that coenzyme Q10 supplements may be useful in the treatment of high blood pressure, muscular dystrophy, heart failure, Parkinson's disease, migraines, certain mitochondrial disorders and HIV/AIDS. However, don't take coenzyme Q10 supplements if you are pregnant or less than 18 years old. In a nutshell, coenzyme Q10:

- Reduces blood pressure
- Is good for the heart
- Energises our cells
- Acts as a powerful antioxidant

In Japan, to reduce both heart disease and high blood pressure, approximately 10% of the population are reported to be talking Q10 medication on the advice of their doctors or medical professionals. If you are stressed or take statins, then you almost definitely would benefit from taking coenzyme Q10.

Combined Multi-Mineral & Multi-Vitamin Tablet

While I always try to eat as healthily as possible, I don't want to risk falling short on any of the minerals our body relies on to function. So for the past two years, I have started to take a combined multi-mineral and multi-vitamin tablet that has been specifically formulated for men over 50. For females out there, don't worry – there are plenty of different options for you too. Why are age-specific multivitamins a better choice? Because as we age, we absorb and process certain vitamins differently and therefore it is necessary to alter the dosages.

Vitamin C

I take one effervescent vitamin C tablet in the morning and use the drink to help take my other supplements. I then have one in the afternoon. As the EU upper tolerance is set at 2grams, that's all I should really recommend. That said, the reality is that I take a lot more. How about this as an interesting fact... According to Dr Suzanne Humphries, a cow makes around 12 grams of vitamin C per day. The average-sized goat produces around 13 grams of vitamin C per day and a sick goat, to fight of toxins, produces up to 100 grams. That's a lot of vitamin C!

In fact, we are one of just a few species on our planet that can't produce it ourselves. Dr Suzanne therefore claims that the amount we are recommended to take by the authorities, is a gross under estimation.

But isn't it dangerous if I take more? To answer this question, I would recommend you watch a video on YouTube by Dr Andrew Saul, where he is giving a lecture at the Riordan Clinic. In it he says that according to the American Association of Poisonous Control Centre, there has not even been a single reported death from over doing vitamin C, even though many people are taking doses 100s of times greater than that recommended by authorities. He then goes on to say that doctors should insist on high dose vitamin C – while they ponder the right medicine for almost any illness.

But please don't rush out and start taking mega doses of vitamin C as you might experience gastric discomfort and diarrhoea. Start with 1gram per day and then maybe extend to two. Beyond that I can't in print recommend that anyone goes beyond the EU's guidelines!

Glucomannan & Inulin (SlimShotz)

When I wrote the first edition of this book, it was prior to us developing the Primal SlimShotz product. While SlimShotz is primarily designed to help people lose weight, regardless of what my bathroom scales are telling me, I take it daily because it both stops me from feeling like I am missing out on snacks and also helps up my fibre intake. Its two main ingredients are indeed fibre superstars.

We have already discussed glucomannan under the subject of fibre. But let me expand on it a little bit more. Glucomannan is an almost magical ingredient from nature. It is extracted from the root of the Konjac plant and has been clinically proven to aid weight loss. In fact, it is the only ingredient to be officially recognised by the EU Commission to contribute to helping us lose weight. A natural plant fibre, in our stomach it expands up to 50 times its weight making us feel full. Taken before a meal it reduces our appetite and for some people, such as me, it completely removes the desire to eat snacks. When we consume more than 4g per day, the European Food Safety Authority also confirm that it helps us maintain normal blood cholesterol levels.

How does it work? Glucamannan is a soluble viscous fibre, which dissolves in water, forming a gel-like substance. Viscous fibres are found in the walls of plant cells and have the ability to expand like a sponge. When you take a SlimShotz drink, followed by sufficient water, the glucomannan gel continues to expand inside the stomach. Our receptors on sensing this fullness, trigger our satiety hormone known as leptin. If we then eat a meal approximately 30 minutes to an hour later, we consume less food as the brain already has received a signal to say its full. Plus, there is physically less room in the stomach too. It's kind of like a natural gastric band! Glucomannan also acts as a prebiotic, feeding our guts friendly bacteria. Furthermore, once past the stomach, and inside the intestines, the fibre slows the process of breaking down food, which in turn reduces the glycemic index of the entire meal, in other words slowing down the release of sugar into the bloodstream. As a result, this means that the body doesn't need to release as much of the fat building hormone insulin.

Now, let's discuss inulin. If glucomannan is king of the prebiotic world, then the god would be inulin. Our friendly gut bacteria are said to have a feeding frenzy when it arrives. They convert it into short-chain fatty acids, which nourish colon cells and provide a multitude of other health benefits. Interestingly, the diverse diets of our cavemen ancestors, included far more roots (the inulin in SlimShotz is from the roots of the chicory plant) and therefore far more inulin was consumed than in the modern diet.

But inulin is far more than just a prebiotic. During Angela Rippon's 'How To Stay Young' programme, they mentioned how inulin helps to reduce internal fats (visceral fats). Then during Dr Michael Mosley's 'Trust Me I'm A Doctor' programme, he discusses how inulin helps us get a good night's sleep.

Psyllium Husk

Just like glucomannan and inulin, psyllium husk is a water-soluble fibre. It is made from the husks of the Plantago ovata plant's seeds, which grows in many countries, but is most prevalent in India. There are numerous health benefits from this fibre; it's another great prebiotic, eases both constipation and diarrhoea, softens stools (very useful if you suffer from fissures or haemorrhoids as I often do), lowers cholesterol, helps to manage blood sugar levels, and improves both heart health and blood pressure.

Can you overdose on fibre? It is very unlikely as your stomach will feel bloated. What I recommend, is not to take your fibre in one hit, but spread it throughout the day. As glucomannan, inulin and psyllium husk all absorb water, it is important to drink plenty of water at the same time. Otherwise there is a danger of dehydrating your digestive tract. Without drinking plenty of water, there is also a potential danger that fibre can swell in the throat and cause choking. You might ask, 'why am I taking even more fibre if I am already taking glucomannan and inulin every day in the SlimShotz? The answer is a simple one. According to the American Journal of Clinical Nutrition, consuming 35g of fibre daily is associated with a 50% lower risk of cardiovascular disease and death from all causes by over a third. These are numbers not to be taken lightly.

While I try and get plenty of fibre in my diet, the fact that I don't eat breakfast cereals, wheat, oats etc, means that my daily input often falls short. I therefore ingest approximately 25 grams per day across glucomannan, inulin and psyllium husk, and get the rest from my nutritious diet.

EXERCISING DAYS

In addition to my daily nine that I try to take religiously, on days when I go to the gym, sprint or play tennis, I either drink a branched chain amino acid (BCAA) shake during my session, or drink a whey protein shake straight afterwards. Even on fasting days, I might sometimes indulge in one of these if I feel low on energy at any point.

Whey Protein

I have weight trained on and off since I was 16 years old, In the early years I was happy with the way I looked, and never took any supplements. Then, at the age of 24, I started my first company and worked day and night, lived off fast food, and was often highly stressed. While I still squeezed in a few weight-training sessions each week, my muscles were constantly covered by a layer of fat. The net result, of course, was that I had no idea what was really happening to my muscles as they were hidden from view.

Then, when I hit 50, with my seventh child on the way, I started to develop and adapt the three core beliefs of Primal Cure – low CARBS, intermittent fasting and high intensity training. The weight literally fell off and I was able to see my muscles for the first time in 26 years. To say I was a little disappointed would be an understatement. It didn't seem to matter how much I trained, my muscles didn't seem to get any bigger. So I decided to purchase some fancy scales to find out if I really was stagnant, or to see if it was more the case of my muscles growing, but I just couldn't yet see them. Sadly, after three months of measuring my muscle percentage, it turned out they just didn't seem to be developing.

Then my personal trainer, Sam, recommended I try a whey protein drink immediately after my workout. After a couple of weeks, I started to notice an improvement. The first powder I tried was bought in a supermarket and was very cheap, but then I started to explore how the powders were produced.

So what is whey? It is a by-product of cheese making. Cow's milk is made up of a lot of water, a tiny bit of fat and sugar (lactose) and a healthy amount of protein. That protein breaks down into 80% casein and 20% whey. Whey contains all nine essential amino acids, making it one of the most nutritional forms of protein we can consume. One of these amino acids is called leucine, which is particularly good to help build muscles. An average serving of whey powder delivers a similar amount of leucine as eating 10 eggs!

I had long read about the difference in nutritional benefits of eating grass-fed beef over factory farmed, grain and hormone-fed meat and then I realised I hadn't questioned the source of my protein drink. From that day onwards, I made sure that my whey protein drinks were derived from grass-fed cows. There are also three different types of whey: concentrate (whey protein concentrate – WPC), isolate (WPI) and hydrolysate (WPH). Concentrate does exactly what it says on the tin, concentrating the formula to try to deliver as high a percentage as possible - but sadly this can range from as little as 40% and goes up to 89%, depending on the brand. Isolate also does what it says on the tin, it's isolating the protein by removing even more of the fat, carbohydrates and lactose, and is more than 90% pure protein.

Both concentrates and isolates are quickly digested by the body. However, if you feel you would like to absorb the benefits even quicker, then go for a hydrolysate. These proteins have already been partially broken down by acid, heat or enzymes and get to work marginally faster. However, the taste can be bitter, and for most people a standard isolate or concentrate will do.

> **PRIMAL CURE ON ESSENTIAL NUTRIENTS:**
> There are nine essential amino acids that we cannot create internally (synthesise) and they therefore must be consumed. A 30g serving of whey protein is normally enough to meet our daily needs.

I prepare mine with water, which I put into a liquidiser with around 20 blueberries (which are naturally high in both vitamin C and vitamin K, as well as being a quality source of fibre). However, if I am going to the gym, and have fasted the day before, I take my whey shake or branched-chain amino acid (BCAA) before my workout, and not afterwards. I find this gives me a much better gain and helps me push harder in my workout. Dr Michael VanDerschelden, in his book *The Scientific Approach to Intermittent Fasting*, agrees too: "These special amino acids have shown the ability to simulate muscle protein synthesis even during times of food restriction or fasting ... Exercising in a fasted state promotes massive growth hormone production as well as optimal fat burning and muscle building".

> ### The Only Recipe In This Book
> Try this out for a really healthy kick start to the day. Add a naturally flavoured whey protein powder, psyllium husk, a tablespoon of coconut oil and a SlimShotz to a blender, add half a litre of water and blend away. Drink immediately and follow by another glass of water.

BCAA

If you want something even more pure protein than whey, then you might want to look at taking a branched-chain amino acid (BCAA). BCAAs contain three essential amino acids – leucine, isoleucine and valine. These are the only amino acids that are not degraded in the liver, meaning that they go directly into the bloodstream and therefore arrive quickly at our muscles. In fact, 35% of our muscle tissue is made up of these three amino acids.

As we age, our body's ability to extract nutrients from food begins to decline. So, while whey protein might be fine in our twenties and thirties, moving to more concentrated forms of BCAAs might prove more beneficial as we get older. My suggestion is, on days when you exercise, try whey for a month or two and see how you get on, and then switch to a BCAA and see which one works best for you. And remember, which one feels right is always the right one.

Even if the positive effect is more of a placebo, it doesn't matter. Plus, it's not necessary to choose one over another – after all it's important to remember that our Primal ancestors ate an extremely varied diet.

But aren't these powders just used by bodybuilders? It's true they are excellent at repairing and building muscles post-workout, but they have also been proven to curb hunger and improve metabolism, therefore helping to reduce weight.

What About All The Other Supplements On The Market?

Remember back to the introduction, where I said that no single approach works for everyone. When it comes to supplements, recognising individuality and not specifying 'a one size fits all' approach is very important. My whole philosophy with Primal Cure is to provide you with knowledge about what we are designed to consume as fuel, so that you can then make informed decisions about your own health and individual circumstances.

> **PRIMAL STEVE:**
> Shortly after writing the first edition of *The Primal Cure*, I started to realise that many of the supplements I was using were being stuffed with all sorts of nonsense. Amongst other nasties, I found some contained sugar, artificial sweeteners and starch. So my amazing team have now developed a very Primal range of supplements and these can be found at both PrimalCure.com and Amazon.co.uk.

THE PILL NATION

There is a famous quote from the father of modern medicine Hippocrates, "Let food be thy medicine and medicine be thy food". It's such a shame that most people living in our ill nation seem to have forgotten this piece of advice. How about this for a frightening statistic: A recent article in *The Telegraph* newspaper titled "Pill Nation", revealed that "half of the nation were now taking prescription medication with rising use of antidepressants fueling a 47 per cent increase in drugs dispensed over the last decade" and that a recent NHS survey showed that, "one quarter of people are on at least three drugs, with millions of pensioners on at least five types of medication".

In her book *Minding My Mitochondria*, author Dr Terry Wahls says, "Universal health care and free medication only treat existing chronic diseases. This is important, but most conventional treatments only control the symptoms of disease. They usually don't reverse damage that has already been done". So, if we combine the wise words of Hippocrates with Dr Wahls, we can draw the conclusion that they are advising that we should use food and nutrition as a prevention, rather than looking to medicine to control and mask symptoms.

Even though living a Primal existence can cure several illnesses, we are all still much better off doing everything we can to prevent health issues occurring in the first place. I want you to consider this for a minute: why is it that we will happily send our car in for a service even when there is nothing wrong with it? Why in business today do we invest more money and effort in preventing problems than we do in building huge customer service teams? Because in everything other than the most important thing of all – our health – we have already shifted our attention to prevention rather than cure.

Due to our present predicament, caused, in my opinion, predominantly by food and pharmaceutical corporate greed and governmental lack of genuine concern, we now have more people that need to be cured than need prevention! And while there are many that criticise our doctors for being too quick to reach for their prescription pad rather than to sit and investigate possible lifestyle changes, I personally don't blame them. I think our doctors are in a really difficult, no-win position. Not only are they overloaded with more and more patients to see each and every day, they are then under immense pressure by being measured and monitored in everything they do. It's far safer for our GP to prescribe a course of approved medicine to help alleviate symptoms, drugs that are produced by the huge pharmaceutical companies paying huge taxes to our government, than to risk sticking their neck out suggesting lifestyle changes that don't make anyone any profits.

While I sympathise with our overworked doctors, I feel the need to scream loudly that too many people are being prescribed drugs to mask symptoms, instead of curing the root of their problems. I often speak to people who are on lifetime medication, when a change in lifestyle would cause the underlying problem to disappear. It drives me crazy that I have got friends on statins, who in my opinion just don't need to be, and even worse when I see antibiotics being handed out for conditions that have nothing to do with bacterial infections.

My lovely wife is beautiful, petite, and for some reason prone to picking up infections. Sadly, over the years, it seems all that the doctors want to do is give her another course of antibiotics. Have you ever heard the saying, 'when all you have is a hammer, everything looks like a nail'? Well, in my opinion, that's what seems to be happening with far too many GPs and their prescription pads, but again it's hard to lay the blame at doctors individually – it's the system that's wrong! Luckily for me, my family and closest friends are now living Primally, and approach illnesses by first listening to the advice of Hippocrates. I hope that you will be successful in convincing your family and friends to do the same too.

> **PRIMAL CURE MOVEMENT:**
> Let us pull together to advocate and campaign on behalf of natural preventative medicine as a first step to wellness, and try as many natural methods as we can before we accept prescriptions for long-term medication.

DON'T RELY ON DRUGS AS A FIX

As you will read in various topics throughout this book, our immune system is very dependent on the health of our microbiome, and every course of antibiotics we take indiscriminately kills off many of the helpful bacteria in our guts along with the bad ones. Even in 1945, when Alexander Fleming won the Nobel Prize in Physiology or Medicine for inventing the first antibiotic – penicillin – he warned, "The time might come when penicillin can be bought by anyone in the shops. Then there is the danger that the ignorant man may easily under-dose himself and, by exposing his microbes to non-lethal quantities of the drug, make them resistant".

In 1942, Anne Miller became the first patient ever to have a course of antibiotics. She became seriously ill after giving birth and was suffering from a raging virus. Within hours of receiving the antibiotics, she started to recover, and the new medicine was heralded a success. But it was so scarce, that doctors actually filtered her urine so that they could recycle it! The reason I mention this story is to show the foresight of its inventor who, even when it was still so rare, was warning of its overuse. Don't get me wrong – without antibiotics the world would be a far deadlier place, but it's the overuse of the medicine that should be of concern.

> **DRUG WARNING:**
> **Professor Peter Gøtzsche at the University of Copenhagen believes that, after heart disease and cancer, prescription drugs are now the third most common cause of death!**

We really have got to the stage where, for almost every ailment, we turn to pills and doctors for a quick fix, rather than trying to eliminate the cause naturally. Over the past few years, whenever I have hurt myself in the gym, pulled a muscle sailing or developed tennis elbow, rather than going to a doctor my personal trainer and his team have solved the problem by identifying the route cause. Some 10 years ago I hurt my knee playing squash, and the result was hospitalisation and a major operation to reconstruct my anterior cruciate ligament. Sadly, my eldest son Matt had the same operation in recent years, but for him two separate on-going rugby injuries led to serious operations on both knees. Having now learnt more from a personal trainer and his team, all three knee operations could most likely have been avoided if we had dealt with the root cause of the issue as soon as we started to feel the symptoms.

In December 2003, Dr Allen Rose, who at the time was the International Vice President of GlaxoSmithKline (manufacturers of numerous drugs for the medical pharmaceuticals industry with a turnover in excess of £81 billion per annum) went public with some alarming statistics. In an article featured on the front page of *The Independent* newspaper he broke the news that, "The vast majority of drugs – more than 90 percent – only work in 30 to 50 percent of the people". That's a huge confession from someone who has been involved with running one of the biggest drug companies on earth.

Then, on the 23rd February 2016, *Mail Online* published an article with the title, 'How Big Pharma greed is killing tens of thousands around the world: Patients are over-medicated and often given profitable drugs with "little proven benefits", leading doctors warned'. It goes on to say, "The Queen's former doctor has called for an urgent public enquiry into drugs firms 'murky' practices". Later in the same article there is a quote from Dr Aseem Malhotra: "There is no doubt that a 'more medicine is better' culture lies at the heart of healthcare, exacerbated by financial incentives within the system to prescribe more drugs and carry out more procedures". Dr Malhorta makes three more, very relevant, comments:

- He accuses the drugs companies of 'spending twice as much on marketing than on research'
- That 'prescription drugs often do more harm than good, with the elderly particularly at risk'
- 'One in three hospital admissions among the over-75s are a result of an adverse drug reaction'

I have got to thank my own doctor, Renee Kellerman, who on more than one occasion over the past 20 years has resisted putting me on a course of drugs, instead explaining the lifestyle changes I needed to make. She has always instilled in me the need for prevention over cure. Much to the disadvantage of the huge pharmaceutical conglomerates, she wants her patients to avoid at all costs any drugs that merely suppress the symptoms of conditions and diseases.

Rather than trying to address the root cause, understandably sufferers often reach without hesitation for medication. What does medication really do for us? It masks the real underlying problems and slows down our immune system's ability to deal with them. They often tell our immune system to stop working quite so hard, and pass the work over to the highly profitable chemical cocktail created by the drug company. This handing over of the responsibility - from the body's natural repair and defence mechanism - to the scientists working for the corporate giants can have numerous harmful side effects for those that rely on certain medicines. Having said this, I fully appreciate there are certain conditions where modern medicines are totally beneficial to the sufferer. My point is more that there are many illnesses where we would be better trying to address the root cause first, rather than being sentenced to a life on medication.

Chapter 8 Highlights

- The European Union NRVs are assembled around avoiding deficiency, not ultimate health.
- Vitamin C is the very best antioxidant of all.
- Avoid crap foods void of nutrition and live longer and happier with natural foods full of vitamins and minerals.
- Let's say one vegetable contains 10 minerals that the body needs, that leaves some 30 to 60 that are missing. The answer is to eat a wide and varied diet of natural organic food, just as our Primal ancestors did and to also take a quality multi-vitamin and mineral tablet.
- Turmeric is one of the most powerful natural medicines we can add to our food.
- Eat foods rich in nutrients and fill any nutritional or vitamin shortfalls with reputable supplements.
- Omega 3. If you don't want to take a supplement derived from fish, then flaxseed oil makes a perfectly good substitute.
- We advocate and campaign on behalf of natural preventative medicine as a first step to wellness, and try as many natural methods as we can before we accept prescriptions for long-term medication.
- Professor Peter Gøtzsche at the University of Copenhagen believes that, after heart disease and cancer, prescription drugs are now the third most common cause of death!

09.
Food: The Superfoods Through To The Ugly

The Primal pantry is absolutely stuffed with healthy and delicious things to eat. In this chapter we discover the organic meats, fruit and vegetables we should be consuming, and more importantly the things we need to avoid.

So, now we arrive at the exciting part. Having got this far, you already have a strong understanding of what steps you can take to cure certain illnesses, what food types can kill you, and what nourishment to consume to prevent many diseases from occurring. As you start going through the Primal Cure list of foods to eat and those to avoid, you might think that you won't be able to afford to fully take advantage of a Primal way of life. However, even though organic foods, quality meats and fish, healthy ingredients and local produce might be more expensive than cheaply prepared and manufactured packaged products, your overall spend might actually go down. Yes, the produce we consume when following a Primal lifestyle is definitely in the main more expensive than the cheaper, highly dangerous foodstuffs, but there are loads of areas where we will be saving money.

Top 10 Big Cost Savings When Living Primally

1. As we intermittently fast, regardless of which approach we chose, we will be eating fewer meals and therefore saving money.
2. No more plastic bottled water. We don't want to ruin our oceans and consume leaked chemicals. Instead we are going to drink readily available, filtered tap water.
3. No need to subscribe to health magazines, as the primalcure.com website and blogs are updated frequently, and completely free.
4. Less time off work through illness. Even if you're paid sick leave, trust me it eventually hurts your career prospects if you are known as 'Sick Note Jo'.
5. No more expensive fast foods that leave us craving more as soon as the sugar spike wears off, often buying more overpriced manufactured snacks from the office vending machine, or even worse, jumping in the car and returning to the fast food drive-through.
6. No more fizzy drinks, which are possibly one of the most profitable and overly priced killers ever invented.
7. No need to sign up for membership of diet clubs. If these things truly worked, then they would have no long-term members at all.
8. By growing some of our own herbs, we won't need to go out and buy expensive, sugar- and salt-laden sauces.

9. Our wardrobe gets cheaper too. The yo-yo dieters constantly need new wardrobes to fit their ever-changing size. Once we have gone Primal, and bought all our new, slimmer clothing, there is little chance we are going to put a lot of weight back on, therefore our clothes are going to last far longer.
10. Other than the quality food we are consuming, all other Primal Cure activities tend to be cheaper than the alternative. We are walking more, exercising more and lifting weights that could be done at home. We are getting more enjoyment out of life, and therefore not indulging in purchases just to make us feel better.

So yes, the food choices are in the main a little more expensive, but overall we can go Primal and actually save money. The only other cost is the time needed to make our selections. But, once we have done it a few times at our local supermarket, then it gets quicker and quicker in the future.

THE TOP 20 PRIMAL SUPERFOODS

While many of the superfoods are individual performers, like avocado, spinach and garlic, others are superfood groups, such as organic meats.

1. Coconut
2. Avocado
3. Eggs
4. Nuts
5. Seeds
6. Berries
7. Cruciferous vegetables
8. Shirataki
9. Spinach
10. Tomatoes
11. Peppers
12. Onions
13. Olives

14. Organic meats
15. Oily fish
16. Garlic
17. Fermented foods
18. Dark chocolate
19. Bone broth
20. Mushrooms

COCONUTS

I have already written a lot about coconuts oils, but let's now look at some other ways to consume this Primal Superfood. Before we get going, I want to touch on a few things first. Recently, coconuts have been receiving a little negative press, with some misguided researchers suggesting their fat content leads to high cholesterol and heart disease.

Sadly, these reports are just recycling old news where they linked saturated fats to heart diseases, which as we have already read has never been established (especially for totally organic saturated fats).

The only warning for coconuts is to be careful when walking underneath these hanging fruits, as apparently 150 people die each year around the world from being hit on the head by them, which is more than the number of people killed by sharks per annum.

> **COCONUT - THE SACRED FRUIT:**
> In Hindu mythology, coconuts are called 'kalpavriksha', which means 'tree that gives all that is necessary for living'.

Coconuts are highly beneficial for our health as they contain vitamins B1, B3, B5, B6, C and E, and come jam-packed with healthy minerals such as calcium, selenium, sodium, magnesium and phosphorous. What's more, they're full of fibre, which today is sadly lacking in most diets in both the UK and the USA.

> **PRIMAL FACT:**
> Coconut is a fruit, not a nut as its name implies. Spanish explorers prefixed their nut with 'cocos' – meaning 'grinning face' – because the three little 'eyes' (known as germination spores or stoma) on their base reminded them of a smiling monkey.

Coconut Flour

Simply a gift from heaven, or at least from some very tall trees. If it wasn't for the holy coconut, making bread without grain flour would be kind of difficult. Derived from the dried flesh of the coconut, this is a flour packed with fibre, protein and healthy fats. It's free of both gluten and grain, and it can be used to make tasty breads or cakes, pancakes and desserts. You can also use it to thicken up sauces and curries, and add it to smoothies to ensure you are getting your daily fix of healthy fat.

Coconut Cream & Milk

Unlike cow's milk, coconut milk is completely lactose free! While Primal Cure is not against organic cow's milk (even though in the true sense it's not really Primal), coconut milk is definitely more beneficial to our overall health. Not to be confused with coconut water, coconut milk and cream is produced by grating the coconut flesh and then soaking it in hot water. The thick cream rises to the top, where it is skimmed off, and the remaining juice can be filtered and bottled as milk. Why is it so beneficial? Well, it's no normal fat. As we discussed earlier in the book, it's the richest source of medium-chain fatty acids (MCFAs), which is the closest thing for sale in a can or bottle to human breast milk! As it's very dense, don't drink it like cow's milk.

Even though we don't count calories, if you do want it as a stand-alone drink, just go for half a glass. Even this small amount will provide you with 25g of healthy fat, plus a good dose of manganese, copper, phosphorus, magnesium and iron. Where I find coconut milk comes into its own is in adding both flavour and thickness to curries. In the summer I have also been known to make a white Russian kahlúa cocktail with it too, but I guess I shouldn't really be mentioning that!

Coconut Water

This is the actual juice extracted from the shell of a young coconut before it develops into flesh. It is naturally sugary and, because of this, you often hear people say you shouldn't drink it if you want to lose weight. Complete rubbish! Well, unless you drink gallons of it. Coconut water contains less than 3g of natural fructose per 100g. Compared to Coke at 11g, it sounds virtually sugar free! And there is less sugar in a glass of coconut water than in an orange! Not only is it an incredibly healthy option when we need to rehydrate our body, in several developing countries, medical centres use it as a treatment for diarrhoea.

As we have already discussed, there are six minerals that together create electrolytes, which rehydrate and recharge our body – which is especially useful after a workout or illness. One of the core six minerals is potassium, of which coconut water is an extremely rich source. In addition, it also contains smaller concentrations of sodium, calcium and magnesium, all of which are also part of nature's electrolyte-hydration formula. Next time you're about to reach for a sports drink to rehydrate during a workout, do yourself a huge favour and replace it with nature's all-natural sports aid, an electrolyte that has been used for centuries by some of the healthiest nations on our planet.

Nutritionally, coconut water is very different to coconut milk. It has zero fat, around 40 calories per glass and contains 10% of our daily vitamin C requirement, plus it's a great source for vitamin B1 (thiamine), vitamin B2 (riboflavin) and vitamin B6. One glass also contains about 11% of our daily dietary fibre, 6% calcium, 15% magnesium, 17% potassium, 11% sodium and 17% manganese. In short, it is full of natural goodness.

> **COCONUT CAUTION: :**
> I found nine different coconut water offerings in my local
> supermarket, but on close inspection only two were completely
> natural. The others had artificial flavourings, additional sugars and
> a whole host of other nasties. As with most foods, make sure you
> always read the label carefully.

Coconut Chunks Or Flakes

Both are great to snack on, put into salads or add awesome flavour to
curries. I will often sprinkle flakes in with nuts or a bowl of berries
topped with probiotic yogurt.

AVOCADO

The avocado is not just a Superfood, it is one of very few Superfruits.
While most fruits have numerous health benefits, they are still
primarily carbohydrates, so not helpful for us when we are trying
to lose a lot of weight, and certainly not good when we consume
too many of them. But the Superfruit avocado is unique in that it is
primarily a fat. There are so many benefits of regularly consuming
avocado that, if I had to pick just one food to take on a desert island, it
would be a toss-up between avocado and coconuts.

Avocados contain an amazing line-up of vitamins and minerals.
First of all, they are 77% heart-healthy monounsaturated fat, 19%
carbohydrates and 4% protein. The majority of fat found in avocado
is oleic acid (also known as Omega 9), which also happens to be the
super ingredient found in olives. Oleic acids provide numerous health
benefits, including helping to reduce inflammation and warding off
cancer. They are full of antioxidants that help, among other things,
to protect our sight. There are lots of white papers and studies that
suggest that having a high intake of potassium helps to reduce blood
pressure (a major factor in heart attacks) and kidney failure. One of
the greatest sources of potassium is avocado.

If we eat both halves of an average-sized avocado, then we will be consuming around 150g of delicious healthiness. Avocados are packed full of vitamins B5, B6, C, E, K, folate and potassium. In addition, they contain copper, iron, magnesium, manganese, phosphorus, vitamin A, vitamin B1, vitamin B3 and zinc, and are also a superb source of fibre, and of its huge fibre content, 25% of it is soluble which allows it to feed our friendly gut bacteria.

EGGS

When I was diagnosed with high cholesterol in my early forties, I was told to avoid eating egg yolks as they were high in cholesterol. So for years, I would spend time delicately removing them before cooking. But now we understand that egg yolks are full of goodness, and even if we are diagnosed with high levels of bad cholesterol, the yolk doesn't actually increase it any further.

Eggs are loaded with quality proteins. In fact, they contain all nine essential amino acids, vitamins A, B12, B2 and B5 as well as lots of minerals. They are full of good fats and many traces of helpful nutrients, such as phosphorus and selenium. I guess when you think about it logically, an egg is full of the greatest ingredients nature could create. After all, each shell must contain all of the essential elements to create new life. Nothing added, nothing taken away. Eggs are full of pure, healthy, life-giving goodness, and each one contains a small amount of almost every nutrient we need.

> **EGG FACT:**
> Omega 3-enriched eggs are created by feeding hens a diet of flax seeds, which themselves are rich in Omega 3.

> **EGG TIP:**
> While a little more expensive, it is crucial to try to buy organic eggs. There is a huge difference in the balance of Omega 3 to Omega 6, with some reports suggesting the difference can be tenfold!

> ## Understanding The Labels On Egg Boxes In The UK
> According to the Soil Association's website (www.soilassociation.org), in the UK we consume 12 billion eggs each year, but sadly only 47% are certified as free range and only 2% are certified organic.
>
> The Soil Association website informs us that standards have been set for organic and 'free range' eggs that stipulate, among other things, flock sizes, stocking densities and how many hens can share a space. Organic standards go further than free-range standards in a number of important aspects:
>
> 1. Soil Association organic standards stipulate smaller flock sizes, and lower stocking densities (the number of birds per square metre). Max 2,000 vs 16,000 in free-range systems.
> 2. Organic farms certified by the Soil Association have to provide more pop holes (exits from the hen house) than free-range farms do, to encourage and promote ranging.
> 3. No beak trimming – this is a mutilation that can be painful and also prevents the hens from expressing their natural foraging behaviour. The vast majority of UK hens kept in free-range systems are routinely beak trimmed.
> 4. Organic chickens are fed a GM-free diet. In the UK alone, more than 1 million tonnes of GM crops are used to feed animals, including some free-range chickens.

NUTS

I remember being in Tanzania, when a Maasai approached my Jeep, clutching a bunch of root vegetables he had just plucked out of the soil. As my friend Mark had lived in the country for more than 20 years, I asked them what the vegetable was. It turned out to be peanuts. "But they can't be," I said, "nuts grow in trees". I was surprised that it turns out that the most consumed nut in the world, the peanut, is not really a nut at all but a legume.

> **PRIMAL TRIVIA:**
> When is a nut not a nut? When it's a peanut (really a pea from the legume family) and a pine nut, which is a seed!
>
> When someone has a nut allergy and is only allergic to peanuts, they don't have a nut allergy at all but a legume allergy! And that label you see on some packs of peanuts saying 'may contain nuts' is therefore, of course, factually incorrect!

Botanically speaking, what defines a nut is a dried fruit with one seed (although on a rare occasion it can be two), in which the seed case wall becomes hard at maturity. In reality, there is very little difference between nuts and seeds. The reason why they are so incredibly healthy is that they all are the inauguration of a plant or tree's life. Just as the yolk of an egg is full of nutrients as it carries all the vital ingredients for a chicken to hatch, seeds and nuts are packed full of both energy and nutrients, sufficient enough to sprout huge trees.

> **PRIMAL THOUGHT:**
> Have you ever stopped and pondered why the word 'nutrition' begins with the word 'nut'?!

Walnuts, pecans, pistachios, Brazil nuts, hazelnuts, macadamias and chestnuts all have numerous health benefits, and can at the same time add real flavour to our Primal lifestyle. "You missed out cashews and almonds", I hear you shout. Well, these are technically seeds and not nuts! That said, as this is a book about how to live Primally and not botanical correctness, for simplicity's sake from here on in we will treat these two no differently and not eject them from the nut family.

Why are nuts in our list of Superfoods? All nuts are rich in protein and healthy oils such as Omega 3. Most of them also contain healthy levels of magnesium, potassium, iron, copper and various vitamin Bs. But with nuts, we do need to demonstrate a little bit of portion control, while we are trying to keep on top of our weight.

You won't be surprised to hear me say that one thing we should try to do is purchase nuts as unprocessed and as organic as possible. Sadly, many branded nuts are over processed, covered in masses of salt and roasted in hydrogenated oils. All that said, when you are out and about and feel the need to eat something, it's still preferable to buy almost any quality of nuts than reach for sweets or packets of crisps. My view is that any negative or toxic affect from eating processed nuts is still going to be less than the benefits you will receive.

> **NUT TIP:**
> **The more you can purchase in the shell, the less harm man**
> **can have done to them. Our time taken extracting them**
> **helps prevent us from eating too many.**

Nuts are really good for us. It's that simple. That said, here are some technical words you might find in articles speaking about nuts and what they really mean:

Phytochemicals
'Phyto' is a Greek word for 'plant'. These chemicals help the plant protect its seeds and nuts from fungi, bugs, germs and other threats. As the word 'chemicals' just sounds too negative, I won't use it in the chart below, but instead replace it with 'phytonutrients'.

Phytosterols
A type of phytonutrient similar in structure to the body's cholesterol. It might sound paradoxical, but when our diet is high in phytosterols, we absorb less cholesterol. In addition, researchers believe that phytosterols may play a role in prevention of Alzheimer's disease.

Polyphenols
A type of phytonutrient with antioxidant capabilities that play an important role in preventing and reducing the progression of cancer, diabetes, cardiovascular and neurodegenerative diseases. They also act as a prebiotic, helping feed the good bacteria in our gut.

Flavonoids

A type of phytonutrient that is an extremely potent antioxidant. More than 4,000 different flavonoids have been identified, and they are accountable for many of the vivid colours we see in fruit and veg.

Lignans

These are chemical that activate our bacteria when we digest them. Lignans are considered a form of phytoestrogens, which, as the name implies, are oestrogens found in plants. Research is starting to suggest that lignans may be anti-cancerous, anti-inflammatory and may reduce the risk of cardiovascular disease.

Nuts - The Excellent Eight

These nuts have been designated as Superfoods because they are high in fibre, packed full of antioxidants, and are all a rich source of minerals and vitamins. Those that make up the 'Excellent Eight' are all available in supermarkets in both the UK and the USA. In all forms, they are better consumed than avoided but, if possible, head down the baking isle and look for nuts that have not been salted, roasted in oils or coated in CARBS and flavourings. And while Brazil nuts in dark chocolate are fine, don't try to sell yourself on the health benefits of nuts coated in crispy sugar!

On 11th June 2015, *The Independent* newspaper in the UK wrote, "Eating just a handful of nuts a day could lower your risk of a heart attack or of dying from cancer and diabetes". They went on to say, "Epidemiologist Professor Piet van den Brandt, who led the study of more than 120,000 Dutch people between the ages of 55 and 69 at Maastricht University, said the findings were 'remarkable', particularly due to the small amount that needed to be eaten daily to make a difference". Find in-depth articles on each of these at PrimalCure.com.

- Almond
- Brazil
- Cashews

- Hazelnuts
- Macadamia
- Pecan
- Pistachio
- Walnut

SEEDS - THE MAGNIFICENT SEVEN

Just like nuts, seeds are in our Superfoods category as they are high in fibre, packed full of antioxidants and offer rich sources of minerals and vitamins. Those that make up the 'Magnificent Seven' are all available in leading supermarkets. As I mentioned with nuts, in most forms they are better consumed than avoided, but if possible head down to the baking isle and look for seeds that have not been soaked in oils and flavourings. Find in-depth articles on each of these at PrimalCure.com.

- Chia
- Flaxseed
- Hemp
- Poppy
- Pumpkin
- Sesame
- Sunflower

BERRIES - THE FAB FOUR

While there are several other berries that are undoubtedly beneficial for our health, including the currently highly trendy acai and goji berries, plus cherries, cranberries and redcurrants, there are four that, for me, stand above all in terms of nutritional value.

Blueberries

Possibly the most highly antioxidant substance you can swallow is the highly praised and delicious blueberry. In a recent study carried out in America, senior citizens were given two and a half cups of blueberries every day for 12 weeks. Dr Robert Krikorian, who led the research said, "Our new findings corroborate those of previous animal studies and preliminary human studies, adding further support to the notion that blueberries can have a real benefit in improving memory and cognitive function in some older adults".

Blueberries are rich in the flavonoid anthocyanin, which is responsible for their vivid colour. The great news is that we can eat them all year round, as it appears that freezing blueberries has no negative effect on their antioxidants.

> **BLUEBERRY ALERT:**
> Only buy organic blueberries, as researchers have proven they contain a significantly higher level of beneficial antioxidants such as malvidin, pelargonidin, cyanidin and peonidis.

Strawberries
Very British, and very good for our health. Full of flavour and fibre, it surprises many people when I tell them how healthy strawberries are. For some reason, many believe they are full of sugar, maybe in a can they can be, but when fresh they are very low in fructose. They are packed with vitamins (especially vitamin C) and minerals, and they're one of the best sources of fruit antioxidants we can consume.

Raspberries
How about this for a key reason to consume raspberries on a regular basis: they are full to capacity with cancer-fighting antioxidants. To put their power in perspective, they are said to be 10 times more concentrated in antioxidants than tomatoes, which in themselves are miracle workers. They boost our mood and help us retain our memory as we age.

Blackberries
I remember as a child picking blackberries from thorny bushes at the end of summer. Just like strawberries, they are naturally very sweet but don't contain many calories. In fact, their nutritional value is tremendously high, with one cupful containing 30% of our daily fibre,

and 50% of our vitamin C requirements. Blackberries are also chock-a-block with lots of other vitamins and minerals too.

THE CRUCIFEROUS FAMILY OF VEGETABLES

The cruciferous (pronounced 'crew-sif-er-us') family of vegetables are descendants of the Brassica genus of plants, famed for their disease-fighting compounds. For more than 30 years, consuming high amounts of cruciferous vegetables has been associated with a lower risk of cancer. Researchers have discovered that it is the sulphur-containing compounds (particularly sulforaphane) that, while giving cruciferous vegetables their slightly bitter taste, are primarily what provide them with their cancer-fighting benefits.

> **PRIMAL GREEN VEGETABLE SAYING:**
> The cruciferous family is so named because they are 'crucial-for-us'.

An increase of cruciferous vegetables in diets has been indisputably linked to a decreased risk in obesity, diabetes, heart attacks and overall mortality. If that's not enough to motivate us to add them to our daily diet, they also make our hair shine and our skin glow, promote strong bones and nails and, above all, pack more nutrients per calorie than virtually any other food. Plus, as I have already mentioned, cruciferous vegetables contain glucosinolates that help to detox the body. Find in-depth articles on each of these at PrimalCure.com.

- Broccoli
- Brussels sprouts
- Kale
- Swiss Chard
- Cabbage
- Cauliflower
- Bok Choy
- Watercress
- Turnips

SHIRATAKI

For someone who believes that CARBS and other sugars are evil, shirataki appears to me as nature's culinary magic trick. The word itself is Japanese for 'white waterfall', which in itself creates an image of health and vitality. Shirataki comes from the konjac plant (also known as elephant yam) and is largely composed of glucomannan, which is a water-soluble fibre. It holds water so well, that when cooked it looks like pasta or noodles, but contains virtually zero CARBS and calories.

Glucomannan is now being heralded as one of the best slimming supplements on the market, as it absorbs water like a sponge, and therefore quickly fills up our stomach and suppresses our appetite. But we don't need to take it as a supplement, instead try it out as a natural substitute for pasta or noodles. There are several shirataki brands starting to appear on the shelves of UK supermarkets. They come in a pouch of water, which you simply drain off, rinse and then cook as normal. While they don't contain any flavour themselves, their fibrous nature means that they easily absorb the taste of the spices or oils we cook them with. I personally love throwing in lots of herbs and seasonings and serving with a Thai curry.

Here is the magical thing – shirataki can take on the appearance of pasta, noodles or tagliatelle, yet a serving contains approximately 10 calories, practically zero CARBS and is gluten free, wheat free, sugar free and normally totally organic!

SPINACH

This Superfood is a terrific source of antioxidants, full of minerals such as iron, potassium, zinc, calcium and selenium, as well as vitamin A, E, K and vitamin B9 (folate). When you next make a salad, chuck in two cups of spinach and you will add just 15 calories. But in return you will receive two wonderful antioxidants by the names of lutein and zeaxanthin, which helps maintain healthy eyesight and promotes a strong healthy heart. As you might expect, with their big green leaves, they are full of phytonutrients that possess anti-cancer properties. In addition, the vitamins in spinach strengthen our bones, prevent anaemia, boost our energy and help us fight infections.

If you would like Popeye-sized biceps, researchers at the Karolinska Institute in Sweden have discovered that nitrate trapped within spinach leaves is the secret behind its muscle-building properties. The nitrate reduces the need for oxygen when exercising, which increases the efficiency of the mitochondria that power our cells. Spinach also contains many flavonoids that help protect our body from free radicals.

As with all big leafy green vegetables, it's absolutely crucial to go organic. With non-organic spinach, just imagine how much pesticide has landed on their huge surface areas. And remember, washing vegetables rarely removes the pesticides. If it were as easy as just rinsing them under the tap, the chemicals wouldn't be able to withstand rain. If you have to purchase non-organic, the only way to remove man-made chemicals is to soak the spinach in a bowl with a few drops of vinegar.

TOMATOES

Tomatoes are believed to contain thousands of different phytonutrients. With more and more research being carried out into how powerful phytonutrients are in the prevention and cure of many diseases, especially in the prevention of cancer, ensuring tomatoes are part of our regular diet makes Primal common sense.

Tomatoes are another excellent source of the double act lutein and zeaxanthin, which have multiple health benefits. The innards are rich in vitamin C, and consuming just two medium-sized tomatoes is sufficient to surpass our RDA for this vital water-soluble vitamin.

The phytonutrient suspended in their vividly coloured skin support a healthy heart, boost our immune system and may even reduce the risk of cancer. Tomatoes have possibly the highest concentration of a super-phytonutrient, known as lycopene. Not only is it the source of their colour, it's a powerful antioxidant that has a number of reported health benefits, longer than your average shopping list!

Firstly, lycopene is possibly the most powerful antioxidant of all. In the Westernised polluted world, even when living Primally, we simply aren't able to avoid all toxins and pesticides. However, a regular portion of tomatoes, naturally loaded with lycopene, helps detoxify the body. Researchers at the University of Portsmouth suggest that lycopene has the ability to slow the growth of both breast and prostate cancers. It's also great for keeping our brain cells connected with one another, and our bones strong too. In many health shops you can now purchase it as a supplement if you don't like the taste but still want to benefit from the miracle cures offered by lycopene.

> **FOOD FACT:**
> **Scientifically speaking, tomatoes are a fruit.**

PEPPERS

There are so many different types of pepper that, at first, it can be a little daunting. If you say the word 'pepper', some people immediately conjure up a hot curry and mad dashes for the toilet, while others think of the big, vividly coloured but mild-mannered bell peppers. In fact, let's separate them into two groups – fiery peppers and mild to sweet peppers.

Mild To Sweet Peppers

It is the fabulously talented bell pepper (also known as capsicum) that led me to adding the pepper family to the Top 20 Superfoods. In the main, I wanted to recognise it as a high source of vitamin C, as a big yellow bell pepper has 341mg of it – that's roughly the same as five whole oranges! One red bell pepper equates to three oranges and the green bell pepper, which is a little less sweet, still contains twice the vitamin C found in an orange.

Green peppers are in fact red bell peppers that have not yet ripened. As they ripen, they become sweeter and the vitamin C content increases. Orange and yellow varieties are specially bred to offer colour variety, and are also sweeter in taste.

Bell peppers aren't just about vitamin C, as just one pepper provides approximately 10% of our daily fibre requirements, plus they also contain vitamin A, vitamin B6, magnesium and potassium.

Pepper Roulette

There is a small green pepper originating from Spain called the Pimientos de Padrón, where nine out of 10 are as mild as green bell peppers, but one out of 10 (and you'll never know which as they all look identical) is as hot as cayenne chilli pepper. They are now starting to become available from a few farms in the UK, and they can make a meal out with a group of friends a lot of fun.

Hot Peppers

Whether you call it sport or a punishment, there are various competitions around the world where slightly insane individuals try to eat the world's hottest chilies. The heat of chilies is measured in Scoville heat units (SHU) named after the American pharmacist Wilbur Scoville, who created the scale back in 1912. The heat in all peppers, regardless of their name, shape or colour, is supplied by the phytonutrient capsaicin, which the plant uses to protect itself from animals, bugs and insects.

As well as proving fun in a curry house, capsaicin offers many health benefits. It has been proven to aid weight loss, cure chronic pain and help fight cancer. In 2006, the UCLA School of Medicine in Los Angeles carried out research to find what effect consuming capsaicin had on prostate cancer. They concluded that it had a 'profound antiproliferative effect'. They also discovered that consumption also significantly stopped the spread of prostate cancer cells. Research in South Korea in 2015 found that it might also be beneficial in helping kill certain breast cancer cells, while in other countries capsaicin is used both in preventing and treating diabetes.

> **HOT PEPPERS AS A MAGIC SLIMMING PILL:**
> It's not quite how they worded it in the American Journal of Clinical Nutrition, but they demonstrated how fiery peppers speed up metabolism and thereby we lose weight by burning more energy.

Capsaicin is also used to treat various skin conditions. Today, its miracle cure is so widely acknowledged that we can purchase it as a supplement or a topical cream that we apply to our skin. The cream is really powerful, extremely Primal and definitely beats toxic deep heat sprays.

> **CHILI FACT:**
> The very component that makes chilies hot – capsaicin – is good for our joints and can relieve certain muscular aches and pains.

ONIONS

Onions, just like garlic, are members of the Liliaceae plant family. After broccoli, Brussels sprouts, shallots and celery, onion is one of the richest sources of polyphenols. These are one of the best types of phytonutrients and include both tannins (as found in red wine), and flavonoids, which are great at protecting against many unhealthy strands of bacteria. A short while back I decided that, with seven children, I had done my bit for the growth of our nation and decided to get a vasectomy. I was devastated when the doctor told me that, as a precaution, he got his patients to take an antibiotic. A few days before my operation, I called and told him that I wouldn't take the antibiotics, and instead was consuming lots of onions on the days leading to the operation, as I felt their natural antibiotic capabilities would suffice. And so they did.

As well as their natural antibiotic powers, onions are thought to help prevent certain cancers and lower the risk of diabetes and neurodegenerative disorders, such as Alzheimer's and Parkinson's disease. They also help protect the heart, help maintain strong bones, and at the same time lower the risk of arthritis and asthma.

Due to their anti-viral and anti-inflammatory benefits, old wives tales recommended tying a bunch of onions around our neck to clear sinuses. While that might not look very elegant, there is plenty of research to suggest eating them helps fend off colds and flu. Plus, when we get a nosebleed, holding an onion under our nostrils should act as a natural coagulant to stop the flow!

While growing in the soil, onions absorb sulphur that later turns into the amino acid sulfoxide. When we cut through an onion this is released, causing the familiar sore eyes and crying. Remember that antioxidants found in fruit and veg were once the plant's self-defence system. With onions, especially larger ones, most of the healthy stuff is in the outer section, so when peeling try not to lose too many layers. They also contain plenty of other antioxidants, with two in particular – quercetin and anthocyanin – known to be extremely beneficial.

Just as the phytochemicals were designed to keep away pests and insects, if we rub onion on our skin or put it in a bowl of water, it helps keeps away mosquitoes. Now that's much more of a Primal solution than spraying toxic chemicals onto our skin while on holiday.

> **ONION FACTS:**
> Dice up an onion and one cupful will provide 20% of our daily vitamin C requirements, 10% vitamin B6, 10% manganese, 8% folate, 8% potassium and 5% vitamin B1 (thiamine).

OLIVES

I am not going to say too much about olives here, as we have already discussed them a lot under the heading of olive oils. Olives and their oil are a staple part of the diet of those living in the Mediterranean, where a combination of lifestyle and food choices dramatically reduces the occurrence of heart attacks, and leads to a disproportionate number of centenarians. Enough said!

ORGANIC MEAT

All organic meats offer a wide variety of health benefits. While bison, venison and goat are available from several supermarkets, I am going to detail the benefits of the most popular three: beef, pork and lamb.

To be Primally acceptable, all meat has to be organic - which means, among other things, that the animals were raised on food they were designed to eat. All those reports about meat being unhealthy might have an ounce of correctness if the researchers were analysing the effect on health of just factory-produced meats. However, when we talk of meats that originate from animals that have lived their entire lives only eating their natural diet, and who have roamed freely, then meat is truly magnificent for our well-being.

Whether it is meat from cows, lambs or pigs, they are all rich in both protein and healthy fats. And to those who suggest all meat is bad for our health; let me say it one more time - you are talking complete nonsense! If we weren't designed to eat meat, then our forefathers would have just gathered plants and vegetables. But they didn't. They spent most of their days hunting wild animals, and when they caught them, they feasted on every part. Without realising it, they gained immense health and brainpower by eating all of the animal's organs, which are without doubt full of the greatest nutrients of all.

When you go to a supermarket, look how cheap all of the organs are. Why is it that I can make a liver pâté for just nine pence per portion, yet the meat is so expensive? The answer is simple – our generation has forgotten how to cook organs and thus there is now more supply than demand. Yet enter a high-end restaurant, and we find plenty of organs on the menu. My local gastropub has kidneys on toast (although I always ask them to remove the toast and to serve them on spinach), homemade pâté and braised ox-cheek pie.

> **PRIMAL CURE MEAT PRINCIPLE:**
> **Always buy organic and local if possible, then be sure**
> **to eat the organs too.**

For a quick overview of the benefits of meat, I am going to assume
that you have bought only organic and totally natural produce. In
other words, it has not been packaged or altered in any way (apart
from butchering). As for the cut of the meat or type of organs, the
age and the location can make a big difference. I won't breakdown the
percentages of NRV as I have for non-animal produce, instead I will
just highlight some of the key nutritional benefits.

Organic Beef Health Benefits

Rich in Omega 3 and an excellent – in fact possibly the best – source
of protein, grass-fed beef also contains a secret healing component
called conjugated linoleic acid (CLA). Early research into the benefits
of CLA revealed how it could reduce tumours by more than 50% in
cancers of the breast, skin, stomach, lung, bowel and colon. CLA is
also said to help sufferers of asthma, lower blood pressure, fight off
cardiovascular disease and reduce the risk of osteoporosis. If you
don't eat meat, then there are now dozens of CLA supplements on the
market, and they seem to becoming hugely popular in both the UK
and the USA. Among their many claims is the ability to help control
type 2 diabetes, assist in losing body fat and then maintaining a
healthy weight by retaining muscle mass.

Pork

When it comes to pork, look for a pack that carries the organic label.
If you want to be put off mass-produced pork forever, make sure you
watch 'Food, Inc.' by Robert Kenner. This 2008 documentary goes
undercover in a huge slaughter house in the US which reportedly
processes more than 32,000 pigs every day, in what appear to be the
most horribly inhumane conditions. It might cost a little more to buy
from real farms rather than animal factories, but it's not just better

for the pig, it's far better for our health too. Let's quickly look at the different labels we might find in the supermarket, and understand what they all mean. These are very similar to what you will find for beef and chicken too, and I have listed them in order of preference.

▶ Organic Pork

The EU has a group of requirements for pork to carry an organic label, but better still, try and find pork with the Soil Association's (www.soilassociation.org) organic label, as this is a stricter standard. All pigs must be fed organic food without antibiotics. To avoid overcrowding and allow access to sustainable food, there is a minimum amount of land that farmers must have per pig.

Free Range Pork

These pigs are born outdoors and stay outdoors their entire life.

Outdoor Bred

These pigs are born outdoors, but tend to be moved back inside at around four weeks old or once they are weaned.

Outdoor Reared

Similar to outdoor bred, but here the piglets get to stay out until they are about 10 weeks old.

RSPCA Assured

Pork carrying the RSPCA's label ensures the living standards of the animal. About 30% of pigs reared in the UK are living a healthier and happier life thanks to the protection of this label.

If pork doesn't carry any of these labels, we shouldn't buy it. Why eat pork? It's an excellent source of vitamins such as vitamin B3 (niacin), vitamin B1 (thiamin), vitamin B2 (riboflavin) and vitamin B6, plus minerals phosphorus, selenium, zinc, iron, potassium and magnesium. Pork offers a great source of protein without CARBS, but is very low in fat compared to other meats.

Lamb

Just like beef, lamb is an excellent source of protein and Omega 3 fatty acids. It's rich in minerals such as zinc, iron, selenium, phosphorus, potassium, copper and magnesium, plus it's a great source of vitamin B12, vitamin B3 (niacin), vitamin B2 (riboflavin), vitamin B6 and B5 (pantothenic acid). Both lamb and beef are regarded as red meats.

Have you ever wondered what meat is? For example, if you saw a diagram of a lamb, you would not see the word 'meat', but muscle and fat, organs and bone. When the animal dies, it's the muscle that becomes the meat that we eat.

Red meat is a great source of iron. If you feel that you are lacking in it, then adding a few lamb dishes to your weekly line-up of meals should prove beneficial.

Lamb is rich in zinc, which among other things provides a boost to our immune system. From some farms, depending on the pasture (and I am assuming of course that we are only buying organic) lamb can actually provide more Omega 3 per gram than beef. It also contains conjugated linoleic acid (CLA), which in some research studies has been shown to fight off breast cancer.

▶ Organic Lamb

The accreditation for organic lamb in the UK is normally carried out by the Soil Association. Unlike cattle, sheep are rarely kept indoors, so the only real question to consider is whether they were reared organically or not. If you see an organic emblem on the packaging, it guarantees that any dips the sheep have been in are organic, and that the soil and therefore the grass they eat is free from pesticides too. The UK government's website states, "Organic sheep must be fed on organically produced feedstuffs. Maximum use should be made of grazing, and all of the feed required should ideally be produced on the farm".

> **PRIMAL LAMB FACT:**
> Pretty much globally, lamb is called lamb if the animal is less than one year old. But when meat is sold in Britain as lamb, the age of the animal must be between five and six months. Meat from younger sheep, from three to five months old, is normally called spring lamb. Meat from sheep more than one year old is called mutton.

Poultry

If it's not both organic and free range don't buy it. Not just for the sake of our own health, but for the sake of the bird too. Only organic birds offer a clean source of protein and healthy fat. In the UK, it is estimated that 46% of the protein of the average Brit comes from chicken, and our small nation consumes a staggering 17 million chickens a week.

Let's explain a few details that you might find on the label. First of all, it's important to cut through all of the nonsense. 'Natural', 'Farm-Fresh', 'Premium Chicken' and 'Country Style' are completely meaningless and just marketing fowl play! They're prominently placed on packaging just to encourage us to pick up the produce and feel good about it. Just as I mentioned regarding the welfare of pigs, if you watch the film Food, Inc., I am pretty sure you will immediately be converted to the merits of organic and free range.

> ### Organic Poultry
> In the UK this is again regulated by the Soil Association, who limit flock size to 1000 chickens. Every bird must have continuous and easy daytime access to outdoor pastures, and each bird should have a minimum of four square metres each to roam freely. The pasture must be covered with suitable vegetation, and the bird must reach a minimum age of 81 days. The chicken must be fed organic foods and antibiotics must not be used at all.

Free Range

Chickens must have outdoor access for at least half of their life, and there must be the equivalent of one square metre of land for each and every chicken. Minimum slaughter age is 56 days.

Freedom Food

This is a welfare scheme run by the RSPCA that can apply to indoor, organic or free-range chickens. It limits how many can be raised in each space and also details such things as how much straw they get, the size of their perch, etc.

Red Tractor

Seems to be nothing more than a paid-up membership for farmers to use the logo, and their website has very little other rules and guidelines beyond what the EU require. That said, it does mean that the food can be traced back to the original British farm ('The Union Jack flag in the Red Tractor logo confirms your food has been born, grown, prepared and packed in the UK').

If you want to see the most detailed report on chicken produce ever, which breaks down the nutritional value between breasts, skin, wings, thighs, whole chickens, drumsticks, drumsticks with skin and much more, then visit www.nationalchickencouncil.org. Alternatively, the following nutritional facts should be enough to encourage you to put chicken on the menu tonight.

Why is it important to buy organic chickens and only eggs from organic hens? Because those that live indoors are often genetically modified to gain weight more quickly, meaning they take less time to mature and therefore are both cheaper to rear and cheaper to sell. By overcrowding indoor sheds, the cost per chicken becomes lower. With such cramped conditions, many companies rely on the heavy use of antibiotics to fight off diseases. So much so, that I recently read an article where it suggested that some indoor chickens end up consuming twice their own body weight in antibiotics during their first 14 days of life. Just think what that does to the poor chicken, but more importantly what effect it will have on the bacteria in our gut.

> **ORGANIC PRIMAL CONCERN:**
> It is said that of the 50 billion chickens farmed around our small planet each year, 70% of them are no longer organic.

THE SLIPPERY SIX - OILY FISH

There are thousands of different edible fish in our oceans and rivers, and the vast majority are healthy to eat. As with all food, there are a few questions we need answering before eating them. After concerns about the environment or sustainability have been met, it's important to check how the fish were caught or raised. One key concern we have with farmed fish is the conditions in which they are kept.

The Food and Agricultural Organisation of the United Nations recently issued a report that stated farmed salmon production had risen 4,000% over the past 20 years, and today most of the produce we are offered in shops appears to be farmed rather than caught. One of the problems with farmed fish, especially those from inland waters, is that the food they are fed is not all natural.

Let's remind ourselves of a Primal Cure mantra here, 'we are what we eat – eats' and if that is pellets full of synthetic foodstuff, it's not really something we want to be putting in our Primal body. I could go on and on about toxins and the huge difference in nutritional value between wild and farmed fish, but let's get on with the positives of eating fish with just one caveat – all comments about the health benefits of the top six slippery fish relate to those that have been caught in the wild. And by the way, I named them the 'slippery six' because the main health benefit linking them together is their richness in Omega 3 oil.

The Omega 3 found in most seafood is derived from small plant life, known as phytoplankton, that the fish feed on. Virtually all fish and shellfish are sources of Omega 3 fatty acids, but their concentrations vary based on the diet of each species, and both the season and location they were caught.

> **OMEGA 3 DEFICIENCY RECAP:**
> If we don't regularly consume enough Omega 3, then we are more prone to suffer from inflammation, arthritis, joint and muscle pains, allergies, digestive disorders, cognitive dysfunctions and have a higher risk of heart disease.

Salmon

Have you ever noticed how some fish becomes dry even if we just slightly overcook it, yet salmon always appears to remain moist? Guess what – that's the Omega 3 holding the fish nicely together in our frying pan. Salmon is one of the richest sources of Omega 3 in both our oceans and rivers.

'Beauty is only skin deep, but ugly goes clean to the bone' might be a phrase that relates to some farmed salmon, but when it's caught in the wild, both the skin and the fleshy meat are full of nutrients. Yes, the skin too. In fact the skin is full of nutritional goodness and I personally love to fry it (in healthy oil of course) until it's really crispy and then serve it separately on a salad.

> ### The Technical Salmon Stuff
> A typical salmon fillet weighs in at about 150g (5.2oz) and provides us with around 20g of healthy natural fat (approximately 70% of our daily requirement of Omega 3), three times our RDA of vitamin B12, one and a half times the vitamin D we need, plus it provides 100% of our selenium requirements and 70% of our daily protein! Wow, all in one small fillet! It also packs in 70% vitamin B3, 67% phosphorus and really big doses of vitamin B6, iodine, choline, vitamin B5, potassium and biotin.

> What does all this mean for our health? Pretty much everything!
> It's simply a miracle food from the rivers. It's good for our
> cardiovascular system, our bones and joints, our blood and our
> immune system, and it participates in the prevention of many
> diseases such as cancer, Alzheimer's and Parkinson's.

Trout

If you are not a big fan of the taste of salmon, then a close relative
that's a lot milder in flavour is trout. Being of the same family, trout
are also rich in Omega 3 and share many of the other wonderful
nutritional benefits that are enjoyed when eating wild salmon.

For a different prospective on the health benefits of oily fish, I thought
I would give you the opinion from the people at www.britishtrout.
co.uk: There is good evidence for reduction in risk of cardiac death
if you eat fish. Evidence also suggests that eating fish is probably
associated with a lower risk of stroke and is possibly beneficial
for mental health, for example to improve mood and help treat
depression. The health attributes of fish are most likely to be long-
chain PUFAs, although other nutrients in fish (e.g. protein, selenium,
vitamin D) may also contribute to the health benefits".

Mackerel

They might taste different, but did you know that mackerel and tuna
both belong to the same fish family? Known as Scombridae, they offer
a full menu of nutrients for the healthy Primal eater.

> ### The Technical Lowdown On Mackerel
> I have used a weight of 80g (2.8oz), as that's the typical size of
> a fillet in UK supermarkets. Each piece will provide us with
> the following amount of the daily recommendations: Vitamin
> D 201%, sodium 148%, vitamin B12 160%, vitamin B6 15%,
> magnesium 12%, potassium 11%, iron 6% and calcium 5%. And
> of course let's not forget why we eat slippery fish, as just one

> small fillet provides us with around 2,900mg of healthy Omega
> 3 fatty acids. That's the equivalent of three of the large Omega
> 3 capsules I take as supplements every day. And for building
> muscles, there's 20g of protein in each piece of mackerel too.

Tuna

In 2014, off the coast of New Zealand, Donna Pascoe caught a bluefin
tuna on her line and wrestled with it for more than four hours. She
eventually hauled it onto her boat, and it weighed in at twice the
weight of a baby elephant at 411kg (906lbs, or 64 stone). It was said
to be so large that it could fill more than 1,700 tins of tuna! However,
you can also find tuna that weigh one or two kilos. While historically
we haven't seen many big examples in UK waters, over recent years the
huge bluefin have started to appear off the coast of Cornwall.

Whether it is in a can or a fresh slice of raw tuna, this fish is full to
the brim with goodness. In fact, let's start with the can. We shouldn't
buy it with added oil, as when we drain it we also drain away a lot
of the Omega 3. If the tuna is canned in water, as water and oil don't
mix, when we drain off the water we retain all of the fish's natural
oil. A typical small can, where the chunks are stored in water, will –
depending on the variety of tuna – provide around 300 to 1,000mg of
Omega 3. While not as potent as salmon or mackerel, it's more easily
consumed when we are out and about and don't have time to prepare
a full meal.

Technical Tuna

As there are various types of tuna, I won't give percentages
for its various nutritional values, but just announce some of
its amazing line-up. Tuna is an excellent source of vitamin B3
(niacin), selenium (an unusual and hugely beneficial type called
selenoneine, which is an extremely strong antioxidant), vitamin
B12, vitamin B6, phosphorus, vitamin B1 (thiamine), vitamin
B2 (riboflavin), choline, magnesium and vitamin D.

Sardines (AKA Pilchards)

The word 'sardines' was first used in England to describe small fish towards the end of the 14th century. Its origin probably relates to the warm waters off the Mediterranean island of Sardinia, where small fish were abundant. There are 21 different species of fish that the World Health Organisation (WHO) allows to be classed as a sardine. While the description sardines and pilchards are often interchangeable, technically speaking sardines are normally under 15cm (6in) in length and pilchards are longer. Small herring, sprats, shad and brisling are all varieties of sardines. One of the great things about sardines is that we don't have to spend time worrying about whether they are farmed or not. All sardines and the bigger pilchards are caught in the wild. They are full of oily goodness and wonderful to eat.

> ### ▶ Sardine Specifications
>
> With sardines varying a lot in size and shape it's hard to work out what measurement to use, so I have opted for 100g (3.5oz) as that's roughly what a Cornish sardine weighs. So, of the Nutritional Reference Value (NRV), just one sardine offers 400% vitamin B12, 101% selenium, 75% phosphorous, 71% Omega 3, 51% vitamin D, 41% calcium and 35% vitamin B3, plus significant portions of iodine, copper, zinc, vitamin B6, potassium, magnesium and choline. How does this translate for our health? Well, you name it, and sardines will pretty much do it for you! They defend against depression, fight against cancers and infertility, improve our moods and memory, protect our heart, stave off Alzheimer's and Parkinson's disease and so much more.

Anchovies

I won't write a lot on anchovies, as I appreciate they are often an acquired taste. I personally love them and confess that when dishing up a salad at home, my plate always contains the most! There are more than 100 different species of anchovies and some of the very best tasting are from the Mediterranean.

They are full of mineral goodness including calcium, selenium, iron and magnesium, plus they're loaded with vitamins such as riboflavin, niacin, folate, vitamin E, vitamin B6, vitamin B12, vitamin A and vitamin K. And of course, they provide a rich source of Omega 3, where in just 100g (3.5oz) of canned anchovies you will find more than 2,000mg of oily righteousness.

GARLIC

I struggled pushing some other foods out of the Top 20 so that I could include garlic. Several friends suggested I should put it under the herb section, alongside ginger and turmeric. Others suggested that, as there are dozens of brands of garlic supplements, it should make its way into those pages. But as garlic is so powerful and so amazing for our health, I felt it needed to take pride of place in the Top 20.

Hippocrates famously said, "Let food be thy medicine, and medicine be thy food", (I love this quote) and he used to prescribe garlic for various ailments. Its use as a medicine has been well documented across many civilisations including the Egyptians, Babylonians, Romans and Chinese. Its main claim to fame lies in its use as an all-natural antibiotic. For thousands of years, people have known about its ability to kill off various unhealthy strands of bacteria and fungi. Its strong aroma comes from a compound called allicin, which provides both its antifungal and antibacterial properties. Garlic is also rich in selenium, vitamins C, B1, B2, B3, and B6, folate, calcium, iron, manganese, phosphorous, potassium, magnesium, sodium and zinc.

Garlic is famed for its ability to lower blood pressure. There is also mounting research that suggests its antioxidant power is one of the best at helping to prevent cancer. For those suffering with spots, eating a few cloves of garlic every day will tackle the root cause of acne and cleanse the skin, from the inside out. For those of us who are a little older, garlic is great for both our hair and skin and slows down our loss of collagen, which is what we need to keep the skin supple and prevent the dreaded wrinkles.

FERMENTED FOODS

In Chapter 7, we discussed how important it is to get our gut in good working order. While there are a whole host of supplements we can take in order to create the right balance in our intestines, one of the more natural processes is to eat fermented produce. While it is true that the fermentation of yeasts is used to convert sugar in grapes into wine, unfortunately I am not suggesting that consuming plenty of alcohol is the right approach for the rehabilitation of our gut's friendly bacteria!

Fermented foods go through a process of lacto-fermentation whereby, in the absence of oxygen, natural bacteria feed on the sugar and starch in the food, creating lactic acid. It gets its name from a specific species of bacteria, Lactobacillus, which was first discovered when studying the fermentation of milk. When it comes to fermenting vegetables, they are normally soaked in salt water or sometimes just their own juice, and given sufficient time the bacteria eats the sugar in the vegetable, turning it into a sour/tart tasting and incredibly healthy lactic acid. But why would we want lactic acid in our gut? It helps our immune system fight off harmful bacteria, acts as a natural antibiotic, defends the lining of our gut and helps control and regulate inflammation, all while protecting our essential levels of vitamins and enzymes.

> **PRIMAL CURE FACT**
> The word 'probiotic' to describe food with beneficial
> bacteria was coined more than 100 years ago by Russian
> zoologist Élie Mechnikov, the father of immunology and the
> 1908 winner of the Nobel prize in medicine.

Fermented foods aren't a new concept, in fact before tinned goods became the norm it was the way that most foods were preserved in jars. Sally Fallon, in her book *Nourishing Traditions*, says, "The proliferation of lactobacilli in fermented vegetables enhances their digestibility and increases vitamin levels. These beneficial organisms produce numerous helpful enzymes as well as antibiotic and anti-carcinogenic substances. Their main by-product, lactic acid, not only keeps vegetables and fruits in a state of perfect preservation but also promotes the growth of healthy flora throughout the intestine". The US publisher Doctors Health Press ran an article in September 2015 stating, "Aside from the high calcium, potassium and B-vitamins, the major benefit to yogurt and kefir is the probiotic content". This is really why we urge everyone to include them in their Primal lifestyle. Probiotics are good bacteria for our gut that provide a number of benefits – many of which are still likely to be unknown. The impact of a healthy and diverse gut bacteria has been tied to many things, including:

- Lower LDL cholesterol levels
- Reduced Alzheimer's risk
- Reduced blood pressure
- Allergy and eczema prevention
- Improved digestion
- Alleviation of bloating and constipation
- Improved mood
- Treating IBS and Crohn's disease
- Treating depression
- Potential treatment and preventative measure for colon cancer

The following are my Top 5 fermented food recommendations:

Yoghurt

Just as wine is made from fermenting sugar in grapes, yoghurt is made by fermenting the sugar in milk (lactose). The fermentation process requires the presence of two friendly bacteria, Lactobacillus bulgaricus and Streptococcus thermophilus. Of course, we should only consume yoghurt from grass-fed cows, yoghurt that's totally organic and contains zero added flavourings. Try to choose a natural plain Greek yoghurt, or for that matter any unsweetened natural live yoghurt (these should contain nothing other than milk and added bacteria).

In 2013, there was a study carried out at the Aristotle University of Thessaloniki in Greece to measure the effects of eating probiotic yoghurt. The scientists split a number of lean mice into two groups. The first group ate nothing but fast food and the other ate fast food and probiotic yoghurt. Those eating just fast food became obese, but the group who ate the same volume of fast food but also probiotic yoghurt remained lean. Their conclusion was that supplementing the diet with probiotic yoghurt inhibits obesity.

Without doubt, a totally natural fermented yoghurt is full of millions of nature's tiny miracles, and adding just a small daily portion to our diet can do wonderful things for our gut flora. But there is just one slight word of warning. A whole cup of yoghurt can contain 10 to 15g of CARBS, and remember we ideally want to stay below 50g a day, especially when we want to remain in ketosis, so don't go mad on it!

Kefir

The fermented milk of cows, sheep or goats. Its texture is like a cross between milk and yogurt and it is a great source of vitamin B12, calcium, magnesium, vitamin K2 and a whole host of healthy bacteria. If we ever get diagnosed with IBS, then consuming half a cup of kefir each day might just provide a natural Primal Cure.

Many experts claim that kefir is actually superior to probiotic yogurt in that it is home to a wider array of helpful bacteria. My advice is that we should use both in our weekly routine and benefit from a dietary double dose!

Non-Pasteurised Cheese

When people ask me what the difference is between the Paleo diet and a Primal way of living, I always start by saying that we love cheese! Cheeses that are made from raw milk and haven't been pasteurised are a brilliant source of naturally fermented goodness. Soft cheeses are especially rich in helpful bacteria and can cure many smaller digestive issues, while at the same time help boost the immune system. But don't rely on cheese at the exclusion of yogurt or kefir, because many of the helpful strands of bacteria can be lost in the production process.

Pickles
Full of vitamins, minerals, antioxidants and friendly bacteria, pickles work wonders for the gut. As always, it is really important to look for an organic jar and don't buy any pickled in vinegar as this kills off the helpful bacteria. It's okay to purchase them in brine, as not only are they great for the gut, they also often provide a rich source of vitamin K that among other things supports both healthy bones and a healthy heart.

Sauerkraut
Dating back more than 2000 years ago, the Romans fermented vegetables to take on long sea voyages. Made from cabbage, sauerkraut is one of the oldest traditional foods available, and is not only a great source of probiotics, but is also rich in vitamin A, vitamin C, vitamin K and vitamin B. In addition, sauerkraut also contains iron, copper, calcium, sodium and magnesium. As well as helping cultivate a healthy gut, it is believed to boost our digestive system, aid blood circulation, give us stronger bones and fight inflammation.

Another popular form of sauerkraut is the traditional Korean dish kimchi. Just like sauerkraut, its main ingredient is fermented cabbage, but it's more flavoursome, with a host of extra spices and seasonings.

10 REASONS TO EAT DARK CHOCOLATE
Before we get carried away with any old chocolate bar, let me set out the rules from the start. What we are after is real chocolate, not highly manufactured, sugar-stuffed chocolate bars. Chocolate is made from ground cocoa beans, which grow on cocoa trees in Central and South America. Around 3,000 years ago, Maya Indians discovered cacao and named it 'theobroma cacao', meaning 'food of the gods'. They didn't start by making chocolate, but a spicy drink called 'chocolatl'. As we have already read in the herbs and spices section, I am going

to recommend that you put cocoa powder in your Primal pantry and make your own chocolate bars and desserts. If you are not a big cook, then purchase bars of dark chocolate where the cacao content is higher than 70%. Most supermarkets have a variety of brands and strengths. Ideally, the closer we can get to 100%, the more beneficial the chocolate will be, but many people find them a little too bitter at first. What you will probably find is that over time your taste buds will change, and you will start to enjoy bars with more than 90% cacao.

> **THE DIFFERENCE BETWEEN CACAO AND COCOA:**
> **Raw cacao powder is made by cold-pressing unroasted cocoa beans. Because it is unroasted, cacao retains more of its powerful antioxidants.**

In his book *Tales From the Medicine Trail*, author Chris Kilham says, "If cocoa were a pharmaceutical drug, it would be hailed the greatest medicine of all time, and its discoverer would reap the Nobel Prize in Medicine". While I agree with this, always remember that it is cacao which is richer in antioxidants. Here are 10 health benefits on offer:

- Increase insulin sensitivity
- Protect against type 2 diabetes
- Lower blood pressure
- Support brain functions such as memory
- Decrease inflammation
- Support our cardiovascular system
- Protect against free radicals, thereby guarding against certain cancers
- Helps restore flexibility to arteries
- Prevents white blood cells from sticking to the walls of blood vessels
- By triggering leptin, the hormone that tells us we are full, it helps us to lose weight

Who would have thought that dark chocolate could actually help us lose weight?

BONE BROTH

We have all heard the description of a cavemen hunkered down around a fire, chewing on a bone and extracting the goodness from it - and if you haven't then I'm sure you have seen a dog engaging in a similar act. It's not that the caveman was lazy and couldn't be bothered to track down another animal, but that there was and still is so much hidden goodness to be obtained from the bones.

It doesn't matter whether we are talking chicken or cow bones, they are all excellent sources of nutrients, minerals and vitamins. They are full of gelatin and marrow that are brilliant for curing joint pains and aiding mobility.

One of the greatest benefits of boiling up bones into a lovely tasty broth is its ability to break down larger protein molecules of gelatin into a specific amino acid, known as collagen. Its name is derived from the Greek word 'kolla', which translates as 'glue'. In many ways, collagen is in fact the glue that holds the human body together. There is a huge amount of it residing on the inside of bones, in our joints and our tendons, and it also provides the elasticity in our skin.

As we get older, our body becomes less efficient at creating collagen, and without boosting it through what we eat we can suffer joint pains and our skin can become wrinkly. Collagen is often used in skin care products to help reduce cellulite and stretch marks, but it's much nicer and more beneficial to consume it in our diet, as that way we avoid all the chemicals that often accompany it in creams and lotions.

Without trying to get too technical, for both completeness and to explain some of the supplements we see in health shops, it's good to understand that collagen is made up primarily of an amino acid called glycine. This is not classed as an essential amino acid as our body is able to create it, but according to recent research, we are not that efficient at synthesising it. Therefore, many people in the medical and supplement world are now calling glycine a semi-essential amino acid.

It's the smallest of all the 22 amino acids and plays an important role in the health of our skin, our digestive system, circulatory and nervous system, muscle growth and repair and in managing our hormones. As you can see, glycine gets involved with pretty much everything that goes on in our body. Glycine also helps our body in synthesising, amongst other things, salt - which might be lacking from our Primal diet because of the high intake of water and avoidance of salt-loaded packaged and processed foods.

Let's get back to our caveman ancestor for a moment, or man's best friend the dog. By sucking on bones they are extracting possibly the most important amino acid of all. However, as we would look pretty weird doing the same in a restaurant, instead we should make sure that we put bone broth on our weekly menu. There is plenty of guidance on the web on how to make it at home, but if we don't have time then there are cubes available that you can add to boiling water.

MUSHROOMS

It should come as no surprise that the ultimate Superfungi, the mushroom, makes its way into our Superfood list, as we can be pretty certain that our Primal ancestors consumed plenty of them. For the past few thousand years, Eastern cultures have literally worshipped the health benefits of mushrooms. They are rich in protein and fibre and an excellent source of water-soluble vitamins B and C. They also contain calcium, vitamin D, selenium and potassium. They support our immune system and, among other things, are said to help prevent certain cancers. In particular, beta glucans - found in the cell walls of bacteria living on mushrooms - inhibit the growth of cancerous cells, so much so they are available in pill form and often prescribed for people not only with cancer, but also sufferers of diabetes, high cholesterol and HIV/AIDS. Mushrooms also contain linoleic acid that helps prevent the production of excess oestrogen, which is one of the prime causes of breast cancer in women after the menopause.

More recently there has been lots of media attention around the positive effect consuming mushrooms has on our cognitive functions. In January 2017, *The Mirror* newspaper wrote an article under the headline, 'Mushrooms could be the newest "Superfood", as study shows they can stave off dementia'.

> **MUSHROOM WARNING:**
> They are super absorbent and will soak up both good and bad chemicals and minerals from the soil. Therefore, it's crucial that we only purchase organic mushrooms. For our health's sake, if it isn't organic we should leave it on the shelf and choose something else.

OTHER HEALTHY FOODS

All the following are excellent sources of micronutrients, and while they just missed out on the Top 20, they made it into the Top 40:

- Shellfish
- Lemon and Lime
- Kiwi
- Celery
- Artichoke
- Peanuts
- Lentils
- Seaweed
- Romaine Lettuce
- Grapefruit
- Pineapple
- Pomegranates
- Asparagus
- Cucumber
- Carrots
- Cheese

SHELLFISH

Because we eat the entire fish, whether it is an oyster, mussel or clam, shellfish are among the most nutrient dense foods we can possibly eat. With shrimps and prawns, just like shellfish, we pretty much eat the entire thing and therefore we are getting a load of bang for our nutritional buck with these small sea creatures. I say small, but let's also include lobsters and tiger prawns in here too, as they are a rich source of selenium and vitamin B12.

LEMON & LIME

If you only put them in gin and tonic, than maybe you're missing the point. Both lemon and limes are packed full of vitamins and minerals. However, with their very strong bitter taste, few will enjoy sitting down to a plateful, and therefore we have added them to the Top 40 for a slightly different reason.

In 1747, Scottish physician James Lind was aboard a navy ship when many of the sailors became very sick. He conducted what many believe to be the first clinical trial ever, when he divided the sick into different groups and fed them different foods. The only group to recover on the voyage exclusively ate oranges and lemons. A century later, the Royal Navy realised that lime was stronger than lemon, and so in order to prevent the spread of scurvy they began adding it to sailor's drinks. This amused the Americans and the derogatory nickname for Brits as 'Limeys' was born. What was it that prevented scurvy? It was the acid in the lemon and limes, an acid that we call vitamin C.

These two citrus fruits really do pack an extremely beneficial vitamin C punch. Their concentration of antioxidants helps prevent free radicals and therefore reduces the likelihood of many cancers. The short sharp flavour, caused by a phytonutrient called limonin, literally can halt inflammation and therefore reduce the effect of many common illnesses. I personally squeeze them into my filtered drinking water, yogurt smoothies and onto my salads. If I am making a curry, I will often slice up a whole lemon and put it into the dish while it cooks, removing the slices just before serving. And the skin of a lime can be grated to produce an authentic tasting Thai curry.

KIWI

One small kiwi provides our entire recommended daily intake of vitamin C, plus a shot of potassium, vitamin A, magnesium and iron. Despite their sweet taste, they are surprisingly low in sugar and their abundant fibres provide a natural counterbalance to the fructose.

With more vitamin C than an orange, the health benefits of a kiwi are huge. Beyond its high concentration of vitamin C, it's brimming with antioxidants and phytonutrients, including carotenoids that strengthen our eyesight, polysaccharides that help our skin to stay youthful by synthesising collagen and it even contains serotonin that helps us get a good night's sleep.

I could list a dozen more reasons why the kiwi fruit is so healthy, but let me headline lutein, for which it is one of the richest sources available outside of supplements. Lutein, also known as a carotenoid vitamin or 'vitamin eye', is said to help prevent age-related macular degeneration (AMD), cataracts and damage to the retina. It is also associated with healthy skin and in preventing various types of cancer.

CELERY

Used for centuries as a medicine, celery contains an array of phytonutrients that help lower blood pressure and prevent heart disease and inflammation. With their high water content and array of minerals, they're full of electrolytes that help prevent dehydration.

Dr Josh Axe, who created one of the most informative natural health websites (www.draxe.com), says, "It can help prevent or reduce the formation of painful ulcers. A 2010 study published in the Journal of Pharmaceutical Biology found that celery contains a special type of ethanol extract that is useful in protecting the lining of the digestive tract from ulcers. Celery extract has the ability to significantly replenish depleted levels of gastric mucus that is needed in the stomach lining to prevent tiny holes and openings from forming".

ARTICHOKE

Not only do they look like the toughest and most sturdy plant we are likely to find on our plate, they are so full of nutrients and goodness that I just had to place them in the Top 40. While most people only eat the heart, the leaves are so full of beneficial antioxidants that we should try to include them in our dishes too. The 'tough guy' image of artichokes is enhanced by their fibrous construction, and their nutritional line-up includes vitamin B12, vitamin K, vitamin C, manganese, magnesium, potassium, copper, iron, vitamin B6 and many other smaller traces of beneficial minerals.

Artichokes are famed for preventing the most serious of Westernised conditions such as diabetes, various cancers and cardiovascular disease. They also help detoxify the liver and help maintain a healthy digestive tract. They contain some pretty powerful phytonutrients including quercetin, rutin, cynarin and gallic acid. These, combined with its high fibre content, have been known to diminish the symptoms of IBS and even cure it.

PEANUTS

I didn't put peanuts in the nut chart, as they are not nuts at all, but legumes. The question still remains: are they good for us? Simply, yes. They are full of monounsaturated fat, which are really good fats, in fact the average peanut is roughly 50% fat and the same healthy type that you find in olives and oleic acid. While legumes as a family didn't make it into the top 40 and, in the main, should be eaten in moderation, peanuts should be considered differently.

> **WHAT'S IN A PEANUT:**
> A large handful of peanuts is roughly 38 peanuts (28g, or 1oz) and will deliver the following percentages of our recommended daily intake: copper 36%, manganese 28%, vitamin B3 22%, molybdenum 19%, folate 17%, biotin 16%, phosphorus 15%, vitamin E 15% and vitamin B 14%.

When it comes to antioxidant content, peanuts are on par with berries and provide a richer array of antioxidant than most fruits. They also have one amazing antioxidant you won't find in other nuts – resveratrol. It's an antioxidant found in red wine and is believed to help prevent both heart disease and certain cancers.

So, peanuts are super healthy, but don't eat too many. Even though they are 50% fat, 30% protein and 8.5% fibre, if you consume too many handfuls, especially while socialising at a bar for example, you will undoubtedly not realise how many you have consumed and are likely to create a huge calorie surplus.

While I really don't want you to count calories at any stage (it's really not a Primal thing at all), just be aware that each peanut, although healthy, is slightly more than four calories each. So our single handful of 38 nuts is delivering 152 calories! That's more calories than a pack of crisps. Please forgive me for comparing nutritional food to unhealthy processed rubbish – I just need you to appreciate that while peanuts are really healthy, we shouldn't over-consume them.

> **PRIMAL FACT:**
> **Ideally we want our peanuts to be unsalted or just lightly salted. Unsalted and roasted are among the healthiest as roasting actually improves the antioxidant levels in peanuts.**

LENTILS

Here's a double-edged sword. Throughout this book, for all of the reasons I have already stated, we have pretty much stayed clear of CARBS. However, I felt it was important to put lentils into the Top 40 for my vegetarian friends, as they offer one of the richest levels of protein we can get from a plant. The CARBS are also very complex, making them fall towards the bottom of GI index. Lentils also contain lots of fibre, folate, iron, manganese, potassium, zinc, phosphorus, magnesium, copper, vitamin B1 (thiamin) and vitamin B5 (pantothenic acid). I don't personally eat them as I get plenty of protein from meat and poultry, but if you are a vegetarian or vegan, then lentils will almost definitely help fill some nutritional gaps in your diet.

SEAWEED

If the only time you ever eat seaweed is when it's holding together sticky rice in a sushi roll, then it's probably not going to prove to be a healthy choice. But served in soups or used to roll up avocado and prawns or salad rolls for hors d'oeuvre, then it's simply magical. Seaweed is pretty much the only vegetables we consume from the oceans, and it's full of calcium, folate, iodine, magnesium and a whole host of vitamin Bs. Recent research from the University of Newcastle upon Tyne suggests that seaweed, which is also full of fibre, is great for our guts and helps slow down digestion making us feel fuller for longer.

ROMAINE LETTUCE

I was originally going to give both Romaine and Iceberg lettuce their own Top 40 listings as both leaves are healthy, but the more I researched the more I realised that Romaine lettuce was the hands-down winner in macronutrients. For example, Romaine has 10 times more vitamin A than Iceberg. So, if we need help in looking after our skin or teeth, then we should choose Romaine over Iceberg. It is also more concentrated in vitamin K, so if we are worried about our bones or developing osteoporosis, or have concerns about cancer, then choosing Romaine over Iceberg would again be a wise decision.

Romaine also wins hands-down in the two super beneficial carotenoids, lutein and zeaxanthin, so to maintain a healthy eyesight, Romaine is the right choice. That said, if you were to count kale as a lettuce and not a cabbage, then it would be king. By way of explanation, I have included kale in the chart below for two reasons. Firstly, it nicely demonstrates the difference between the Top 20 and Top 40 Superfoods, and secondly, even though kale is technically a cabbage, I personally interchange the two in salads and neither my family or friends rarely spot the difference. I use 150g (5.3oz), because that's approximately two small cups of chopped lettuce, which is close to what I put in a salad at home.

PER 150g	KALE	ROMAINE	ICEBERG
Calories	75	25	21
Vitamin K	1,500%	198%	45%
Vitamin A	462%	261%	15%
Manganese	58%	12%	9%
Calcium	21%	5%	3%
Vitamin B6	21%	6%	3%
Copper	21%	3%	2%
Vitamin C	18%	3%	0%
Potassium	15%	8%	5%

GRAPEFRUIT

Oh, how a little knowledge can be a bad thing. One message remains clear to this day as I left hospital after having kidney stones, 'don't eat grapefruit'. Yet medical research in the USA now suggests that it helps to prevent kidney stones. The citric acid in it is believed to bind with calcium in the kidneys, helping the body flush it out. In addition, the citric acid increases the pH in our urine, which is also believed to help in preventing kidney stones.

Grapefruit's somewhat bitter taste is full of antioxidants and fibre, making it one of the healthiest citrus fruits we can eat. It's rich in vitamin A and C, plus smallish concentrations of various beneficial minerals. Several reports are emerging that suggest that it might help in preventing cells from becoming insulin resistant, therefore preventing type 2 diabetes.

PINEAPPLE

How can something so tasty be so good for us? It's rich in vitamin C and an excellent source of manganese, but most importantly, it's the richest source of bromelain, a mixture of enzymes that are anti-inflammatory and which animal studies suggest protects against tumour growth and cancer. Its ability to reduce swelling makes it an excellent choice for sufferers of arthritis, plus it can cure certain muscle injuries and soreness. Bromelain is also heralded as a natural anticoagulant, therefore can play a role in the prevention of strokes and heart attacks.

The only slight negative is that the pineapple is fairly heavily-loaded with sugar, but that said, one portion still contains fewer calories than an apple and way less than a banana. If you are trying to lose a lot of weight quickly, or abstaining from sugar completely, or maybe you're just not a fan of the tropical taste, today there are dozens of brands of bromelain supplements on the market.

POMEGRANATES

It wasn't until recently that my family added pomegranates to the fruits that fill our fridge. Today, you can buy them in small trays from the supermarket, and they are great to add vital nutrients to a morning yogurt, or to toss into almost any salad. Their health benefits lie in their incredible line-up of antioxidants and other beneficial compounds. When you stop to think about it, they are a cross between a seed and a fruit, and therefore we get a double serving of healthiness.

Rich in vitamin C, vitamin K and potassium, studies have shown that pomegranates may help reduce the risk of cancer and all kinds of inflammation. They are also said to help treat high blood pressure, reduce oxidative stress and hyperglycemia. They have also long been recognised as an aphrodisiac and a recent study at the Queen Margaret University in Edinburgh suggested pomegranate juice lowered cortisol levels, which can lead to an increase of testosterone not just in men, but in women as well.

ASPARAGUS

I placed asparagus after pomegranates as it is believed to be the finest aphrodisiac wrapped up in a vegetable. The Kama Sutra advised that it should be consumed as a paste, and the Greeks linked it to love in poetry. In history, the French would include it in all meals leading up to a wedding in the belief that it increased libido and therefore prevented embarrassing moments on wedding nights. However, my own story has nothing to do with sex drive. When I had a kidney stone, my lovely wife did lots of research on how to break the stone up naturally. As I had to check myself out of hospital to attend an important meeting in Hong Kong, and before the doctors who had procrastinated for two days had a chance to zap it, my wife made me eat lots of mushed-up asparagus. Within 48 hours the pain had eased, and when I returned to the UK the doctor was amazed that it had completely vanished. It appears that its high concentration of potassium helps to cleanse both the kidneys and the urinary tract - and literally caused my stone to disintegrate.

But back to increased libido, which is frankly far more interesting than kidney stones. Asparagus contains aspartic acid, which can neutralise the excess ammonia in our body which is often a root cause of a drop in libido. On top of busting kidney stones and increasing our sex drive, from its tip to stem asparagus is loaded with other nutrients too.

CUCUMBER

There are three nutrients in cucumber that aren't mentioned anywhere else in this book, and that are all very beneficial to our health. Lariciresinol, secoisolariciresinol and pinoresinol are antioxidants that support our immune system and are excellent for balancing hormone levels. These three phytonutrients are said to reduced the risk of cardiovascular disease as well as several types of cancer, including prostate, breast and ovarian. Cucumbers also contain another nutrient called fisetin (also found in strawberries), that helps keep the brain in good working order and has slowed down the development of Alzheimer's in laboratory experiments with mice.

Other than its unique phytonutrients, cucumbers have a huge list of beneficial minerals and vitamins, but due to the fact that they are 95% water their concentration is very slight. That said, the reason why you often see therapists placing them on eyes during a beauty session is that they possess effective anti-wrinkling nutrients known as ascorbic and caffeic acid.

CARROTS

They really do help us see in the dark, honestly! They are rich in beta-carotene that the liver converts into vitamin A. When vitamin A reaches the retina, it is further converted to rhodopsin, a pigment that helps enhance night vision. Beta-carotene is also associated with preventing certain cancers, specifically lung, colon and breast. Vitamin A also slows down the ageing of our skin, while boosting the quality of our hair and nails too.

A study at Harvard University found that people who ate five or more carrots each week were less likely to have a stroke, while other research has found that most foods that contain carotenoids are associated with a lower risk of heart diseases. When it comes to vitamins and minerals, by far its highest concentration is vitamin A, where just one cupful will provide more than four times our RDA.

CHEESE

While cheese does not feature in a strict Paleo diet, I believe that, as long as you follow a few guidelines, it fits perfectly well in a Primal lifestyle. Firstly, I am not talking about mass-produced factory cheeses in brightly coloured wrappings. These are often produced and enhanced in ways that make them not fit for human consumption, or at least Primal consumption. Secondly, it's really important to ensure the cheese is organic. The last thing we want to be putting in our mouths is cheese that originated from the milk of a cow that was pumped full of antibiotics.

But isn't cheese full of lactose and isn't lactose essentially sugar?

Here is the good news for cheese lovers. The fermentation process that turns milk into cheese significantly reduces its lactose (sugar) content. Indeed, the longer a cheese is aged, the more time it provides the healthy bacteria to ferment even more lactose. Brie, feta, goat's cheese, blue cheese, cheddar, Camembert, Gruyère, Edam, Roquefort, mozzarella and Parmesan all have less than 4% CARBS and in moderation they are healthy additions to a Primal lifestyle.

While a lot of people sing the praise of cottage cheese, they tend to have a higher CARB content. As always, avoid any cheeses that say low or reduced fat, as these are most likely pumped with added sugar, sweteners or other such additives to make up for the lack of natural healthy fat.

COFFEE

Coffee is rich in caffeine. The coffee plant produces caffeine in its seeds to defend itself from predators who, if they do have a nibble, go weak, lose their alertness and either fall from the plant, or are easily swallowed up by prey that know better than to consume it. Now it might not send us humans weak at the knees, but it does stimulate our central nervous system. I like to have coffee when I am weight training as it unlocks fat in the bloodstream and turns it into energy.

Some people are more sensitive to the effects of caffeine than others. Personally, I can take a big mug to bed and it has no effect at all on how long it takes me to fall asleep, while others find its stimulation of the nervous system too much and it prevents them from sleeping. As we know already, sleep is really important, so if you find coffee keeps you awake, then as a bedtime drink why not have a herbal tea with ginger, which helps aid sleep. In his book *The IF Diet*, Robert Skinner explains coffee's effect on sleep brilliantly, "Throughout the day, a chemical called adenosine normally builds up, hour by hour. Adenosine dampens down brain activity, eventually allowing us to drift off. Caffeine causes mischief – because it looks like adenosine and jumps into the places where adenosine normally builds up. With the spaces blocked adenosine can't get in to tell your brain 'dim the lights' and we stay… unsleepy".

A slight downside of caffeine is that it's a diuretic, which means it tells our kidneys to pass water. So coffee will dehydrate us a little. As a result, either before or after a coffee I personally try to remember to drink a similar amount of plain water just to balance it out.

A study in Finland of 1,409 people, aged between 65 and 79, found that those who drank more than three to five cups of coffee a day were a staggering 65% less likely to fall victim to Alzheimer's disease, compared to those that drank either no coffee at all just one or two cups a day. How is this possible? It is to do with the effect coffee has on our microbiome. In the Journal of Agricultural and Food Chemistry, researchers reported that gut-friendly bacteria, in particular bacteroidetes and prevotella, receive a 60% growth boost for up to 24 hours after coffee fibres enter the gut. Coffee isn't just great at reducing the risk of mental diseases, its high concentration of polyphenols make it a great antioxidant too. If you don't like coffee you can also get polyphenols in red wine, tea, vegetables and dark chocolate too.

TEA

Tea has for centuries, especially in the East, been regarded as good for health, happiness and wisdom. According to the hugely popular website WebMD, "Studies have found that some teas may help with cancer, heart disease, and diabetes; encourage weight loss; lower cholesterol; and bring about mental alertness. Tea also appears to have antimicrobial qualities". Let's divide tea into two camps – green and all other types.

Green Tea

This is possibly the healthiest natural drink you could have, and is created by drying leaves from the tea plant Camellia sinensis. It's full of epigallocatechin gallate (ECGC), which speeds up our metabolism while at the same time suppresses hunger. With every cup we get a double dose of goodness. It increases the hormone adrenaline, which in return produces heat. For the body to produce heat it has to burn energy and of course burning energy causes us to lose weight.

Green tea is not just about ECGC, there are numerous other phytonutrients and antioxidants that boost the immune system, acting as natural antibacterial and antiviral compounds. Its ability to protect us from free radicals and therefore certain cancers is well documented, as too is its ability to prevent symptoms associated with colds and flu. Green tea is so beneficial for our health that, for those who don't like tea, there are plenty of brands (including Primal Cure) that make ECGC supplements.

Other Teas

One day, for a bit of fun, my daughter Jessica and I went to our local supermarket to count how many different flavours of tea were on sale. We found a staggering 97: from ginger with cranberry, rose and sweet vanilla to oat flower with lavender and limeflower. From a tea infused with chamomile that claims to stop us from snoring, lemon balm and lavender to a palate-refreshing triple mint tea containing peppermint, spearmint and field mint. My current favourite is green tea infused with ginger. On the isles of Ikaria and Okinawa, both regions of extraordinary longevity and very good health, drinking organic and local tea is part of their daily ritual.

As someone who has always slightly overindulged in alcohol (although as I write this chapter I am currently on a dry month), I find flavoured teas a great replacement, especially in the evenings. On my fasting days, where I stay alcohol free, if I feel the urge for a gin and tonic or a glass of red wine, I can always put my alcohol monkey (if you have read *Chimp Paradox* by Steve Peters you will know what I mean) back in its box and satisfy my craving with a flavoured tea. And as a way of keeping tea drinking interesting and varied, I sometimes even put two different bags in the same cup to create different tea cocktails.

According to Dan Buettner in his brilliant book *The Blue Zones*. which features on its cover the subtitle "9 lessons for living longer, from the people who have lived the longest", while discussing the incredible number of centenarians on the island of Ikaria he says, "Ikarians drink herbal teas made from wild oregano, sage, and rosemary – all of which lower blood pressure. How they drink them is important too: They drink these daily but rotate the flavours".

THE 'OKAY IN MODERATION' STUFF

Legumes

Did you know that a mollusc is a sea creature that has a shell that opens and closes on a hinge? Legumes are plants where the fruit is contained in pods, which are casings with two halves that - just like molluscs - often hinge! Legumes are to the land what molluscs are to the oceans. The legume family is normally subdivided into beans, lentils, peas and peanuts.

One of the areas that Primal Cure differs from the Paleo way of living is in our views on legumes. Firstly, there is growing evidence to suggest that our Primal ancestors consumed certain beans and other legumes, such as peanuts, as part of their diverse diet. As a result, I don't think it will be too long before those practitioners of strict Paleo diets begin endorsing them!

Plus, even though I suggested in Chapter 1 that CARBS is an acronym for Carbs Are Really Bad Sugars, it was more to highlight the fact that the body eventually turns all CARBS into sugar, rather that we should banish them completely. While it is true that we could survive without ever consuming a single carbohydrate, avoiding them completely would mean missing out on many fruits and vegetables.

Living Primally isn't about total CARB abstention, but avoiding those that are devoid of health benefits, such as the white and brown category of CARBS including rice, sugar, bread, pasta and potatoes.

So, with healthy foods, where CARBS are wrapped into the package as a side macronutrient, we need to evaluate each one on its own merits.

> **LEGUMES FACT:**
> If we abstained from legumes, we couldn't have dark chocolate – and who would want to miss out on dark chocolate? And a chilli con carne would not be a chilli con carne without kidney beans. Plus, I would personally find it too difficult to live life without the occasional handful of peanuts.

While most legumes do contain CARBS, they are rich in protein and fibre and are often very advantageous to the bacteria in our microbiome. Many are full of vitamins and minerals, making them highly nutritious. One of the reasons legumes sometimes receive a bad press is because they often contain the anti-nutrient phytic acid, which binds minerals together in our digestive system resulting in lower quantities being available for the body to absorb.

> **DIGESTION SCIENCE:**
> Legumes, nuts, seeds and grains store the mineral phosphorus in the form of phytic acid. When phytic acid bonds with a mineral it is known as phytate. Even though there are drawbacks of having too much phytate in the body, allowing some useful minerals to be excreted rather than being utilised, some experts suggest that phytate itself may contain protective properties against cancer, diabetes and cardiovascular disease. With the jury still out, my advice is to consume legumes in sensible quantities.

Let's just pick on one legume, the kidney bean, to highlight why at Primal Cure we are happy to consume them in moderation.

Kidney Beans
Named because they look similar to our kidneys, kidney beans are a great source of minerals, vitamins, proteins and fibre. Yes, they do contain CARBS, but at least they are of the complex form.

Like other beans, kidney beans are a rich source of flavonols. These are a group of phytonutrients that our body uses as antioxidants to fight against inflammation and also to neutralise free radicals. As a result, researchers believe beans are beneficial in helping to treat and even prevent certain types of cancer. Along with several others, they are said to reduce the bad LDL cholesterol without impacting the good HDL. Research has also demonstrated that kidney beans can reduce insulin levels and therefore help in fighting diabetes.

Kidney beans – in fact pretty much all legumes – help release short-chain fatty acids, which strengthen the cells in our intestines, thereby helping us to better absorb micronutrients. Recent research has shown that they also help us to feel full quicker, so are therefore beneficial for those who want to lose weight.

One of the few downsides of beans is that they do tend to make us pass wind. The culprit is a certain sugar called oligosaccharide which, unlike other sugars, is not absorbed into the bloodstream. It's oligosaccharide that causes the beans to become musical in our gut, fueling their embarrassing tunes that we all know tend to announce themselves at the most inappropriate time. Technically this happens as the sugar arrives in the colon, where our bacteria begins to ferment it, a process that unfortunately produces a lot of gas. But, other than the embarrassment of letting one go in public, take pleasure in the knowledge that it's our good bacteria that are getting fed.

Potato VS Sweet Potato

Firstly, this is only a brief overview on potatoes. With more than 5,000 different varieties of sweet potatoes and 4,000 varieties of regular potatoes, we could talk about them all day long. With more people on the planet now being overweight than malnourished, it's important to start with a CARBS warning. Both types of potatoes are loaded with them. If your weight is of no concern to you and you baked either a medium white or sweet potato, this is what you would be getting:

	Potato	Sweet Potato
Calories	153	98
Protein	4g	2g
CARBS	35g	23g
Fibre	4g	4g
Glycemic Load (Baked)	17GL	10GL
Vitamin A	0%	416%
Vitamin C	26%	35%
Manganese	18%	26%
Vitamin B6	25%	15%
Potassium	25%	14%
Vitamin B3	11%	8%
Phosphorus	11%	6%
Vitamin B9	11%	2%
Vitamin B5	7%	9%
Iron	9%	4%
Copper	9%	9%

As you can see they both contain a lot of CARBS, but the sweet potato is approximately a third less. Plus, while both types of potato have a reasonable line-up of vitamins and minerals, just one sweet potato can provide four times our daily requirement of vitamin A. Personally I avoid potatoes as they seem to travel straight to my waist. But if you just can't give up on them completely, then try to find a variety of sweet potato that you like and boil or bake them.

Salt

Just like fat, salt has had a bad rap over the past few decades, but it is in fact essential to our health. The best salt of all is coarse sea salt. As we begin to follow the principles of Primal Cure, we will be drinking more water and eating less processed foods. Therefore, we might need to check whether we are actually consuming enough salt. It is certainly unlikely on a Primal Cure lifestyle that we will be taking in too much.

This is especially true if we workout a lot in the gym and build-up a sweat, or on days when we are sprinting or playing a game of tennis or golf, when we might find that we need to deliberately top up our salt intake. If you feel that you are not taking on board enough salt (sodium) and don't like adding it to food for the rest of the family, then add one or two stock cubes (or if you are in America we mean bouillon) to a glass of boiling water and enjoy a quick broth. With your newfound knowledge in nutrition, spend a little time studying the different ingredients from the top brands of stock cubes and you will be surprised at how healthy some of these can be.

> **PRIMAL CURE ON SALT:**
> Because of its dramatic overuse by the packaged and fast food industries, salt has for several decades been incorrectly vilified. If you eat Primally and avoid food where salt has been unnaturally added and you are not sensitive to it, then there is plenty of medical research to suggest that using salt more liberally should not lead to health issues.

Fruit

Berries made it onto our Superfood list because they are simply awesome, so too did the amazing avocado (which is technically a berry as well). Most other fruits are also healthy, but because of their high sugar content just be sure to eat them in moderation.

Does organic fruit make much difference? I want you to answer the question yourself after considering the following; other than those at the very top of the food chain, all animals and plants have predators, and all animals and plants have developed certain tools to defend against these predators. Most fruits and vegetables too are full of a variety of antioxidants to defend against predators such as animals, mould, insects and too much sun. Our Primal ancestors use to eat lots of natural fruits and our body started to use these antioxidants to defend against various illnesses. When we eat organic fruits, our body puts these antioxidants to work. They form a first line of defence against many internal enemies. However, when we consume fruits that are not organic, that have been developed and modified rather than grown exclusively by nature, many of their natural antioxidants are diminished and in some instances removed completely.

Think about it like this. An organic fruit or vegetable that manages to survive its harsh environment must be full of powerful antioxidants. Those that aren't wither and die and are therefore never consumed. But when a fruit or vegetable is protected by pesticides, their natural antioxidants aren't necessary and don't develop. What's worse, their artificial life support machine means that they reach their ripening age and can make it all the way to our dinner plate without any antioxidants at all. Various experts have written articles on the differing quantity of antioxidants found in fruits that are organic compared to semi-manufactured varieties, and I put the median average of all their reports at about 9:1. In other words, on average an organic fruit is nine times more beneficial than an enhanced fruit. In *The Disease Delusion*, author Dr Jeffry S. Bland writes, "Organic fruits and vegetables have a higher phytonutrient index than their non-organic equivalents. Remember that an organic vegetable or fruit has to work harder to defend itself from the stress of its environment. It therefore manufactures more phytonutrient stress-fighters than do foods coddled by pesticides, herbicides and fungicides that do the stress-fighting for them".

ORGANIC FRUIT TIP:
On average an organic fruit is nine times more beneficial than an enhanced fruit.

WHAT TO AVOID

As a general rule we should be aiming to eat naturally and not artificially. We should only be looking to consume foods that our body has evolved to eat, and therefore we must avoid anything that has been altered or manufactured by humans since the end of the Stone Age.

Sugar

For the sake of our health, we must avoid sugar wherever possible. Study food labels, where any ingredient ending in '-ose' should in my opinion come with as big a health warning as we now quite rightly slap on a packet of cigarettes. Here we are going to look at just one example: high fructose corn syrup, also known as HFCS, but the same avoidance advice applies to all sugars. I have already mentioned this earlier in the book, but food containing HFCS poses a real problem for those of us looking to live a long and healthy life.

In her exposé of the food industry's biggest secrets, *Swallow This*, Joanna Blythman says of fructose, "While the fructose in whole fruits comes hand-in-hand with fibre which slows and reduces the body's absorption of sugar, this is not the case when fructose is added in a highly refined, 100 per cent purified form, as it is in processed food. When Mother Nature designed fruit, she thought it through properly. The potential poison in it (fructose) comes in the same wrapper as the antidote (fibre), which seems to prevent the former having any negative effects on our metabolism".

HFCS is used in packaged foods because it is cheaper than regular sugar and, as it is a syrup, it's easier to handle. Fructose syrup in packaged food is not only a major contributor to obesity, but also has been linked to type 2 diabetes, hypertension and something I have witnessed my father and father-in-law suffer in great pain with – gout.

Artifical Sweetners

So if sucrose, fructose corn syrup and pretty much everything ending in '-ose' are all unhealthy, what about all of the artificial sweeteners such as aspartame, acesulfame and sucralose? Have you seen how tiny these things are? One tiny little pill, less than quarter the size of a Tic Tac, makes our coffee or tea taste like we have put several spoons of sugar in it. In fact, they are all said to be more than 100 times sweeter than corn syrup and the NHS website reports, "Acesulfame potassium, also known as acesulfame K, is a calorie-free sweetener up to 200 times sweeter than sugar and as sweet as aspartame". The fact that these artificial pills are so tiny yet so powerful immediately suggests that something can't be right with these lab-engineered alternatives.

Caveman never ate anything manufactured in a laboratory, so do you really think we are designed to eat anything artificial? The European Food Safety Authority recognises that sweeteners are potentially toxic in larger quantities but has stated that all products it permits for sale are safe for normal consumption. But, as far as I am concerned, we are back to the magician tossing coins and getting 10 heads in a row! According to Joanna Blythman in Swallow This, "Studies have linked artificial sweetener consumption to a variety of negative health effects: migraine, epilepsy, premature birth and brain cancer".

It is also believed that artificial sweeteners cause untold damage to our microbiome, causing good bacteria to run for the hills and leaving the bad guys to flourish. Plus, while the liver is dealing with inbound artificial sweeteners, it has to temporarily suspend producing the satiety hormone leptin.

Processed Food

Caveman didn't have anything processed at all. Everything was fresh, almost fresh or rancid. But even if it was rancid, at least it was 100% natural. I went to a supermarket with four of my children and asked them to spend an hour thinking about what percentage of food in the shop was processed. It's not that my kids are all geniuses, I wanted to see how well they were understanding the Primal Cure approach, and to try to figure out how much stuff was truly natural compared to what percentage of food was manufactured. Together, we arrived at a figure of 92% of all the food on sale being processed. So, based on my family's research, more than nine out of 10 items of food in a supermarket are indeed processed.

But is that a problem? Of course it is, because we are not designed to eat processed food. Let's take bread for example: as it is pure sugar once digested, it doesn't sit well with a Primal lifestyle. However, if you bake a loaf at home, while it is still 'one level of evil', it's nothing compared to supermarket bread, which is in fact the devil in disguise. Did you know supermarket bread contains on average seven times more salt than home-baked bread? "A large proportion of the bread we buy is bleached, blanched and nutrient stripped," reported nutritionist Vicki Edgson in an article on the Mirror website in March 2012. "It's made from processed wheat and as well as containing salt and preservatives, some loaves also contain sugar."

Packaged food can last weeks, months, sometimes years before it needs to be consumed. How is that possible? They stuff it full of nasty preservatives. Generally speaking, the longer the shelf life, the more preservatives are in the food. While these preservatives might provide extended shelf life, they tend to kill the helpful bacteria in our gut. Think about it, how do you extend the shelf life of food? You add chemicals that kill off bacteria. However, there is no safety mechanism in these foods to make sure they exclusively kill off bad bacteria. Woefully, once they enter our gut they kill millions of healthy bacteria that, over thousands of years, nature has ensured we keep alive in our body to fight off both diseases and infections.

Jen Whitington in her brilliant book *Fixing Dad*, explains why, "The dilemma for the food manufacturers or supermarket is a big one: if you make efforts to substantially reduce the levels of sugar, salt or saturated fats in foods you run the risk of altering flavours too much and losing your customers. Sugar, salt and saturated fats make up the holy trinity of palatability in processed foods; if you reduce one you must increase the other to compensate". So what Jen Whitington is warning is that if we purchase a zero fat or low-fat version of a regular product, then it must have extra sugar or salts stuffed into it. Jen, whose husband cured his own father's diabetes by putting him on a low CARB diet and the right exercise program, goes on to say, "These high sugar foods that we have lived on for years and grown accustomed to – even dependent upon in our cravings for them – are massive drivers of insulin. Remember this is a fat-storing hormone".

Dr Dan Maggs

"Low fat or zero fat? Simply avoid them both. Fat is not the enemy."

Genetically Modified Organisms

How un-Primal are genetically modified organisms (GMO)? Did our ancestors sit in caves with a chemistry set gluing together different bits of plants in an attempt to produce strawberries in December? Of course not, they were simply too busy hunting and gathering! Don't confuse GMOs with crossbreeding. What is happening in the designer dog world, with a never-ending creation of goldendoodle (golden retriever and poodle), labradoodle (Labrador retriever and poodle) and cockapoo (cocker spaniel and poodle) etc, is very different to artificially messing with the DNA of plants and animals.

How common are GMO foods? Regrettably very! Simply type into Google, 'Top 10 GMOs' and you will find hundreds of different lists. Nearly all websites quote corn, soy and sugar to be the most widely consumed genetically modified foods. The statistics are staggering. In the USA 95% of sugar, 94% of soybeans and 88% of corn is from modified crops. In total it is estimated that more than 80% of packaged food in the USA contains GMOs. In Europe the situation is much healthier, with many GMOs banned from sale and others having to be declared on food labels.

There have been thousands of studies over the past three decades into whether GMOs are safe or not, with much of the recent consensus being that there is no proven difference between GMOs and organically grown crops. But I don't believe this for one minute.

While there is no concrete evidence of the ill effect of GMOs compared to non-GMOs, allow me to make three observations:

1. One of the main reasons for their invention was to make crops more robust to pesticides. So, a GMO product is more likely to be sprayed with toxins that we really shouldn't consume.
2. Any toxins sprayed onto food to protect it, reduces the crop's inherent self-defence mechanisms, thereby reducing the amount of beneficial anti-oxidants we receive when consuming it.
3. The top three GMO crops – sugar, corn and soy – are not recommended to those living Primally. So a GMO label on packaged food might just be alerting us to the fact that we shouldn't be consuming it anyway.

Fish & Chips

I wasn't going to give this traditional British dish its own heading, but the other evening a good friend of mine began to argue that a Primal lifestyle should allow us to eat fish and chips as they have been part of our heritage for over 150 years. He further pushed his case by telling me that Winston Churchill called them 'the good companions'. But as I reminded my friend, even though Churchill was a brilliant leader he was also very overweight! "But Steve, they are just vegetables and fish, both of which you preach we should eat", he continued.

> **PRIMAL FISH SAYING:**
> **It's the batter that makes you fatter!**

So, I explained that while 'fish like cod is god', the way it's cooked is evil, and I told him that potatoes, if he were to pay a little more attention to the details, were not a very healthy vegetable as they were loaded full of CARBS.

> **PRIMAL ACRONYM:**
> **'CHIPS' stands for Carbohydrates Hidden In Poisonous Substances, referring to the fact that most chip shops use cheap chemically enhanced oils.**

Quinoa - The Jury Is Still Out

As it's not technically a grain, there has been so much hype and confusion around quinoa over the past decade. Yes, it's not a grain, so yes it doesn't therefore contain gluten, but it's still not on the Primally acceptable list. While some researchers believe quinoa is exceedingly healthy as it contains Omega 3 and all nine essential amino acids, others say it drives the gut crazy! I can understand the reasons behind the claim as quinoa contains saponins, which could potentially damage our microvilli. Saponins got their name because, just like soap, they lather up in water. But at the time of writing this book, the quinoa jury is still outside debating if it's friend or foe.

Chapter 9 Highlights

- To be Primally acceptable, all meat has to be organic - which means, among other things, that the animals were raised on food they were designed to eat.
- Always buy organic and local if possible, then be sure to eat the organs too.
- It is said that of the 50 billion chickens farmed around our small planet each year, 70% of them are no longer organic.
- If we don't regularly consume enough Omega 3, then we are more prone to suffer from inflammation, arthritis, joint and muscle pains, allergies, digestive disorders, cognitive dysfunctions and have a higher risk of heart disease.
- Just like fat, salt has had a bad rap over the past few decades, but it is in fact essential to our health.
- As a general rule we should be aiming to eat naturally.
- We should only be looking to consume foods that our body has evolved to eat, and therefore we must avoid anything that has been altered or manufactured by humans since the end of the Stone Age.
- Caveman didn't have anything processed at all. Everything was fresh or almost fresh.

10.
Diseases That Plague Britain & How To Avoid Them

In this chapter, we will look at the main causes of illness, disease and even death in Great Britain and reveal some of the secrets of how to try and avoid them.

All of the illnesses and diseases we discuss in this chapter are Westernised (influenced by the cultural, economic or political systems of Europe and North America) diseases. In other words, they all begin with either the food we eat, the way we eat it, our exposure to pollution and toxic chemicals and our lifestyle in general. As I firmly believe these have to be the root cause of them all, you will unavoidably find a little repetition in both the causes and the solution. Despite this, if you are particularly concerned about a specific medical condition, or simply want to discover more, then I am sure you will find the information more than useful.

FREE RADICALS – THE AGEING THEORY

Just like everything else in the universe, our body's cells are made up of atoms and groups of atoms called molecules. Each cell is said to contain more than 100 trillion atoms, which by coincidence is approximately the number of cells in the body!

After we have fully digested our food, the excess energy in our body is stored as adenosine tri-phosphate (for simplicity let's just call it by its abbreviation ATP), and the task of its production is primarily handed over to the mitochondria within our cells. If they are in good condition, and fed plenty of vitamins and nutrients, our mitochondria can remain very good at their job and can convert virtually the entire incoming glucose molecules into ATP. However, if they are not fit and well they end up creating quite a lot of waste.

When oxygen interacts with this waste, our cells create what is known as free radicals. So, while oxygen is vital to all life, it can have a harmful effect on unhealthy cells (known as oxidative stress). The process goes something like this: the waste becomes oxidised, which creates free radicals – these attack the mitochondria and they are no longer able to turn glucose into ATP. Once the free radicals are done with damaging all the mitochondria (there are normally several hundred in each cell), they turn on the nucleus. As the nucleus holds the blueprint for the cell, the entire cell becomes damaged.

Free radicals are highly contagious, and often start a chain reaction that turns their neighbouring molecules into free radicals too. Free radicals eventually cause so much damage inside the cell that the mitochondria send a premature message to the nucleus, telling it to kill off the entire cell - and that's what causes premature ageing. Free radicals can also be a direct cause of cancer, strokes and various illnesses relating to the brain.

One of the fundamental reasons why Primal Cure does not recommend lots of endurance exercise is that it can massively increase the levels of oxygen utilisation in the cells. This can then lead to the generation of free radicals that damage muscles and other tissues. In his book, *The Low Carb Athlete* (a great read if you are doing lots of sport and are still not convinced that you don't need to CARB load) Ben Greenfield says, "When glucose is used to create energy, a high number of free radicals are produced. Free radicals are dangerous molecules that can damage normal cellular processes. The burning of fat for energy does not create this same cellular damage. In an athlete who is already creating a high number of damaging free radicals from exercise, further damage from high blood glucose levels becomes a nasty one-two combo".

But it's not all bad news. If the right antioxidants are present in our body, they interact with the free radicals and halt the chain reaction before too much damage is done. Fruit, vegetables, nuts and seeds often contain several different types of antioxidants. The strongest antioxidants are vitamin C, vitamin E, carotenoids, beta-carotene and selenium, but as we have already learnt there are hundreds more.

In addition to making sure we eat plenty of colourful fruit and vegetables rich in antioxidants, there is something else we can do to constrain our free radicals. It's to not rely on CARBS and other sugars as our main source of fuel. Remember what was said towards the beginning of the book – sugar is seen as a poison inside the body. One of the reasons for this is that glucose produces more oxygen interaction. If instead of constantly using glucose as our fuel, which free radicals feed off, we burn our own body fat, then it can only be a good thing. But of course it's a balancing act. To burn our stored fat, we need to intermittently fast, and by doing so we might end up consuming a smaller quantity of helpful antioxidants. This is why when we do intermittently fast, the quality of the small amounts of food that we consume is very important. No matter which type of intermittent fasting we undertake, if we break our fast with a pre-packaged meal or fast food, then we might do more harm than good. But if we end our fast with nuts, eggs, colourful fruit and vegetables and organic meat, we should be able to keep our free radicals under full control.

> **PRIMAL CURE TIP:**
> **By intermittently fasting we can reduce the accumulation of free radicals, therefore reducing the catalyst to many diseases – oxidative damage.**

I mentioned intermittent fasting and its beneficial effects on slowing down the ageing process above. By now, I bet you can guess what goes hand-in-hand with fasting. What can prevent cancer and inflammation and of course radically prolong the onset of ageing? It's moving our body into a state of ketogenic metabolism as frequently as possible.

INFLAMMATION AND AUTOIMMUNE DISEASE

If you have ever suffered a sports injury, I'm sure you have experienced swelling or inflammation around the joint or muscle that you hurt. This is the body's self-defence system that protects the damaged area. Inflammation occurs when the body's immune system dispatches white blood cells (plus a few other substances) not only to protect the injured part of the body, but also to create barriers against viruses and bacteria and other stuff it just doesn't understand. Although the science is only just beginning to emerge, it appears that the bacteria in our microbiome play a large role in the creation and control of inflammation. Our good bacteria is acting as the fire brigade and putting out the flames, while our bad bacteria act like Guy Fawkes on a mission to set alight the entire internal infrastructure of our body.

Sometimes Guy Fawkes wins and tricks the immune system into an inflammatory response when there was no need for one. This misinformed inflammatory response is known as autoimmune disease. It is a disease of the protective immune system, causing it to damage its own tissues rather than protect them. For example, arthritis – which affects a staggering 350 million people worldwide – is a form of autoimmune disease. But inflammation isn't just restricted to autoimmune conditions. Inflammation can be a silent killer, and can progress over years and years without you even realising it. Inflammation is associated with many different modern world diseases. From Alzheimer's to cancer, from heart disease to strokes, from multiple sclerosis to ADHD, inflammation is a root cause of the vast majority of diseases of the Western world.

Think about it logically – if we are living a lifestyle very different to the one we were designed to live, it is going to put a huge amount of stress on our immune system. The immune system is a complex network of cells, tissues and organs that work as a team to protect our body. But like a modern car with electrical sensors for literally everything, when they go wrong they can go really wrong. Our body was designed to hunt and gather, to eat healthy foods and to move around more. The immune system was developed to protect against viruses and bacteria. It wasn't created to deal with a daily overdose of sugar, an onslaught of toxins, repetitive over frequent eating patterns and all while sitting on our backsides for 14 hours a day. The immune system has tried to do its best, but it's fighting a battle on multiple fronts that it neither understands or is equipped to deal with!

AVOIDING TYPE 2 DIABETES

Let me start this Primal Cure piece of advice by reminding you that I am not a doctor, and don't have a single letter after my name. But by reading hundreds of books and lots of white papers on health, I have gained a reasonable understanding of diabetes. While there are undoubtedly a lot of people suffering from type 1 diabetes due to genetic reasons, type 2 diabetes is not only often avoidable, in many cases it is reversible. As I have already mentioned you could view type 2 diabetes as an equation:

> **Refined CARBS lead to too much sugar in the blood, which creates too much insulin**

Looking at the above equation, it's logical to arrive at the conclusion that type 2 diabetes is in fact an intolerance of carbohydrate overloading! Of all the diseases we are about to cover, type 2 diabetes is in some respects one of the more straightforward to suggest a potential cure. Cut out all CARBS and other sugars from anything other than vegetables. If you have diabetes, or are close to someone that suffers from this Westernised disease, please buy the book *Fixing Dad*. It's wonderfully written and explains the journey the Whitington family took to rid their father of the condition.

CANCER

I was going to start this piece by saying something like, "Cancer has only been around for a few hundred years and therefore it is in the main caused by all of the chemicals that are being injected into packaged foods". Then I came across some research where, in a Scythian burial site in Russia, they discovered the 2,700-year-old human remains of a man whose bones were riddled with tumours. But the more articles you read by experts in aetiology and pathogenesis (the study of the history of illnesses), it seems that while cancer may have been around for a very long time, it was extremely rare until the last century. My theory would be that in these rare cases of caveman cancer, they were most likely caused by them being lousy cooks and constantly burning their food (burnt food can be carcinogenic).

In *Prescription for Nutritional Healing*, which has sold more than 8 million copies, author Phyllis A. Balch writes, "When burning fat drips onto an open flame, polycyclic aromatic hydrocarbons (PAHs) – dangerous carcinogens – are formed. When amino acids and other chemicals found in muscle are exposed to high temperature, other carcinogens, called heterocyclic aromatic amines (HAAs), are created". Now the worrying thing is not only are these the likely cause of caveman cancer, but these very same chemicals caused by overcooking proteins are actually used to generate cancer in animal laboratories!

> **BARBECUE WARNING:**
> **Don't burn your poultry or meat when having a BBQ.**

Back to my main point. The current growth rate in cases of diagnosed cancer is nothing short of a pandemic. According to Cancer Research UK, one in two people will now at some time in their life be diagnosed with cancer. They do state that the recent move from one in three people to one in two is partly because we are living longer, and they do go on to say that through advancements in healthcare 50% of people with cancer beat the illness, but the growth in numbers is still concerning. Cancer Research UK state on their website, "More than three-quarters of all people diagnosed with cancer in the UK are over the age of 60". So, it seems quite logical that the older we become, the more precautions we should take to avoid this horrible disease.

In *The Scientific Approach to Intermittent Fasting*, Dr Michael VanDerschelden shares some alarming growth in cancer rates. He says that in the early 1900s only one in 20 people developed cancer. This grew to one in 16 by the 1940s and one in 10 by the 1970s. He finishes by saying that, "Today, a whopping one in three develop cancer!" And of course we have read above, that with an ageing population there is now a one in two chance that we will develop cancer at some point in our life, most likely after we are 60 years old.

I don't mean to frighten you with the bleak picture painted above, but I do intend to shock you into realising we need to do everything we can to reduce the likelihood of being in the wrong 50%. I lost both grandfathers, my wonderful grandmother and my amazing auntie Avis to cancer. I am sure you have had similar tragedies. So let's focus really hard right now on what we can do to increase our odds. Do I really think it's possible? Absolutely. If cancer is growing at an alarming rate, there has to be a cause. If our Primal ancestors rarely suffered defeat to cancer, if it affected only one in 20 some 100 years ago, then surely we can change our odds from one in two back to better than one in 20 by adopting a lifestyle and diet from a bygone age.

But what is cancer? While they are all slightly different and can form almost anywhere in the body, in all cases they begin when some of the body's cells start to divide and multiply and spread (metastasise) into surrounding tissues. Under normal conditions, when our old cells die in a natural process known as apoptosis (around 10 billion per day), new cells grow but only when the body requires them. If this orderly process breaks down, cancer may develop. Once cancer starts to develop, old or damaged cells survive when they should die, but at the same time extra new cells that should replace them continue to form. This leads to abnormal growths known as tumours. When tumours are malignant they can spread into surrounding tissues. Often they can break off and travel via the blood or the lymph system to other parts of the body. Even after removal, there is a potential that they may return. Benign tumours are contained and do not spread. When benign tumours are removed, they usually don't grow back.

Compiled from the in-depth research I have done, here are the top 14 things I believe we can all do to best defend ourselves against the terrible disease that is cancer:

1. Don't smoke. Period!
2. Intermittently fast. Frequently put our body into repair mode.
3. Don't consume CARBS and other sugars. This isn't news, 75 years ago Dr Otto Warburg won the Nobel Prize in Physiology for discovering it. He explained, "Cancer, above all other diseases, has countless secondary causes. But, even for cancer, there is only one prime cause. Summarised in a few words, the prime cause of

cancer is the replacement of the respiration of oxygen in normal body cells by a fermentation of sugar".

4. Avoid packaged foods, hydrogenated fats and processed meat (trust the cow, not the chemist).
5. Eat organically and avoid poisonous pesticides.
6. Avoid poisons/toxins. We shouldn't put anything onto our skin that we wouldn't be happy to eat.
7. Don't burn food as it can be carcinogenic.
8. Move more, exercise regularly and get active. Adopt the Primal Cure principles of MOMMS.
9. Avoid stress. If we are stressed, then we must invest time reading and researching what we can do to reduce it.
10. Make it a habit to get between 7 and 9 hours sleep.
11. Don't consume too much alcohol.
12. Try to tune our body into a ketogenic fat-burning machine (remember that cancer needs sugar to develop and grow).
13. Get a regular check-up. While this won't help avoid cancer, most cancers are now treatable if caught early.
14. Avoid obesity. According to Cancer Research UK, obesity is the second biggest preventable cause of cancer in the UK.

Other than in the listing above, I haven't yet talked about how a ketogenic diet could help prevent and possibly cure certain cancers. If you have been keeping up with me so far, you might not be surprised by this statement, as going keto means avoiding the very thing that cancer thrives off, sugar. Admittedly, at the moment there isn't heaps of scientific evidence to prove my hypothesis.

However, in *Keto Clarity*, author Jimmy Moore quotes scientist John Kiefer, "I've worked with a woman who had stage IV cancer. She was told to go and see her friends right away, because she had less than three months to live. That was six months ago, and now she has a clean bill of health… The power of ketogenic diets is simply astonishing. More accurately, it's astonishing to see how poisonous carbohydrates can be".

THYROID PROBLEMS

It is believed that around one in 10 adults in the Western world suffer with some kind of thyroid problem. But as synthetic thyroid hormone tablets are now the number one best seller in both the USA and most of Europe, sadly very little is being done to solve the root cause of the disease. With so much money being made, in my opinion, thyroid sufferers are facing the same onslaught of misinformation as those with elevated levels of cholesterol have been subjected to by huge pharmaceutical companies and brainwashed into a lifelong commitment to statins.

After the birth of our second child, and the stress caused by the breakup of her parents, my wife Sarah suffered from illness after illness in a short space of time. At one point her entire face swelled up so badly she was admitted to hospital, where they labelled the infection as elephantiasis! Next, chunks of hair started to fall out and she was constantly battling with fatigue. After six months of problem after problem, Sarah was diagnosed with an underactive thyroid. She was told there was a tablet called levothyroxine and as long as she took it daily and had regular blood tests, everything would be okay. Surprisingly, even though she was being informed that she was officially ill and needed to take drugs every day for the rest of her life, the fact that there was a solution meant she took the diagnosis positively. At the time, we never thought to ask what was actually causing the problem and sadly back then we never looked into natural ways to fix the disease.

When we eventually started to look into underactive thyroids (known as hypothyroidism), we learnt that it is far more common in women and tends to first surface at either puberty, pregnancy or perimenopause (the years leading up to the menopause).

So, let's look at the three most common issues people face with their thyroids, underactive, overactive and Hashimoto's disease. Actually before we do: what is the thyroid, where does it live and why do we need one anyway? Our thyroid is situated to the front of the windpipe, and its butterfly shape is about 3–4cm (1–1.5in) in length. As the thyroid is a gland, its job is to release hormones into the body. Thyroid hormones are incredibly important, and send messages to virtually every single cell in the body. They help regulate our heartbeat (irregular heartbeats were a symptom of my wife's condition), metabolism, breathing and body temperatures – my wife regularly suffered from cold feet and hands and much more.

Underactive Thyroid (Hypothyroidism)

Insufficient thyroid hormone production = underactive thyroid. If we suddenly start putting on weight and haven't changed our diet, then it might be a sign that we have developed an underactive thyroid, which is slowing down our metabolism. Other symptoms include sensitivity to cold, feeling tired and weak, forgetfulness, loss of hair, constipation, depression, muscle aches and cramps.

Overactive Thyroid (Hyperthyroidism)

This is pretty much the exact opposite of an underactive thyroid. With an overactive thyroid, the gland pumps out too many hormones into the body. While an underactive thyroid makes us sluggish and slows everything down, an overactive thyroid speeds everything up. It increases our metabolism, meaning that we might be losing bodyweight unintentionally. Other symptoms caused by an overactive thyroid include anxiety and irritability, palpitations, difficulty in sleeping, swelling in the neck, mood swings and while underactive thyroids lead to sensitivity to cold, an overactive thyroid may make you sensitive to heat.

Hashimoto Thyroiditis (Lymphocytic Thyroiditis)

Named after Japanese physician Hakaru Hashimoto who first described the condition in 1912, Hashimoto's disease is a condition where the thyroid fluctuates between being underactive and overactive. While its name and its condition both sound extremely rare, most people suffering with a thyroid problem actually have

Hashimoto's disease! Before I explain what the condition is, it's important to explain that as the condition is a fluctuation of the thyroid being underactive and overactive, the symptoms can be that of either condition.

When my wife was diagnosed as having an underactive thyroid, most people we spoke to who had any knowledge of medicine or biology didn't believe us. Everyone thought that an underactive thyroid always made the sufferer overweight. But actually, Sarah has always been blessed with a beautiful lean figure. We even had one local doctor tell us that we must have heard it wrong and that Sarah must in fact have an overactive thyroid! So it turns out, just like most people with a thyroid problem, Sarah actually has Hashimoto's. Dr Izabella Wentz, in her book *Hashimoto's Protocol*, explained that she had the very same experience as my wife. She writes, "Because of the autoimmune nature of Hashimoto's, it operates by its own rules – which can confuse not just people with the condition, but doctors as well".

Trying to keep it as simple as possible, effectively Hashimoto's is a precursor to an underactive thyroid. If we suffer with an underactive thyroid, our immune system sees the gland as an intrusive foreigner and begins to attack it. This self-destruction fuelled by the autoimmune system eventually grinds down the thyroid and can severely restrict its ability to produce sufficient hormones. Hashimoto's is therefore the disease that leads to the development of an underactive thyroid (hypothyroidism). But while the attack is happening and the thyroid is being assaulted it becomes inflamed. At this point, it starts to pump out even more hormones and the body is temporarily in a state of hyperthyroidism (overactive).

During this transient state the hormones levels can become toxic and the sufferer becomes diagnosed with either Hashitoxicosis or thyrotoxicosis. Once the toxins pass through the body, then either the thyroid gets inflamed again and the sufferer stays in a state of Hashimoto's, or it passes and they end up with an underactive thyroid.

If you take levothyroxine for either Hashimoto's or hypothyroidism, the key thing to remember is that you are not fixing anything, you are just regulating your thyroid. What you are also doing is masking the root cause of whatever is going wrong with your immune system.

As we know, most modern Western disease are all linked to just one or two root causes and once you suffer one disease, if you don't address the real cause you are more susceptible to developing another. If you have Hashimoto's or an underactive thyroid, you are at a far higher risk of developing a whole host of autoimmune diseases such as celiac disease (gluten intolerance), rheumatoid arthritis, type 1 diabetes, multiple sclerosis and many more. I highlight this not to frighten anyone, but to encourage sufferers to start looking for the root cause to their condition and not just mask it with levothyroxine, carbimazole or propylthiouracil.

So, let's see what causes thyroid diseases to occur. Firstly, remember it's a problem with the immune system and as we have already discussed, the immune system, is pretty much controlled by the small and large intestines. Current research suggests that three separate things need to happen for someone to develop any one of the many autoimmune diseases.

1. The intestines must have developed a leak. A permeable leaky gut prevents the immune system from balancing itself and sends it out of kilter.
2. A person must be susceptible to developing an autoimmune disease.
3. Something needs to trigger the event.

What can we take from the three-step process? The good news is, just as we mentioned in Chapter 1, even if our DNA makes us more susceptible to a disease, it still doesn't mean we will contract it, especially if we look after ourselves Primally.

In particular there are three things we must do:

1. Avoid stress. In research carried out by Dr Izabella Wentz with more than 2,000 of her Hashimoto's patients, 69% of patients said they were stressed before they started to develop symptoms, 23% had recently had a baby, 20% put it down to moving home and 17% experienced the death of a loved one.
2. Look after our gut via a healthy Primal diet.
3. Avoid toxins. How do we avoid toxins? Make sure we only use organic creams, toothpaste, shampoos etc. Use a water filter and try as best as we can to avoid air pollution. I have also read that too many dental X-rays could be a trigger for thyroid disorders.

So now we know the cause, let's break down what we can do to either prevent thyroid conditions from developing, or if you have a thyroid problem already how you can start to tackle the root cause and hopefully either reverse it completely, or at least prevent other immune disorders from occurring.

Let's start by looking for clues in what food might be causing the condition and work out how we then rebalance the gut. This is pretty much the same advice as Primal Cure recommends for most disease and conditions relating to the immune system.

If you suffer from any type of thyroid problem, then I fully recommend you purchase a copy of Dr Izabella Wentz's book *Hashimoto's Protocol*, which carries the subtitle, 'A 90-Day Plan for Reversing Thyroid Symptoms and Getting Your Life Back'. In this life-changing book, Dr Wentz also explains that there are so many other aspects of this disease that we might not at first realise, such as, "A less obvious but equally important dysfunction in Hashimoto's is related to an impaired ability to detoxify".

Another approach to curing thyroid disorders might be to go on a ketogenic diet. In *Keto Clarity*, author Jimmy Moore includes a quote from Stephanie Person, whose mother was diagnosed with a terminal brain tumour and given just six months to live. She then went on a ketogenic diet that completely cured her terminal illness. Stephanie says, "Gluconeogenesis provides all of the glucose you need to restore thyroid function and heal the thyroid when you are in ketosis. Several of my keto clients have now thrown away their thyroid medication".

Make no bones about it, what Stephanie is suggesting is that going on a ketogenic diet might cure thyroid disorders. While I have no proof that this might work, it does make a lot of sense for two reasons. Firstly, we know that consuming too many CARBS cause all sorts of harm in our body, and secondly, we understand that ketones are a preferred source of energy for many functions within our body. Therefore, it might just be the case that going keto could provide a cure for many thyroid sufferers.

OSTEOPOROSIS

Around 10 years ago I started to do quite a lot of work for the National Osteoporosis Society (NOS). I ran several marathons on their behalf and when their President, the Duchess of Cornwall, asked what I could do next, one of her senior members of staff jumped in and suggested that I should walk to the North Pole. Two years later, I stood at the top of our planet in order to raise money for the society. The reason I got so involved with NOS was that one of my team members at work told me a story about how all her senior female family members were suffering with the disease. So I started to research osteoporosis, a condition at that point I had never heard of, let alone be able to pronounce properly (being dyslexic I still can't). I was flabbergasted at just how prevalent it was. It is estimated that more than 200 million people suffer from this debilitating disease. In the UK and the USA, approximately 30% of all postmenopausal women have osteoporosis. Of those that have the disease, at least 40% will sustain one or more fractures as a result.

Osteoporosis is a medical condition where bones become brittle and fragile from loss of tissue, typically as a result of vitamin D deficiency, hormonal changes or a lack of calcium. So how do you avoid it? Let's deal with the easy part first: get out in the sun and make sure you are not deficient in vitamin D, or if that's not possible, start topping up your levels with a supplement. One of the main hormonal changes that triggers osteoporosis is an increase in insulin levels. And as you are fully aware by now, to reduce insulin levels you need to eat Primally, severely restricting CARBS and substituting them with healthy fats and proteins. The deficiency of calcium is actually linked to insulin too. You see, when insulin levels are too high the body often excretes the stress hormone cortisol. The two hormones then work together to leech calcium from our bones. In addition, women who do a lot of long intense cardio sessions put themselves at higher risk as this also causes cortisol levels to rise significantly.

Many people who suffer with osteoporosis are also at a high risk of cardiovascular disease. The reason for this is that when bones start to leach calcium, while some of it exits the body in urine, a high proportion becomes stuck to the lining of the arteries.

Can living Primally and eating the same diet that our ancestors ate in the Stone Age reverse osteoporosis? While most of our bones completely replace themselves every 10 years or so, as we get older the rate of replacement dramatically slows down. So if we are aware of the disease at an early age and if we truly live Primally, it is possible to cure the disease, as we will by regenerating our bones through the presence of the right levels of vitamin D and calcium.

COELIAC DISEASE

More commonly known as gluten intolerance, coeliac disease is, in some ways, the body's self-defence system informing the sufferer that CARBS in the shape of wheat and barley are not what they are dressed up to be, and are in fact poisonous. Gluten is the protein found in grain and for some people it triggers an autoimmune reaction in the small intestine.

Several years before we started living Primally, at the age of six, my daughter Jessica was described by our doctor as being sensitive to gluten, and we were recommended to cut bread and cereals from her diet. While it is estimated that only one in 100 people suffer from coeliac disease, being sensitive to gluten appears to be far more common. As grains weren't part of our ancestral past and were first farmed just 12,000 years ago, I would argue that, in some sense, all humans are sensitive to gluten but we don't all demonstrate symptoms.

The website celiac.org introduces the disease as follows, "Coeliac disease can develop at any age after people start eating foods or medicines that contain gluten. Left untreated, coeliac disease can lead to additional serious health problems. These include the development of other autoimmune disorders like type 1 diabetes and multiple sclerosis (MS), dermatitis herpetiformis (an itchy skin rash), anaemia, osteoporosis, infertility and miscarriage, neurological conditions like epilepsy and migraines, short stature and intestinal cancers". For the sceptics out there still struggling to come to terms with the fact that most neurological conditions start in the gut, hopefully the above description should act as further proof that what we eat affects far more than just our waistline.

When people with coeliac disease eat grains, their body mounts an immune response that attacks the small intestine. These attacks damage the villi inside the gut. When our villi becomes damaged, whether from gluten or other diseases or intolerances, the gut is unable to properly digest nutrients and therefore we open the door to an onslaught of health problems. In his book, Brain Maker, neurologist Dr David Perlmutter says, "My patients often reach me only after they've been to a slew of other doctors and have 'tried everything'. Whether they're suffering from headaches or migraines, anxiety, ADHD, depression, memory problems, MS, ALS, autism or just some odd set of neurological symptoms with no definite label, one of the first things I do is prescribe the total elimination of gluten from their diets. And I continue to be astounded by the results".

Of course, one of the simplest ways to avoid gluten is to live Primally and eat as they did in the Stone Age. As you have already discovered in this book, our gut and brain are inextricably linked. Taking good care of our microbiome is like taking out insurance for the brain. 'Avoid gluten and mass-produced packaged foods stuffed full of high fructose corn syrup' was the first dietary advice I gave my two grown-up children when I started to take my own health and longevity seriously. And, it's a great bit of advice for people who prefer bite-sized chunks of information rather than fully diving in.

NEUROLOGICAL DISEASES

My good friend Glenn Lehrer's mother is 103 years old and Glenn describes her as 'bright as a button'. Why is it that some people can keep their brain in excellent working order for their entire lives while others, including some of the most intelligent people on our planet, have their brains start to fail at a very young age? Before I jump into the detail, I would like to thank Dr Perlmutter for the vast amount of research he has done connecting so many neurological disorders and diseases with what goes on in our gut. I found his first book, *Wheat Belly*, extremely informative and brilliantly researched, but his subsequent book *Brain Maker* ranks as one of the most insightful and life-changing books I have ever read. The fact you have read this far tells me that you are serious about your health, and therefore let me recommend that you get hold of a copy of these books, in which you will discover exactly what goes on inside our guts.

As a neurologist, on a daily basis Dr Perlmutter is confronted with the outcomes of Westernised brain disorders. He has the devastating task of informing patients about their diagnosis. Through his research and subsequent books, he works relentlessly to try to prevent disorders of the brain from causing more damage. He is very open about what fuels his desire to rid the world of these debilitating diseases as his own father, who himself was a neurologist, is now suffering with advanced Alzheimer's. For me, a highly qualified expert in a field, driven by such personal emotional connection, is the ultimate individual to take advice from.

In *Brain Maker*, Dr Perlmutter writes, "New, leading-edge science coming from the most well-respected institutions around the world is discovering that to an extraordinary degree, brain health and, on the flip side, brain diseases, are dictated by what goes on in the gut". Yes, you read that right. Science is now connecting our gut with the vast majority of disorders and diseases of the brain. From multiple sclerosis to schizophrenia, from bipolar disorder to migraines, from ADHD to Alzheimer's, from headaches to Parkinson's, from autism to depression, scientists are now starting to look at the gut as the primary root cause and the place to start the fight back against these potentially avoidable conditions. In the USA, more than one in four adults suffer with a diagnosable mental disorder, and globally the number one disability is said to be depression. What's extremely worrying is that the number of people being diagnosed with depression and being put on medication is spiralling out of control. Some go as far as saying it is one of the fastest growing illnesses ever!

We have already discussed that we can remove brain fog by limiting our CARBS, intermittently fasting and by exercising. But here I want to go beyond a foggy brain and look a little deeper. Let's first start by looking at a protein that is synthesised (created) in the brain, called brain-derived neurotrophic factor (BDNF). While it was once believed that we are born with all of our brain cells and we can't make more of them, BDNF is able to make them grow and help them better connect with one another. A better-connected brain makes us more intelligent and helps improve our memory. The best ways to support our brain's production of BDNF is:

- Intermittent fasting
- A good night's sleep

Why does intermittent fasting synthesise BDNF? It's logical really. Picture the scene: caveman is sitting in his dwelling getting more and more hungry because he hasn't been able to gather any food, and he has also forgotten where he last saw that apple tree. He's been moving around a lot recently and his mental mapping of his surrounding is a little hazy. Now Mother Nature doesn't want him to go hungry, so as he sleeps he begins to connect more and more cells together, and when he awakes he experiences a eureka moment and remembers where he last saw the tree. It's not that Mother Nature doesn't want our caveman to starve, but unless he is of older years, she needs him to still create offspring – if he were to starve then the species would soon die out. When he is awake and sitting down chomping on a bone or eating his hoard of apples, nature has no concerns about our caveman fulfilling his procreation duties and switches her attention from brain-building to digesting food and extracting nutrients.

> **PRIMAL CURE PRINCIPLE:**
> **If you want to be smarter and remember where you left your car keys, make sure you intermittently fast and get a good night's sleep too.**

10 Primal things to keep our brain in good working order:

1. Intermittent fasting – increases neurogenesis.
2. Use it or lose it – cognitive stimulation increases neurogenesis.
3. Eat berries – especially blueberries that are rich in the flavonoid anthocyanin, which increases neurogenesis.
4. Omega 3 – whether it is from organic oily fish or a quality supplement, Omega 3 is simply food for the brain.
5. Exercise – follow the MOMMS principle to keep the brain healthy.
6. Dark chocolate or a glass of red wine – both are rich in healthy flavonoids.
7. Turmeric – is said to help in the regeneration of damaged brain cells.
8. Coffee – contains polyphenols that are powerful antioxidants that increases neurogenesis.
9. Green tea – the epigallocatechin gallate (EGCG) found in green tea increases neurogenesis.

10. Go out in the sun – vitamin D increases levels of BDNF in our brain.

If you go to PrimalCure.com or our channel on YouTube, you will find a fascinating interview that we conducted with Dr Emer MacSweeney who is CEO of Re:Cognition Health.

ALZHEIMER'S

Alzheimer's is a horrible debilitating disease. My good friend Chris' father was a rocket scientist, and not in the hypothetical sense – a real life rocket scientist. Sadly, he was recently diagnosed with Alzheimer's. This disease of the brain can truly affect anyone. Over the past five years, my mother has started to repeat herself many times during the same conversation and often can't remember what we talked about two minutes earlier. As a result I have spent many hours researching this ruthless degenerative disease of the brain. While we still don't know exactly what triggers Alzheimer's, Dr Shivapour, who is a Professor of Neurology at the University of Iowa, believes that, "Too many physicians do not understand the critical role nutrition plays in brain health". What many scientists are starting to suggest is that regular eating and not allowing the body to self-detox (autophagy) might be a contributing factor. So intermittent fasting might be a way to prevent the disease from occurring, or at the very least delay its onset. Recent research has shown that many people suffering from Alzheimer's and many other brain disorders have a very low level of BDNF (brain-derived neurotrophic factor), and once again diet – in particular ensuring sufficient levels of Omega 3, intermittent fasting and exercise – are all recommended to boost BDNF.

But without doubt, of the mass of research papers I have studied, the one recurring belief that seems to now crop up in almost every single white paper on Alzheimer's, is that there is a direct correlation between high blood sugar levels and this awful debilitating disease. In a study of more than 2,000 individuals with an average age of 76, the University of Washington measured the sugar levels of participants over a period of seven years. They found that there is a direct correlation between blood sugar levels and the onset of dementia. Put simply, if we eat too many CARBS and other sugars, our chance of developing dementia, Alzheimer's, Parkinson's disease and many more neurological dysfunctions, not to mention cancer and diabetes, increase dramatically.

On the flip side of the coin, there is now plenty of research that suggests that those of us in our more senior years that consume healthy oils such as coconut, olive and avocado oil, plus those that eat plenty of organic nuts and seeds, are less likely to suffer neurological diseases than those that eat lots of CARBS and other sugars and avoid fat. Let me make this very clear, my mother was a huge believer in low-fat everything since it was heavily promoted as a health benefit some 40 years ago, and now she will remind me five times in as many minutes that the hospital I was born has been pulled down.

Alzheimer's and dementia is caused by inflammation in the brain, which is caused by the brain becoming insensitive to insulin. This is so similar to type 2 diabetes - where the liver becomes insensitive to insulin, leading to many other cells locking the door as well - that many researchers and scientists are now referring to Alzheimer's as type 3 diabetes. But what happens if we change our body from a sugar-burning furnace into a ketone lean machine? Dr Perlmutter, author of Grain Brain, tells how research has uncovered that in some patients suffering from mild Alzheimer's, an increase in ketones led to an improvement in cognitive function. When you think about it, this makes complete sense. Just like cancer growths begin to stagnate with the absence of sugar, the development of type 2 diabetes and type 3 (Alzheimer's) must be disturbed if insulin is reduced by the body changing fuel supply from glucose to ketones.

But why does Alzheimer's creep up on people? It turns out that, while the brain is always quick to inform us about problems in all other regions of the body, it doesn't possess any pain receptors in its own backyard. Many researchers are now citing excess sugar and gluten as the most likely root cause of Alzheimer's. Yes, that right – this disease of the brain begins in the gut. Excess sugar molecules in our bloodstream can bind with protein molecules or fatty acids molecules, creating new molecules that can best be described as deformed or irregular. You might have heard of AGE and wondered what they are. AGEs stands for Advanced Glycation End products, and this is simply the name given to these proteins or fatty acid molecules that become glued (glycated) as a result of exposure to sugar. The body doesn't recognise AGEs as being normal, so creates inflammation as a response. And as we don't have pain sensors in the brain itself, AGEs can play havoc before we witness any symptoms.

Let me say it one more time. Now that scientists have recognised that Alzheimer's relates to an overload of sugar in the bloodstream, many are referring to the disease as type 3 diabetes.

If you are worried about neurological diseases, or know someone who appears to be showing signs of dementia, please purchase a book titled *Alzheimer's Disease: What if There Was a Cure?* It's passionately written by Dr Mary Newport, whose husband was diagnosed with the disease and who through several steps, primarily removing starchy white carbs from his diet and encouraging ketosis through the use of my beloved coconut oil, managed to reverse her husband's condition.

> **PRIMAL CURE FACT:**
> Elevated blood sugar dramatically increases the risk of
> developing Alzheimer's, as it does many other diseases.

One final thought. In one of my favourite books ever written on health, *The Orthomolecular Treatment of Chronic Disease*, which carries the subtitle, "65 experts on therapeutic and preventative nutrition", the collective opinion of the authors conclude on Alzheimer's, "It has been known for over a century that aluminium is a neurotoxin. The uncomfortable truth that its widespread use is the major cause of Alzheimer's is now unavoidable. For the sake of your brain, please go and throw out your aluminium foil and cooking pots."

DEPRESSION

It's really important that we see depression as a disease, and not the fault of the person who is suffering from it. I remember years ago, arriving home from Madagascar and explaining to my children how strange it was that everyone I met, regardless of how poor their plight, all seemed happy. I had been in the bush for 10 days with people that had no possessions, no running water or toilets and who lived with their huge families in tiny mud huts. Even though most were very undernourished, they all had one thing in common: a big heartwarming smile. Yet back in the UK, I would get annoyed at how many people I saw who had so much to celebrate – meals on the table, a roof over their heads and a comfortable existence – but were depressed. What was wrong with these people?

It turns out that depression is caused by a hormone imbalance, and what causes this? Our food. One of the first imbalances to address is the Omega 3:6 ratio. Scientists have discovered that those suffering from depression have a low level of docosahexaenoic acid, which is an Omega 3 fatty acid. If we ever find ourselves becoming a little moody and are not sure why, we should quickly rush to our local health shop and purchase an organic, cold-water source of Omega 3.

In the UK, millions of people now suffer with depression, and in the USA, one in four middle-aged women take antidepressant drugs. The epidemic is spreading so quickly, that the World Health Organisation (WHO) suggests that depression is now the leading cause of disability in the world! If the main cause is diet, why on Earth isn't everyone aware? With the drug companies in the USA raking in more than $12 billion of sales each year from doctors prescribing their antidepressant suppressants (and that is all they are – something to suppress symptoms rather than fix them), we can bet that they will do everything possible to keep the truth a secret. If we start to feel down, we should act quickly by trying to get our gut in good working order.

MIGRAINES AND HEADACHES

Dr David Perlmutter informs us, "Headaches, including migraines are among the most common disorders of the nervous system; nearly half of the adult population wrestles with at least one headache a month". He then goes on talk to about how the pain killers people take in the USA to simply mask the pain and not cure the root cause of the problem leads to about $30 billion (£24 billion) a year in sales. Hopefully, you will understand why, in my opinion, none of the big pharmaceutical companies want to tell us the secret of what causes headaches in the first place!

As I have previously mentioned, science is just starting to come around to the idea that many diseases and disorders of the brain are related to the gut. While the pain of the headache appears inside our skull, the root cause is most likely to be in the gut.

Chapter 10 Highlights

At Primal we believe the root cause of nearly all illnesses in Great Britain can be traced back to:

- Imbalance of macronutrients (fat, CARBS, protein).
- The poor state of our gut's microbiome.
- Toxins (not just eaten but absorbed through the skin).
- Lack of fasting.
- Lack of certain vitamins and minerals.
- Sedentary or incorrect exercise.
- Stress and lack of sleep.

All seven of these are because we no longer live our lives in the way us Homo Sapiens have been programmed. We are no longer staying true to our Primal design.

11.

The 7-Day Weight Loss Programme

In this chapter we explain the quick and effective Primal way to start burning body fat, which also for many sufferers, could fix their IBS.

What follows does repeat a good chunk of the first part of the book, but I know lots of you will refer to this chapter time and time again, so I've made it nice and easy for you to have everything to hand to accelerate your weight loss.

Before we get to the conclusion of the book, I have added this chapter to address two of the most common questions that we receive at Primal Cure. The first one normally goes along the lines of, "How do I get my weight under control quickly" and the second "I have IBS and nobody seems to be able to help me". As well as adding a few new learnings, this chapter in the main recaps a lot that we have already discussed throughout the book. Hopefully for most people it will answer these two common questions and I have written it in such a way that the chapter can also work standalone. Why have I done this? Because if you know anyone who needs to lose weight or suffers from IBS, you can simply photograph these few pages on your mobile phone and email it to them (or use a good old-fashioned photocopier). Don't worry about all that copyright stuff you normally get at the front of the book, we really do want you to help us spread the word and help us restore the health of our great nation.

OVERWEIGHT? IT'S NOT YOUR FAULT!

Your Primal needs aren't being met by the modern diet, which has strayed way too far from our genetic requirements. You have to cut through all of the marketing hype and corporate brainwashing and get back to the natural diet enjoyed at the origin of our species. Put simply, your diet needs to return to what your body is designed to eat. And to that end, you need to start eating Primally.

If you follow the advice throughout this book and especially in this chapter, then you can lose weight for good. There is only one requirement... forget everything you previously thought you knew about how to lose weight! Remember, much of what you currently think about food has been shaped by misguided research, bad information, corporate greed and crazy government advice. Over the past 60 years we have been fed inaccurate information from a variety of sources, leading us to become misinformed about food and our dietary requirements. For example, in the 1970s, the Sugar Council of America repeatedly ran an advert with the statement, "If sugar is bad for you why don't you ever see fat kids?" – seriously, they did! Yet less than 50 years later, globally in 2016, 41 million infants and children were overweight or obese. We have seen equally stupid advertisements here in Great Britain, but for now let's forget how we got here and move on to the solution.

The 7-Day Weight Loss Programme Overview

This programme is about spending as much time in fat burning mode - as opposed to fat storing mode - as possible. Why just seven days and not more? Because within just seven days you will definitely see results. Then it's up to you. You can decide to reintroduce a few more food types or carry on with the rapid weight loss programme. While many people will say rapid weight loss is bad for you, they're simply misinformed. Besides, this isn't a crash diet, this is kick-starting both a new habit and way of life.

Psychology in weight loss is half the battle. After just seven days of experiencing great results, both your level of comprehension and willingness to commit to living more naturally, seeking out whole foods and going out of your way to avoid packaged foods, fake foods and other sugar-loaded rubbish will increase. Plus, if you currently suffer from symptoms like IBS, bloating, headaches, depression, anxiety etc, there is every chance these are connected to your diet. You may not be intolerant to something you are currently consuming, but you might well be sensitive to it. Any offending food usually leaves your system within five to seven days and within seven days, their effect on allergies should have disappeared. If you are still experiencing allergy-related symptoms after going strictly Primal for seven days, then seeking medical assistance is highly recommended.

The *7-Day Weight Loss Programme* does five things:

- Dramatically restricts CARBS
- Removes common foods that people are sensitive to
- Helps detox the body
- Provides education and awareness for future health
- Helps seriously lose weight by burning fat

Is this not just another diet, you ask? That depends on your view of what a diet is. The word 'diet' is derived from the Greek word 'diaita' – meaning 'way of life' – and in this respect it is the ultimate diet! But it is definitely not the modern interpretation of a diet book. Living our daily lives more Primally is enjoyable and provides a long-term approach to sustainable health. There is no calorie counting or any strict recipe regimen. I also don't believe that one approach to health fits all. We are all biologically different, we all have different genes and we all live different lifestyles. So, once you are past the first seven days, you might want to tweak things and experiment with a few of our guidelines. If you choose to experiment a little and start to regain weight or any of your previous ailments reappear, with the insights you're about receive, you should be able to pinpoint the cause.

Introduction To The 7-Day Weight Loss Programme

Let's remind ourselves of some horrific Great British statistics that relate to our poor diet:

- The average adult weighs 2.5 stone (15.8kg) more than just 50 years ago
- The rate of diabetes is growing at 2% per annum
- Two out of three adults are overweight, and one in three are obese
- During their lifetime, one in two adults will now be diagnosed with cancer

I truly believe that the above four statistics are almost entirely down to diet. Why? Because I've spent time with tribes in Kenya and Tanzania, communities in the Arctic and travelled through northern Siberia, where I have yet to witness any of these problems. The absence, I am convinced, is due to their Primal diet.

Regular diets fail because they typically focus on calorie counting, which in the long run is boring and impossible to maintain. Many also focus on telling you what to eat and what not to eat, but the fundamental problem is this: they never explain WHY!

Unless you really understand the basics of food, then you will never permanently get your weight to where you want it to be. That's why, in Great Britain, where we don't have to hunt for our food and it's readily available 24/7, two thirds of the adult population are now fat! Once you understand about food and nutrients, you'll see how you can effortlessly lose weight by burning body fat, through cooking and eating gorgeous Primal foods.

The Biology Of Why We Put On Weight And How To Lose It

There are seven critical things to understand about body fat:

1. It is caused by carbohydrates
2. It is impossible to 'lose' weight, we have to burn it
3. It is impossible to burn body fat when there is sugar in the bloodstream
4. All carbohydrates (with the exception of fibre) turn to sugar in the body
5. Excess sugar in the bloodstream is poisonous and detrimental to our health
6. While sugar does provide energy, it is totally void of any other nutritional benefit
7. It is not fat that makes us fat, but carbohydrates (OK, this is the first point repeated, but it is crucial you understand it)

Over the next few pages, I am going to explain how carbohydrates alone make us fat. Fat does not make us fat and protein rarely does (although be aware that protein can be converted into sugar when consumed in excess).

It's now time to get a glass of water, a cup of black coffee or green tea, switch off your mobile phone and pay attention. If you really want to lose weight permanently, you must fully understand the next few pages. It might need reading a few times, but I guarantee it's 100% worth it for the sake of your health. A small investment of your time spent concentrating right now will yield huge results forever, and will help prevent you from being part of the 50% of the population who will shortly be obese (a prediction made by our NHS).

Understanding Macronutrients

Nearly all ingredients of virtually everything we eat are made up of carbohydrates, fats and/or proteins. These three substances are known as macronutrients – derived from the Greek word 'macro', meaning large. Most natural whole foods are made up of just two of these macronutrients.

If the food (or drink) is derived from something that once had a face, it is made up of protein and fat, the exception being a small amount of carbohydrate in eggs and milk. If the food came out of the ground, it generally consists of protein and carbohydrates. Note how everything has protein! This is because protein is the building block of life.

A few exceptions to the two macronutrient rule are nuts, seeds, milk and avocados, which feature all three macronutrients. There are also a few foods made of just one macronutrient: table sugar (although it's less a food, more poison) is made up of just carbohydrate, and oils such as coconut and olive are made from just fat.

What Do Macronutrients Do?

In all humans and animals, all three macronutrients can carry out energy-related roles:

- Carbohydrates – are converted to sugar for energy
- Fats – are converted to fatty acids, in the main to repair cells or to use as energy
- Proteins – are converted to amino acids, to repair and rebuild cells or to use as energy

Carbohydrates

All carbohydrates (which we're calling CARBS as an acronym for Carbohydrates Are Really Bad Sugars), whether they are simple or complex, unrefined or refined, eventually become sugar in the body. Without debating that some are worse than others, we need to understand that all CARBS – even those that are complex and unrefined – will at some point become sugar once digested.

Potatoes, pasta, bread and rice are all converted to sugar in the body. To our body, sugar is either used as an immediate source of energy or it is poison! They might be dressed up in fancy packaging and often carry labels with misleading health benefits, but we need to realise our body was never needs to consume them. There is one exception to the rule though. Our Primal ancestors were designed to eat fruit in the autumn as a means to store body fat for the winter (the fridge hadn't yet been invented). But at this point I believe you are reading this chapter because you want to lose weight, not pile it on for the winter months! This is why during the *7-Day Weight Loss Programme*, I am actually going to ask you to avoid most fruit, other than the 'fab four berries'. These are blackberries, blueberries, raspberries and strawberries, which contain less sugar and are packed with vitamins and antioxidants. Don't worry, once you are fully Primal, there are plenty of other fruits you can start to reintroduce, as long as they are organic, and consumed in moderation.

Let's not beat about the bush. CARBS fulfil no purpose other than to provide energy or to store energy in the form of body fat. They don't help the body repair or rebuild cells and they possess zero nutritional value. Yes, ZERO! They don't contain any vitamins or minerals and they have zero benefits associated with them. In fact, quite the opposite, as all CARBS once in the body turn to sugar and too much sugar in the bloodstream KILLS!

Dr Dan Maggs

"The most nutritional part of a donut is the hole. Processed/refined CARBS and sugar are void of nature's nutrients, minerals and vitamins."

Sugar Explained

Let's look at the three sugar groups. All the sugar groups are a type of 'saccharide' – the Latin word for 'sugar'.

Monosaccharide (pronounced moh-no-sack-a-ride): a single molecule. These simple sugars include glucose – found in fruits and grains – and fructose (found in fruit).

Disaccharide (die-sack-a-ride): a double molecule. These include sucrose, such as table sugar, and lactose which is found in milk.

Polysaccharides (polly-sack-a-ride): including glycogen, which is how humans and animals store energy in the liver and muscles. Also starch, which is how plants store energy. The indigestible form of polysaccharides is fibre, which cannot be broken down in the body. There are two forms of fibre: insoluble and soluble. Although a carbohydrate, fibre is non-digestible and is the one exception to the rule as fibre does not have a negative effect on the body. In fact, sufficient consumption is crucial to our health and well-being.

It infuriates me that governments and much of the medical profession still recommend a balanced diet to people that are overweight, obese or type 2 diabetic. This is utter rubbish! As I've already stated, CARBS serve no purpose other than as an energy source. If we are fat and overweight, we have plenty of stored energy in our body. We simply need to know how to unlock it and consume it.

The body can survive, indeed thrive, without CARBS. If it couldn't, how did the human race survive through the ice age, when little or no CARBS were available? Or how can my friends the Maasai survive when living off nothing but livestock? The Maasai consume virtually no CARBS, except for a little dairy and the occasional orange berry. But I can tell you from personal experience, these berries contain very little sugar and are very bitter indeed. Likewise, the Inuit of Greenland

and Canada live off the land and sea, consuming whales, seals and Arctic foxes. Furthermore, I've met people in the remotest parts of Siberia who eat barely anything other than reindeer. Their CARB free diets not only keep them slender, but athletic and strong too.

Dr Dan Maggs

"CARBS do nothing for the body other than to provide it with energy. And excess energy is stored as fat."

Protein

Protein comes from the Greek word 'prota', meaning 'of primary importance'. All proteins get converted into amino acids inside the body. There are 22 different types of amino acids, all created from the elements carbon, hydrogen, nitrogen or sulphur.

Our body can make all but nine of these amino acids, and these nine are extremely important for our health. That's why they're called the 'essential proteins', and we must make sure they form part of our regular diet. Without consuming these, the ability of our body to repair itself and rebuild cells and organs will be compromised.

Fats

Fat does not make us fat! Fat has been demonised for far too long. It is not the villain. The villain who broke in and messed up your slender body was Mr CARBS.

Just like there are those nine essential amino acids that we need to consume in order to survive, it is also essential that we consume both saturated and unsaturated fats/oils.

Whilst what follows over the page is slightly geeky, it really helps if you can take a little time to understand it.

▶ Technical Stuff

There are two types of fat inside our body. Fats that are ready to be burned as energy are known as fatty acids, and fats that are stored as body fat are known as triglycerides. They are known as triglycerides because they are simply three (tri) fatty acids bonded together by glycerol (pronounced gliss-er-roll).

Fat can only enter or leave cells when broken down to the smaller fatty acids. Body fat (accumulated by too many CARBS) – the fat we are battling to lose – can only be stored as triglycerides and these can only form in the presence of sugar (glycerol – the glue - can't form without sugar).

In the words of Dr Zoë Harcombe, "If we make more glucose available to fat cells, more glycerol can be made. If more glycerol can be made, more fat is stored in the fat cells".

Fats, also known as lipids, are all insoluble. Fats and oils are exactly the same thing, but those referred to as fats are normally solid at room temperature, whereas oil tends not to be.

Saturated fats: which in the main are solid at room temperature, have their bonds filled with hydrogen (i.e. they are literally saturated). Despite all that you have read and heard, saturated fats cannot be bad for us because breast milk – without which many of us wouldn't be here right now – is rich in saturated fats. So too is my beloved coconut oil!

Unsaturated fats: include the hugely beneficial Omega 3 and olive oil. They're not unhealthy either. These can be further broken down into monounsaturated and polyunsaturated:

Monounsaturated fats/oils: (usually liquid at room temperature) have one double bond of hydrogen missing. As long as they are natural, these aren't unhealthy either. They can't be, as all health-conscious individuals will be aware of the many benefits of both avocados and nuts.

Polyunsaturated fats/oils: (usually liquid at room temperature) have two missing bonds (I know 'poly' normally means many, but when it comes to fat, it means just two). The hugely beneficial Omega 3 is indeed a polyunsaturated fat/oil.

In principle, all fats are incredibly healthy, as long as they are real fats and not manufactured fake fats, which can be very toxic and dangerous. The health concern should not be whether a fat is saturated or not, but whether it is real or manufactured. Seriously, you don't need to concern yourself with which type of fat you are consuming, as long as you ensure it is real!

Stick to the healthy (i.e. natural) fats and you'll be living Primally.

Trans fats: be extremely cautious of trans fats. While natural trans fats are produced in the guts of some animals, such as beef, lamb and some dairy products, the vast majority of trans fats are artificial fats, hydrogenated to make them last longer. If the ingredient list says hydrogenated or partially hydrogenated, then it's not a healthy fat and should be avoided! Artificial trans fats or hydrogenated oils are toxic, ugly and deadly.

So let's get this cleared up once and for all. Fat doesn't make us fat on its own. It's sugar that makes us fat. We can eat as much natural fat as we want and if there is no sugar in the body, it can't create glycerol and therefore we can't store it as fat.

Insulin: The Fat Building Hormone

Let's start with a basic understanding of insulin. When our blood sugar (glucose) levels are too high after eating CARBS, the pancreas releases a hormone called insulin, which binds to the liver and muscle cells, signalling them to remove glucose (the liquid form of sugar) from the bloodstream and store it as insoluble glycogen (a solid form of sugar). The problem is, depending on our build, our liver and muscle stores combined only hold around 300 to 500g of glycogen, which in terms of calories is just 1,200 to 2,000, and therefore all excess sugar gets stored as body fat (also known as adipose tissue). Before we start to look down on insulin, we should remember that the hormone is only doing the job nature intended! Insulin is one of the most critical hormones in the metabolism of food and our cells are unable to process sugar without it. As long as we don't overload on CARBS, our insulin system will function perfectly - just as it has for our ancestors for more than two million years.

Glucagon: The Slender Hormone

Glucagon works in the opposite direction to insulin. When our blood sugar levels are too low, the pancreas releases a hormone known as glucagon, to break down insoluble glycogen (solid sugar) into liquid sugar. This allows it to be released into the bloodstream where it can be used as energy. When all the glycogen has been consumed, guess what? Glucagon begins to break down our stored body fat and only now do we start to burn body fat.

Remember, there is no such thing as losing body fat/weight, we have to burn it.

Now, there is bad news for those of us who like to drink the odd glass of beer, or in my case wine. It's not just the empty calories in alcohol that makes us fat. Alcohol inhibits and restricts the release of glucagon. So even if we have very low blood sugar, alcohol will inhibit glucagon from turning our stored fat back into energy. This is also the reason why we get the munchies when we drink alcohol. As the body can't call on its fat reserves to put sugar back into the system, it tells us to eat more. We eat late night kebabs not just because of an alcohol-induced lack of willpower, but a lack of energy caused by us restricting the creation of glucagon.

Alcohol deals a double blow. We can't burn fat while it's in the system and because we can't burn fat, if we need energy our body tells us to consume more food. Even worse, it's possible the hormone even instructs the brain to eat CARBS so that it can unlock energy more quickly.

Recap Of Insulin & Glucagon

Insulin transports sugar to the fat stores and glycerol welcomes it with open arms. This warm greeting is because it needs sugar to bind fatty acids together to make even more body fat. And Nature wants us to store more body fat as a precaution in case we can't gather or hunt more food in the coming days. Nature does not know about supermarkets, restaurants or Just Eat home delivery!

No sugar, no glycerol and no accumulation of fat. This is why calorie counting doesn't work. We could eat copious amounts of healthy fats in a day, and as long as we didn't eat CARBS, our body couldn't convert it to triglycerides and we wouldn't put on weight.

How do we burn fat? It's actually quite simple. We need to remove sugar from the bloodstream so our body has to break down glycogen for energy. Once this has all gone, the pancreas will direct glucagon to our rolls of body fat to break up triglycerides back to fatty acids for fuel. It really is that simple.

Recap Of Glucagon & Glycogen

When we eat CARBS/sugar, the pancreas creates insulin to get rid of the excess sugar in the bloodstream and insulin converts glucose (the liquid form of sugar) to glycogen. If the two glycogen stores are full (the liver can store approximately 400 calories and muscles around 2,000 calories) excess CARBS/sugars are converted to body fat. On the flip side of the coin, if there is too little sugar in the bloodstream, the pancreas creates a different hormone called glucagon which does the opposite to insulin: it informs the liver to convert stored glycogen back to glucose and then stored fat back into usable energy.

They sound ridiculously similar, but it's crucial to remember the difference between glycogen and glucagon:

Glycogen (pronounced gly-co-jen) – is a type of solid sugar (a starch/polysaccharide) and is the first storage form of sugar in the body. It is stored in the liver and muscles.

Glucagon (glue-ka-gone) – is a hormone sent to the liver with an instruction to reconvert solid glycogen to liquid glucose. Glucagon performs the opposite task to insulin.

NINE THINGS TO DO ON THE PRIMAL 7-DAY WEIGHT LOSS PROGRAMME

1. Learn the basics about macronutrients
2. Eat only Primal foods
3. No snacking
4. Get a good night's sleep
5. Coconut oil
6. Drink plenty of water
7. Eat plenty of fibre
8. Vitamin C
9. Ignore Mr Ghrelin

Learn The Basics About Macronutrients

Congratulations, if you have so far read and understood this chapter and have gained a general understanding throughout the book, then you already have this one nailed. Just six more steps to go...

Eat Only Primal Foods

For seven days, try to only eat the foods listed below. Yes you guessed right; they are just an expansion of the top 40 foods from the previous chapter, For seven days please ensure they are organic. We have cut out fruits that are heavy in sugar such as apples and oranges. You can reintroduce these once you reach your desired weight. We have included cheese, milk and eggs, but if you are suffering from illnesses such as IBS and want to find out what is causing it, then I would recommend you don't eat these during the programme.

Meat & Poultry

Beef
Bacon
Chicken
Duck
Ham
Kidney
Lamb
Liver
Pork
Turkey
Venison

Fruit

Avocado
Blackberry
Blueberry
Cherries
Coconut
Cranberry
Goji berry
Gooseberry
Grapefruit
Kiwi
Lemon
Lime
Olives
Passion fruit
Pomegranates
Raspberry
Strawberry

Fish

Anchovies
Bass
Cod
Haddock
Herring
Mackerel
Monkfish
Perch
Red Snapper
Salmon
Sardines
Trout
Tuna

Oils & Fats

Avocado Oil
Coconut Milk
Coconut Oil
Ghee
Macadamia Oil
Olive Oil
Organic Butter

Dairy

Kefir
Organic Eggs
Full Fat Cream
Yoghurt (probiotic)
Cheese /Soft Cheese (organic)

Shellfish

Clams
Lobster
Mussels
Oysters
Prawns
Scallops

Nuts & Seeds

Almond
Brazil nut
Chestnuts
Chia Seeds
Flax Seeds
Hazelnuts
Hemp Seeds
Macadamia
Mixed Nuts
Mixed Seeds
Pecan
Pistachio
Poppy Seeds
Pumpkin Seeds
Sesame
Sunflower Seeds
Walnuts

Vegetables

Artichoke
Asparagus
Avocado
Bean sprouts
Bell Peppers
Bok Choy (Pak Choi)
Broad beans
Broccoli
Brussels Sprouts
Cabbage
Carrots
Cauliflower
Celery
Chives
Courgette
Cucumber
Fennel
Garlic
Ginger
Green beans
Horseradish
Kale
Leek
Lettuce
Mangetout
Mushrooms
Onions
Parsley
Peas
Peppers
Romaine Lettuce
Runner Beans
Shallot
Spinach

Herbs & Spices

Basil
Bay Leaves
Black Pepper
Cardamom Pods
Cinnamon Sticks
Coriander
Crushed Chillies
Cumin Seeds
Curry Leaves
Curry Powder
Dill
Fennel
Lavender
Lemon Grass
Mint
Mustard Seeds
Nutmeg
Oregano
Paprika
Parsley
Rosemary
Sage
Star Anise
Tarragon
Thyme
Turmeric

Spring Onion
Tomato
Turnip
Watercress
Tomato
Turnip
Watercress

Other

Bone Broth
Cacao Powder
Coconut Flour
Coconut Water
Coffee
Kefir
Pickles
Salt
Sauerkraut
Seaweed
Shirataki
Tea
Vinegar

No Snacking

Eating "little but often" is very unhealthy and definitely not what our bodies were designed to do. Especially if snacking includes CARBS. If it does, you're screwed!

Remember it is impossible to burn fat when there is sugar in the system. Let's repeat it again, as it is fundamental to understanding how to lose weight. Here is the body's preference for fuel: it burns sugar first, not just because it is easy to burn, but because it's poisonous and needs to get rid of it. Secondly, it burns glycogen, because this is also a form of sugar, albeit a complex sugar (polysaccharide). Finally, it will turn on body fat. While fat is in fact the preferred source of fuel for many parts of the body, it's harder to access. View it as the body leaving the best until last. One of the reasons I haven't mentioned fasting here is that until you stop craving sugar, fasting is just miserable. But once you kick the sugar addiction, fasting is not just easy, many (including me) actually find it enjoyable too. For now, though, only eat two or three times a day. If you get hungry in between meals, drink plenty of water or take a meal replacement such as a Primal SlimShotz. Of course, if you can get to just one meal per day, you will reap the rewards tenfold!

Get A Good Night's Sleep

There is now plenty of research to suggest that if we don't get at least seven hours of sleep, our body will struggle to lose weight. So, on the Primal *7-Day Weight Loss Programme*, there's no getting up early to go jogging. Just get as much sleep as you can.

Coconut Oil

It might have been a while since you have burnt your own body fat for fuel and believe it or not, the longer you are burning your endless supply of CARBS, the longer it takes for your body to remember how to burn its stored fuel.

There are several thermogenic supplements you can take that turn you into a fat burning machine, but one of the most effective fat burning triggers is simply coconut oil. Coconut is a saturated fat and also an MCT (Medium Chain Triglyceride). It sometimes gets bad press because it is a saturated fat. But now that you are Primally trained, you know that saturated fats aren't evil, we just wouldn't exist as a human race if that was the case. MCTs are the fats that just keep on giving! When consumed they turn almost immediately into fuel, help the body convert body fat into energy and help suppress hunger. Although we don't count calories when living Primally, it's interesting to know that MCTs have a lower calorific content than other fats. Not only are they low in calories and provide almost instant energy, they actually help the body burn its own fat stores in a process called 'thermogenesis'. MCTs are so good for our body that they are starting to be used in treatments for cancer, obesity, Alzheimer's, Parkinson's and other diseases. I personally put a teaspoon in my morning black coffee for a great kick start to the day. If you can find coconut oil that is cold pressed at a very low temperature, then you will love the taste so much you can eat it straight from the spoon.

Drink Plenty Of Water

It is crucial to stay hydrated when we are trying to lose weight. The best water is natural mineral water supplied in glass bottles, or filtered tap water. As I have already mentioned earlier in the book, drinking from one-time use plastic bottles is not healthy. Some of the toxins from the plastic can leach into the water and potentially harm your body. The main culprit is a compound called BPA (bisphenol A), which the European Food Standards Agency (EFSA) have already banned from being used in polycarbonate infant feeding bottles. But as yet neither the UK's Food Standards Agency nor the EFSA have banned it from being used in any other products, from food packaging to disposable water bottles.

Eat Plenty Of Fibre

The more fibre you can eat during the Primal *7-Day Weight Loss*

Programme, the easier you are going to find it. You will also be feeding your healthy bacteria with the food of their choice and they will reward you by letting a lot of the incoming calories slip straight through to the toilet, thereby accelerating your weight loss.

My favourite three fibres to take are glucomannan, inulin and psyllium husk. All three are soluble viscous fibre, which dissolves in water, forming a gel like substance. Viscous fibres are found in the walls of plant cells and have the ability to expand like a sponge. When you consume these fibres with plenty of water, the gel continues to expand inside the stomach. Our receptors on sensing this fullness, trigger our satiety hormone known as leptin. If we then eat a meal approximately 30 minutes to an hour later, we consume less food as the brain already has received a signal to say its full. Plus, there is physically less room in the stomach too. It's kind of like a natural gastric band! Many people have had great success taking our very own SlimShotz product, which features both glucomannan and inulin. In fact, glucomannan is the only ingredient officially scientifically proven by the European Food Standards Agency (EFSA) to aid weight loss.

Vitamin C

Take plenty of vitamin C, as it will further aid your weight loss and detox week. It's especially beneficial if you are trying to solve IBS.

Ignore Mr Ghrelin

Unless you are on any prescription medicine (in which case you should not undertake any programme without seeking medical advice), ignoring the hungry hormone ghrelin should do you no harm at all. You might feel a little light-headed at times, and until you get used to the tummy rumblings they might feel a little strange. But if either of these happen, just congratulate yourself on boosting your immune system and taking back control of your weight. If they get too uncomfortable, then rather than reach for a snacking CARB, take on board a little coconut. The fast acting MCT will give you an almost instant energy boost, without any danger of it ending up in your fat stores.

WHAT YOU MUST NOT DO ON THE PRIMAL 7 DAY WEIGHT LOSS PROGRAMME

1. Don't eat CARBS
2. Don't eat a 'balanced diet', just eat quality fats and protein
3. Don't jog, do cardiovascular exercises or take long bike rides
4. Don't drink alcohol

Don't Eat CARBS

The only food you should eat is listed in the approved foods section. For seven days, you absolutely need to avoid anything on this list, or made of any of the following ingredients:

Barley	Flour	Rice
Bread	Grains	Rye
Cakes	Oats	Spaghetti
Cookies/Biscuits	Packaged Food	Sweets
Chocolate	Pasta	Vegetable Oils
Cereals	Potatoes	Wheat
Corn	Processed Foods	

Don't Eat A 'Balanced Diet', Just Eat Quality Fats & Protein

I find it extremely frustrating how even though virtually everyone's aware that sugar is responsible for the obesity issues in our society, the government still recommends a balanced diet, simply promoting the reduction of calories to lose weight. It's totally nonsensical, total bulls**t and it just doesn't work. If you want to lose weight and are not diabetic, then don't balance your diet, stick to the guidelines above.

Don't Jog, Do Cardiovascular Exercises Or Take Long Bike Rides

Firstly, in the Primal *7 Day Weight Loss Programme*, try and do as much standing up and not sitting down as possible. Then try and walk as much as you possibly can. Simply put, I want you to MOVE MORE. But DON'T go jogging or on any long bike rides. Why? Because at this point, you are probably not yet an efficient ketosis burning machine. And therefore, if you burn lots of calories quickly, your body will want to replace them with CARBS and of course that's exactly what we are trying to avoid. Once you've completed the Primal *7 Day Weight Loss Programme*, and rid your body of poisonous sugar (instead allowing your body to burn fat), you can start introducing the Primal Cure MOMMS exercise principles (Max Out – Move More – Sprint).

Don't Drink Alcohol

During the Primal *7 Day Weight Loss Programme*, we shouldn't drink alcohol as this inhibits the pancreas from creating glycogen, which is needed to turn our body fat back into energy. Once you are fully living Primally, you should find you can add in the odd drink or two… or you may decide to cut the booze out completely!

Final Thought

Just like I tell my friends who want to stop smoking – not to see it as giving up but escaping – we must feel the same way about CARBS, junk food and toxic packaged food.

You're not giving anything up, you're instead escaping the corporate trap of addictive sugar and toxic infused mass-produced rubbish. Once you have kicked the sweet tooth syndrome into touch, your new treats become whole natural foods, flavoured by herbs and spices. You'll see from our recipes and blogs on PrimalCure.com that you can still enjoy puddings and snacks, but preferably only those made with 100% Primal ingredients. Recipes include raspberry protein brownie bars, coffee banana bread, energy balls and one of my favourite recipes, my CARB-free Primal Spaghetti Bolognese.

Give up the CARBS and other sugars for just seven days and see what happens. Once you have started, I promise you that you just won't want to stop.

12.
Primal Living: Conclusion

Calling this chapter a conclusion goes against the grain a little (if you'll pardon the pun), as it is in reality just the end of the beginning of a wonderful journey.

Let's start by first summarising the principles of living Primally. Let's from now on in call these our 'Caveman Primal Principles':

1. Eat a diet that is low in carbohydrates
2. Intermittently fast
3. Drink plenty of water
4. Move more
5. Lift weights
6. Sprint occasionally
7. Sleep – get lots of it
8. Stress – avoid it
9. Sunshine – embrace it sensibly

Then there are three more principle that we have to undertake that are kind of post-Primal. In other words, Primal man didn't have to concern himself with these, as they relate to protecting our body against the effects of our current environment.

Let's call these our 'Life Beyond the Cave Principles':

1. Toxins and poisons – avoid them
2. Toxic medicine – if possible try to go natural first
3. Gut – look after it because the soil and environment no longer do

IF IT'S TO BE - IT'S UP TO ME!

I am very fortunate to have a father that instilled a can-do attitude in his children. While we often hear parents telling their kids what they can't do, my dad has always told us to pursue our dreams. At the age of 14 when I started sailing, I told him that one day I wanted to be a champion. He told me that anything was possible, but to be a champion I would have to give up lots of things I liked doing and really dedicate myself to the challenge. If I wanted to be a champion all I had to do was to try harder than everyone else.

It was at this early point in my life I learnt the phrase 'if it's to be it's up to me'. I learnt that anything is possible if you set yourself a target and commit everything to achieving it. I learnt the more we give up, the more we discover how deep our passion is. I learnt that you have to give to get.

It's true that every action has an equal reaction, for example:

Eat bread = get fat
Eat protein = get strong
Eat probiotic yogurt = healthy gut
Intermittently fast = putting body into recovery mode

The more Primal principles we are prepared to adopt, the more we will control our own health and happiness.

Getting our health back on track is never plain sailing, there are going to be bumps in the road and times when we want to pack it in. But with an overriding 'if it's to be it's up to me' attitude, we will discover that these storms make us stronger. If we really want to be healthy and to live a long happy life, then by and large our destiny is in our own hands. Nobody is going to do it for us, nobody is going to force us to take control and start steering our ship to the destiny we want to reach – we have to make the decision ourselves. As was said in the film The Shawshank Redemption, "get busy living or get busy dying". I know that may sound a little harsh for a health book, but this isn't a dress rehearsal, this is it. Either make the most of it and really live your life or just slowly move inexorably towards death.

My six older children must be sick of hearing me constantly muttering, 'if it's to be it's up to me'. I am a real believer that those of us who have been fortunate enough to be born with good health and in a land that is prosperous, all have the ability to control our own health, happiness and longevity. The question I encourage everyone who asks for my advice is 'where is your attitude going to take you?' We all need to understand that our current situation bears a direct correlation to our past attitude. Where we find ourselves today in terms of our health and physique is simply an accumulation of our past attitude. Unfortunately, before you read this book, your past attitude was largely shaped by misinformation and brainwashing from corporate advertising.

Helping Others Live Primally

Our health is worth fighting for, right? But with all the brainwashing we have endured over recent decades, with all the advertising by food giants, the ill-funded research and the onslaught of fast food and packaged food with their highly addictive ingredients, going Primal is sometimes not easy. What's more, many of your friends and relatives just won't grasp your new approach to health as they will still be suffering from corporate indoctrination. It really is going to require willpower and determination.

As the principles of Primal Cure go against much of what we have been brainwashed with over the past six decades, it is unlikely that we are going to convince all of our friends, colleagues and loved ones to join us on our Primal journey. Therefore, forget all the copyright stuff, feel free to pass this book around your family. Ensure your family and friends read it cover to cover. Not only will you be helping them prevent certain illnesses and maybe even cure a few, by sharing the principles behind our new lifestyle you will be making your own journey an easier and more rewarding one.

Willpower & Determination

First of all, this Primal lifestyle works. Not just a little bit – a lot. I didn't set out to write this book for your benefit, but for my own family. I was fed up (pun intended) of seeing them being held hostage by the big food corporations and had to write down my findings. As a result, my 13-year-old daughter, Jessica, has transformed her eating habits to the Primal way of living and is reaping the benefits with her body image, ability to concentrate and increased energy levels, simply by cutting out cereal for breakfast and exchanging it for fermented yoghurts and berries. Going Primal really works, we just need determination and willpower to get through the first few weeks, and after that it really becomes both enjoyable and rewarding. As soon as you start seeing results and start feeling healthier, I promise you that you will no longer need determination and willpower – you will simply just love the new you.

But getting through the first few weeks is going to take guts and a thick skin. The new you begins when you, and only you, make the decision to give it a go and make it a habit.

Habit

When learning new things, it is necessary to go through an intense period of conscious self-training, constantly evaluating if we are moving towards our aim of perfecting that element of our skill set. Eventually everything will become second nature; eventually everything will become a habit.

It's like learning to ride a bike for the very first time. Remember how hard it was and how hard we had to concentrate to keep our balance, but once we have learnt we no longer have to think about it, we have learnt the habit of how to ride a bike. To create or change a habit there are three important steps: awareness, knowledge and desire. We first need to be aware of our current habits, then gain the knowledge of how to change them and finally have the motivation and desire to act upon them as if it is a matter of life or death.

The good news is you are already two-thirds of the way there! You are already aware of your current eating habits, you have now gained the knowledge of how to look after your body and take control of your health – all you need next is a strong enough desire. I'm not trying to sound like the cover of a conventional diet book with a '14-day plan' or 'lose 12 pounds in 12 days' type of message, but as soon as you have seven days where you can focus on your diet, just give it a go. Give up the CARBS and other sugars for just seven days and see what happens. Once you have started, I promise you that you just won't want to stop.

Placing People & The Planet Before Profit

For decades, the core motivator for starting a business was to create personal wealth. Almost at any cost to fellow human beings and the environment, business leaders would push their businesses to the max in order to create wealth and recognition for their achievements. I am glad to say the tide is turning. I believe two events are converging. Firstly, the world is becoming more connected and more and more people are becoming aware that there is a serious imbalance: that while 3.5 billion of us live in a world of excess, 3.5 billion barely have enough to survive. Secondly, many business leaders are starting to wake up to the reality that it is not governments that are going to solve the problems our planet is facing, but business leaders themselves.

As consumers we are starting to become more aware of the issues facing our health and the well-being of our small planet. I also believe this is just the start of the consumer revolution and I pray that in the very near future, us consumers become even more demanding and increasingly influential, both in what ingredients go into the food we eat and saving the planet via our purchasing decisions.

> **PRIMAL CURE REQUEST TO BUSINESS LEADERS:**
> **Put the public's health and the wellbeing of the planet before profits.**

I hope that one day stock markets and governments find a way to measure the social impact that businesses have, and that this – combined with all of us consumers voting with our wallets, choosing the good over the bad – will help the good companies prevail. I would like to believe that 20 years from now, profits will no longer be the main driving force behind businesses, but viewed equally alongside both the health of people and the planet. Especially here in Great Britain, all corporates need to do their part in restoring the health of our nation.

HAPPY PRIMAL LIVING

When you have got your weight and health back on track, please email steve@primalcure.com with your story, along with a before and after photo if possible (please go take one today, because you are about to change your shape permanently).

Primal Scoring System

In this final section, we are going to explain how to track your Primal journey through either our mobile app, or Primal Cave Cards.

How Primal are you? We all know that you can't manage what you can't measure, but at the same time we also appreciate that none of us want to spend too much time logging and recording every little detail. The Primal Scoring System is not like counting calories which is time consuming and as you know by now pretty pointless. It's a way of quickly checking and monitoring your Primal progress. On the following page there is a simple Primal Cave Card, which is essentially a paper version of the Primal Cure App. You can photocopy and duplicate it as many times as you like. The Primal Cure App is available as a free download for both iOS (Apple iPhones, iPads etc) and Android devices. The app has been created in line with the same guiding principles adhered to throughout *The Primal Cure*, designed to be simple and easy to use. You can also find a video on YouTube called "How To Use The Primal Cure App".

HOW TO USE THE PRIMAL SCORING SYSTEM

The aim of both the Primal Cave Card and the app, is to record how Primally we are living. The closer we can get to our top score of 10, the healthier and more enjoyable life will be. If you use the Primal Cave Card instead of the app, I recommend you get a folder and store them. This way you will be able to track your progress and see how your scores correlate to both your health and happiness. Regular app users should absolutely download it now. Obviously I am a little biased, but what the Primal team have built is simply brilliant. And remember, it's totally FREE!

So here is how it works. Each day you score the three core areas of living Primally: Nutrition, Environment and Lifestyle (NEL). There are no rights or wrongs, you just need to score your own performance as openly and honestly as possible. Some aspects such as nutrition and exposure to toxins, are of course subjective. However, as long as you approach them in a consistent manner, over time you will be able to track your changes.

Nutrition, Environment & Lifestyle (NEL)

Diet/Nutrition – Record how Primally you ate. The score ranges from -3 to +4. Don't go cheating yourself, try and be as honest as you can. Only go +4 if you 100% ate Primally and got plenty of nutrition (either from food or supplements), -3 would be a day of takeaway or processed foods and stuffed with CARBS (but you wouldn't go doing that now, would you?!)

Fasting – If you fasted, whether it be 5:2 or an 18 hour fast, click the fasting button on the app or add one point to your Primal Cave Card.

Water – Water is crucial for good health, click either the "Less than 1.5 litres" or "More than 1.5 litres" button on the app. On Primal Cave Card add one point if you drank more than 1.5 litres and minus one if you didn't.

Alcohol – There are no positive points to earn, but if we take the NHS guidelines as a general rule, then as long as you had no more than 2 drinks, there is no need to record a negative score. For every extra drink above two, calculate one negative point. So 3 alcoholic drinks is -1, 4 alcoholic drinks are -2 etc. If for some reason you had 5 or more, even though that's very naughty, the worst score you should give yourself is a -4. We restrict it to this so that your total Primal Score ranges from -10 to +10.

Toxins – Did you use any shampoo, antiperspirant, make-up with chemicals? Did you have your mobile phone up to your ear all day? If you are unsure how to rate your day, be sure to read Chapter 6: Primal Environment. If you are confident you made a conscious effort to avoid toxins, give yourself one point.

Other - Use this to record other things that influence your well-being. If you had a bad night's sleep, you might want to put in a negative score, if you managed to get some good sunshine you might want to add one point. If you are stressed, you might want to put in a negative score, but if you are feeling blissfully happy might want to add a point. (Please note that the maximum here is plus two or minus one point.)

Once you have completed the above six questions, you should have a Nutrition, Environment and Lifestyle (NEL) score of somewhere between -10 and +9.

Exercise

When it comes to recording exercises, this is where the app comes in to its own. It's absolutely fantastic at recording workouts and tracking your progress. The three areas where you can score points, relate to the principle of MOMMS (see Chapter 4 to learn more about MOMMS – Max Out – Move More – Sprint).

Max Out – If you go to the gym or perform a workout at home, depending on how hard you felt you worked out, score yourself up to 4 points on your Primal Cave Card. In the app, there are plenty of videos and help tools explaining how to properly max out. Once you have found the exercise you want to do, press the start button and record your time. The app will allocate relevant points automatically.

Move More – If you went for a walk, played tennis, golf, went swimming etc, then give yourself one point for every 20 minutes of exercise. Again, if you use the app, it will allocate points automatically.

Sprint – Before you attempt to do any sprinting please read the sprinting section in Chapter 4 or for more information on how to sprint safely, visit primalcure.com. For every sprint you do, regardless of whether it's on foot, on a bike or a rowing machine, add yourself 1/3 of a point. If you complete 3 sprints then give yourself 1 full point.

Exercise Total – Each day you can allocate a maximum of 5 points for exercise. The reason? Because, remember what Dr Shan says, "You can't out exercise a poor diet." And we would also add, you can't out train a poor environment and lifestyle. So, if you had a terrible day with your food intake and exposed yourself to lots of toxins, your NEL score could be, say -10. Then if you add in a maximum of 5 for your exercise, your Primal Score is still only -5. If this happens, you'll see why we stress the importance of your diet and environment.

Total Score – Add your NEL Score to you EXERCISE Score. Please note if this is more than 10, then, whilst applaudable, please just add a maximum of 10. Even if you are doing well with your nutrition, environment and lifestyle, we don't want to encourage people to over train. If you use the app, it automatically calculates all of this for you.

Extra Features On The App

The app is designed to integrate with our Primal Bathroom Scales where you can view measurements such as weight, body fat, BMI, muscle %, water % and more! You can also enter lots of measurements manually, and log photographs charting your journey. Make sure you always measure yourself at the same time of day, ideally as soon as you wake up.

PRIMAL CAVE CARD

CIRCLE YOUR SCORES AND ADD THEM TOGETHER

NUTRITION, ENVIRONMENT AND LIFESTYLE (NEL)	DATE:
DIET / NUTRITION (This is how Primaly I ate)	-3 -2 -1 -0 +1 +2 +3 +4
FASTING	0 +1
WATER	-1 0 +1
ALCOHOL	-4 -3 -2 -1 0
TOXINS	-1 0 +1
OTHER	-1 0 +1 +2
TOTAL NEL SCORE Score ranges from -10 to +9	
EXERCISE	
MAX OUT	0 +1 +2 +3 +4
MOVE MORE	0 +1 +2 +3 +4 +5 +6
SPRINT	0 +1
TOTAL EXERCISE SCORE Maximum 5 (round down if necessary)	

BODY WEIGHT	BODY FAT %	**PRIMAL SCORE** Add NEL score to EXERCISE score (Maximum 10)

INDEX

1:1 Diet, 142
18 Hour Fast, 142
3 or 4 Day Fast, 142
5:2 Diet, 141
A New You, 29
Acesulfame, 355
Acne, 154, 191, 226, 279, 327
ADHD, 78, 84, 237, 259, 365, 377
Aerobic, 169, 178
Akkermansia Muciniphila, 247
Alcohol, **211**, 407
Algae, 96
Allicin, 327
Almonds, 41, 61, 256, 266, 304
Alternate Day Fasting, 142
Alzheimer's, 118, 237, 273, 315,
    329, 381
Amino Acid, 152, 253, 260, 285
Anabolic, 163, 216
Anaerobic, 169, 174
Anchovies, 277, **326**
Anthocyanin, 108, 308, 315
Anthropometric, 72
Antibacterial 226, 239, 248, 327, 347
Antibiotics, 234, 248, 290, 314, 320
Antioxidant, 258, 259, 273, 279, 306,
    315, 337
Antiperspirant, 3, 222, 224, 229
Anxiety, 235, 269, 371, 377, 389
Arteries, 332
Arthritis, 84, 93, 118, 279, 315, 342,
    365, 373, 430
Artichoke, 240, 247, **338**
Artificial Sweeteners, 23, 289, 354, 355
Asparagus, 240, 260, **343**
Aspartame, 355
Asthma, 194, 237, 265, 315, 317
ATP, 362
Atrophy, 165
Autism, 197, 237, 377, 379
Autoimmune Disease, 63, 239, **364**,
    372, 377

Autophagy, **138**, 381
Avocado Oil, 103, 382
Avocado, 256, 259, **301**
Bacteria, **46**, 232, 238, 341, 322, 329,
    346, 349
Bacteroidetes, **45**, 230, 240, 246, 247
Baked Beans, **40**
BCAA, 288
Beansprouts, 40
Biomolecules, 52
Biotin, **260**, 323, 338
Bipedal Apes, 25
Blackberries, 109, 117, 257, **308**
Blackcurrants, 257
Blood Pressure, 145, 154, 191, 317, 327,
    329, 332, 342
Blueberries, 108, 117, **307**, 380
BMI, **69**
BMR, 143
Bok choy, **309**, 402
Bone Broth, 333
BPA, **122**, 221, 229, 404
Breakfast, 22, **112**, 115, 137, 285
Breast Cancer, 314, 319, 334
Broccoli, 41, 61, 151, 257, 259, 260,
    264, 309
Brussels Sprouts, 257, 260, 270, 309
Butter, 32, **97**, 266
Cabbage, 41, 264, 309, 331, **340**
Cacao, **273**, 332
Caesarean, 238
Calcium, 57, 130, 190, 254, **263**,
    265, 280
Calorie, **75**, 144, 148, 150, 164, 181, 212
Cancer, 193, 237, 306, 257, 308, 309,
    334, **366**
Capsaicin, 272, **313**
Carbage, 152
Carbocoaster, 34
Carbohydrates - complex, 35
Carbohydrates - refined, 36
Carbohydrates - simple, 35

Carbohydrates - unrefined, 36
Carbohydrates, 33, 53, 146, 301
Carcinogenic, 224, 227, 329, 369
Cardiovascular, 4, 47, **61**, 178, 234, 265, 406
Carotenoids, 108, 344
Carrots, 40, **344**
Cashews, 40, 304
Cat Naps, 203
Catabolic, 163
Cauliflower, 263, **309**
Celery, 41, 77, 314, **337**
Cellulite, 119, 333
Cereal Killer, 112
Cereal, 113, 149, 285
Cheese, 129, 243, **330**, 344
Chia, 307
Chickpeas, 40
Chips, 358
Chloride, 269
Chlorophyll, 108
Chocolate, 267, 273, **331**, 246
Cholera, 78
Cholesterol, 23, **57**, 101, 329
Chromium, 268
Circadian, **197**, 201
Citric Acid, 341
Clothes, 224
Cobalamin, 261
Coconut Chunks, 301
Coconut Cream and Milk, 299
Coconut Flour, 299
Coconut Oil, 50, 94, **96**, 383, 396, **403**
Coconut Water, 300
Coconut, 95,151, **298**
Coeliac Disease, 376
Coenzyme Q10, 276, 279, 281
Coffee, 95, **345**, 380, 404
Cold Temperature, 216
Colds, 257, 315, 347
Collagen, 119, 327, 333, 337
Colon Cancer, 263, 329
Concentration, 145, 213
Copper, 267

Corn Oils, 100
Corn Syrup, 354
Cotton, 100
Cranberries, 108, 307
Crohn's Disease, 329
Cruciferous, 309
Cucumber, 343
Curcumin, 108, 229, 272, **278**
Cycling, 178
Dairy, 127
Dandruff, 227
Darren Brown, 81
Deodorant, 223
Depression, 235, 237, 273, 329, **384**
Detox, **228**, 237, 309, 312, 338, 374, 381
DHA, 97, 277
Diabetes, 306, 309, 314, 332, **365**, 373, 382
Diaita, 18
Disaccharide, 394
DNA, 63, 232, 373
Dysentery, 78
Eggs, 23, 32, 60, 194, 243, **302**
Electrolytes, **268**, 300
EMF, 227
Endurance Sports 18, 62, 157, 169, **176**
Enzymes, **48**, 287, 328, 342
Evolution, **25**, 52, 64, 134, 223
Fasting, **134**, 285, 347, 364
Fat, **31**, 90, 395
Fatty Acids, **52**, 226, 253, 299, 399
Fermented Foods, 128, ,230, 280, **328**
Fibre, **46**, 85, **115**, 283, 394, 404
Firmicutes, **45**, 234, 240
Fish, **322**
Fizzy Drinks, 111
Flat Feet, 210
Flavonoids, **314**, 380, 306
Flavonols, 350
Flaxseed, 277, 294, 307
Flu, 315, 347
Fluoride, 266
Folate, 260

Free Radicals, 143, 165, 179, 256, 336, **362**
Free-Range, 105
Fructose, 245, 354
Fruit, 56, 352, 393, 400
Fungus, 210
Gallbladder, 257
Galt, 244
Garlic, 61, 240, 247, 314, **327**
Gas, 350
Gelatin, 333
Genetics, 46, **64**, 66
Ghee, 97
Ghrelin, **42**, 85, 201, **405**
GI tract, **48**
Ginger, **272**, 278, 327, 345, 347
Glucagon, **53**, **398**, 399
Glucomannan, 115, **283**, 310, 405
Gluconeogenesis, **152**, 176, 375
Glucose, **53**, **152**, 173, 264, 362, 396
Glycemic index, 37
Glycerol, 31, 396, 399
Glycogen, 53, 152, 165, 169, 394, **399**
GMOs, 357
Gout, 64, 77, 84, 354
Grains, 35, **106**, 132, 377, 406
Grapefruit, 40, 257, 341
Green peas, 40
Gum Disease, 237
Gums, 225
Hair, 225, 227, ,327, 260, 309, 371
Hara Hachi Bu, **41**
Hashimoto, 371
HDL, **58**, 101, 154, 350
Headaches, 265, 377, 379, **385**, 389
Hemp, 307
Herbs, 270, 296, 402
Hereditary, 22
HGH, 44, 137
High Blood Pressure, 78, 192, 237, 257, 281, 342
HIIT, 163, 183
Homo Sapiens, **25**, 56, 84
Homogenisation, 130

Hormones, **42**, 56, 105, 119, 136, 175
Hydrogenated Oils, 97, 100, 128, 369
Hyperthyroidism, 371
Hypertrophy, 165
Hypothyroidism, 371
IBS, **246**, 329, 338, 388, 401
Ibuprofen, 273, 279
Immune System, 62, 224, 235, 249, 405
Inflammation, 145, 201, 364
Insulin, **53**, 397, 399
Intestines, **49**, 50, 235, 350
Inulin, 283
Iodine, 267
Iron, 266, 319
Jogging, 176
Kale, 257, 259, 309
Kefir, 330
Ketogenic, 146
Ketones, 146
Ketosis, 146, 183, 375, 407
Kidney Beans, 349
Kidney Stones, 341
Kimchi, 331
Kinesthesia, 168
Kiwi, 257, 337
Labels, 77
Lactose, 110, **129**, 287, 329, 345
Lamb, **319**
LDL, **58**, 101, 329
Legumes, 348
Lemon and Lime, 336
Lentils, 339
Leptin, **42**, 242, 332, 354
Lettuce, 340
Leukemia, 273
Libido, 343
Lignans, 306
Linoleic Acid, 106, 317, 319, 334
Liver, 4, 49, 223, 355, 382, 394, 398
Lutein, 107, 311
Lycopene, 312
Lymphatic System, 50, 52
Macadamia, 41, 92, 103, 304, 401
Mackerel, 324

Macronutrients, 30, 392
Magnesium, 96, **264**, 269, 276, 279, 300
Makeup, 222, 223
Maltose, 110
Manganese, 267
Max Out, 163
MCT, **94**, **95**, 150, 404
Meat, 104, 241, **316**
Medication, 4, 28, 60, 118, 290, **291**, 379
Memory, 145, 308, 326, 332, 377
Meningitis, 78
Metabolic, 135, 147, 155, 171, 182
Metabolism, 23, **51**, 135, 188, 210, 233, 266, 346
Microbiome, **44**, 84, 120, **231**
Microtrauma, 169
Migraines, 84, 118, 265, 281, 377, 379, **385**
Milk, 129
Misrepresentation, 81
Mitochondria, 49, **62**, 173, 280, 362
Molybdenum, 268
Monosaccharide, 394
Mosquitoes, 315
Multiple Sclerosis, 63, 78, 84, 189, 192, 237, 273, 365, 373
Mushrooms, 26, 334
Neurological diseases, 109, 377, 378, **382**
Niacin, 259
NRVs, 254
Nucleic Acid, 52
Nucleotides, 52
Nucleus, 63, 362
Nuts, 303
Ob/ob mice, 242
Obesity, 12, 45, **67**
Oestrogen, 122, 214, 306, 334
Okinawan, **41**
Oleic Acid, 98, 106, 226, 301, 317, 338
Oligosaccharide, 350
Olive Oil, 92, 95, **98**, 396

Olives, 315
Omega 3, **92**, 276, 302, 319, 325
Omega 6, **93**
Onions, 108, **314**
Orange, 257
Organelles, 62
Orthomolecular, 275
Osteoporosis, 189, 265, 317, **375**
Ovarian Cancer, 192, 342
Oxygen, 165, 169, 362, 368
Pantothenic Acid, 259
Paraffin, 224
Parkinson's Disease, 84, 237, 265, 273, 281, 315, 382
Parsnips, 40
Peanuts, 40, 338
Peppers, 312
Phosphorus, 264
Phytochemicals, 107, 305, 315
Phytonutrients, 108, 305, 337
Phytosterols, 58, 305
Pickles, 331
Pigs, 90
Pilchards, 326
Pineapple, 342
Poisonous, 101, 137, 223, 275, 358
Polio, 78
Polysaccharides, 394
Pomegranates, 342
Poppy, 307
Pork, 317
Potassium, 269
Potato, 350
Poultry, 320
Probiotics, 233, 239, 276, 279, **280**
Prostate cancer, 190, 192, 312, 313
Protein, **32**, 395
Psyllium husk, 276, 284
Pumpkin, 307
Pyridoxine, 260
Quercetin, 108, 315
Quinoa, 359
Rapeseed, 100
Raspberries, 257, 308

Riboflavin, 258
Safflower, 100
Salmofan, 106
Salmon, 243, 256, 261, 277, **323**
Salt, 352
Sarcopenia, 166
Sardines, 326
Sauerkraut, 331
Scoville, 313
Seaweed, 340
Seeds, 307
Selenium, 268
Serotonin, 243
Sesame, 100
Sesame, 307
Shampoo, 223, 226
Shellfish, 335
Shirataki, 115, 310
Skin, 222, 225, 327
Sleep, **195**, 403
SlimShotz, 283
Smallpox, 78
Sodium, 269
Soy beans, 40, 100
Spices, 270
Spinach, 310
Sprinting, **172**
Stains, 290
Sterols
Straight Back, 210
Strawberries, 40, 108, 257, 308
Stress, 204, 235, 243
Strokes, 71, 138, 257, 342, 363, 365
Sucralose, 355
Sucrose, 110, 354, 394
Sugar, **109, 354**
Sunbathing, **188**
Sunbeds, 192
Sunflower, 100, 307
Supplements, 32, 93, 115, 124, 132,
    143, 252, **274**
Sweating, 229
Swiss Chard, 309
Tannins, 314

Tea, 346
Teeth, 225
Thermogenesis, 216
Thyroid, 370
Tomatoes, 257, 311
Toxic, 228
Toxins, 220, 279
Trans fats, 90, 100
Triglyceride, **95**, 396
Trout, 324
Tumeric, 273, 276, 278
Tuna, 325
Turnips, 309
UHT, 130
Vegetable Oil, 101
Vegetarian, **124**
Vitamin A, 255
Vitamin B, 258
Vitamin B1, 258
Vitamin B2, 258
Vitamin B3, 259
Vitamin B5, 259
Vitamin B6, 260
Vitamin B7, 260
Vitamin B9, 260
Vitamin B12, 261
Vitamin C, 257, 282
Vitamin D, 188, 256
Vitamin E, 256
Vitamin K, 256
VLDL, **58**
Waistline, **70**
Water, **116**, 404
Watercress, 309
Watermelon, **40**
Whey, 285
Whooping cough, 78
Worry, 204, 205
Yoghurts, 129, 329
Zeaxanthin, 311
Zinc, 266, 319

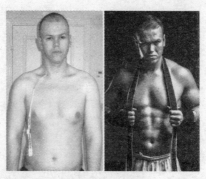

JAMES WELLS' TESTIMONIAL
General Manager, Primal Cure

As an elite Karate athlete and two-time cancer survivor, I believe in maximising our full potential and that not a single day in life should be wasted. A chance to change our own lives for the better should be grasped with both hands and the opportunity to make a real, tangible difference to others shouldn't be missed.

So when Steve Bennett asked me to manage Primal Cure, it was an absolute no-brainer. I saw it as the chance of a lifetime and an opportunity to change the world for the better.

I've competed in the sporting arena and I've competed with cancer… Whilst winning silverware at international level, I spent 286 days of my young life in hospital battling Acute Myeloid Leukaemia. I had 111 days of Chemotherapy, Total Body Irradiation and a stem-cell transplant from my sister… Few people are better placed than I am to talk from experience about mainstream health advice given in the UK.

The bulk of my sporting victories have been achieved after beating cancer – AFTER being told I wouldn't be fit to fight again due to the affects of intensive treatment. But I was able to defy the odds by going against mainstream advice and living life naturally; training and eating like our caveman ancestors.

Perhaps I'm living proof of *The Primal Cure*? Long before I ever read the book, I'd been adopting Steve's ethos and adhering to his principles before our paths had crossed… Our ambitions align seamlessly and we share a similar psychology. Because I firmly believe that living life the Primal way aided my response to treatment, improved my subsequent recovery, enabled me to achieve success as an athlete, allowed me to enrich people's lives as a motivational speaker and ultimately put me on the path to become a force for change at the forefront of this incredible movement.

Through the power of correct exercise, healthy nutrition and organic living, free of artificial rubbish and poisonous toxins – the way nature intended – we can embrace a cleaner lifestyle, free of the stress and disease that plagues western society today… Cancer is one such illness I believe could be averted, if we make only minor adjustments.

Owing to the challenges I've faced, I feel that life is our most precious gift and that time is our most valuable commodity… One body. One world… As individuals, we shouldn't abuse our bodies. Collectively, we share responsibility to encourage healthy living so we can all live longer together.

Our physical, mental and social health suffers as a consequence of the pressures we all face in the modern world. Corporate agenda blinds us from the truth and we're restrained by irresponsible marketing designed to steer us away from making healthy choices for the sake of profit, at the expense of our well-being.

But rest assured, *The Primal Cure* offers solutions to the problems we face and I believe that Steve has exposed the truth. His book is my gospel; one I was preaching without realising. Now, I'm fortunate enough to act as a voice for it and you could do the same.

The foundations are in place for you to turn your life around and maximise your potential. Take the first step and start something great. Join the movement. Read *The Primal Cure* and turn your life around for good.

READER & JOURNALIST TESTIMONIALS

By following the Primal principles
I have managed to keep the
weight off and never even feel like
I am actually on a diet.
Nick

Steve's book is a real eye-opener.
Stephen

Worthy coffee table book by entrepreneur and global
adventurer Steve Bennett on his personal journey to fitness.
Great intro from Richard Branson... I'm putting the book in
front of my husband, who chomps on cereal every morning.

Denise Barrett
Freelance Writer and Member, Guild of Health Writers

My name is *Valerie*, I am 73 and have had a number of serious,
complex health conditions. The worst is called Spinal Canal
Stenosis... It is a particularly nasty result of arthritis and I
have been in crippling pain for the last eight years. Due to *The
Primal Cure*, I have changed my diet and lost some weight,
taking magnesium, zinc and green tea. After about six days
of taking the supplements I suddenly realised that I was free
of back pain for the first time in eight years! I have even been
trying to do some cleaning etc round the house rather than
leaving it to my carer/cleaner... I am almost back to my old self,
and this is nothing short of a "miracle".

As a nutritionist and keen promoter of the low carb and sugar free way of eating, I have no hesitation in recommending the book *The Primal Cure*. The book is bursting with everything you need to know about changing your health for the better.

Sarah Flower
Freelance Journalist

The best health book I've ever read! Full of factual information that really works; this is my new bible for life.
Review from an Amazon customer

I have now recommended six people to *The Primal Cure* as I want to share my "find" with family and friends.
Avalin White

I have been living as near to Primal as I can; especially the low carb scenario. But here is the amazing bit... Aside from regular hip pain, I typically have high readings in both cholesterol and a poor liver count. Recently I had my three month MOT (blood tests, etc). When I phoned up, they said, "All fine and no further action needed". So I decided to request a phone call from my doctor - having lost just under two stone and feeling great - just to see if my readings had altered in any way. God, am I glad I did! Let's just say, he mentioned the word *BRILLIANT* six times! "You must be on a good diet," he said. So I endeavoured to explain *The Primal Cure* and my new low carb regime... We have decided to bring me off my cholesterol pills for the next three months 'til my next MOT. So it goes without saying I have been on cloud nine. I'm keeping the two stone off, not counting calories and simply living Primally. That suits me.
Dayne Johns

Having suffered with thyroid disease - both over/under active for more than 25 years and conditions like carpel tunnel, ME and diabetes - I have always looked at my diet to reduce my medication through detox. However, these conditions have always re-appeared. Never one to give up, I always believe in the concept of fight or flight; and I fight! By chance, I came across *The Primal Cure* and the rest is history... I am now off all medication except for Thyroxine. With the support of my doctor (who is very forward thinking) I am working on coming off drugs altogether.

Jayne Bagnal

I am a 100% convert! *The Primal Cure* is brilliant. Bye bye Slimming World. Thank you Primal Cure.

Elizabeth

The Primal Cure is brilliant. Although I'm generally a sceptic, this book is packed full of interesting facts and research references. It has really changed the way I think about the food on my plate.

Kate

Wow!! What an incredibly informative book this is.

Gerard

With the recent news that four out of five Brits face an early death due to health factors, I think this book is even more timely than it otherwise would be! I am on a major weight loss programme at the moment. I can't quite believe how much info *The Primal Cure* contains. It's quite incredible and proving very helpful to me at this time.

Jo Lamiri
Freelance Journalist and Editor for the Independent